SPORTS DRINKS

Basic Science and Practical Aspects

NUTRITION in EXERCISE and SPORT

Edited by Ira Wolinsky and James F. Hickson, Jr.

Published Titles

Exercise and Disease,
Ronald R. Watson and Marianne Eisinger

Nutrients as Ergogenic Aids for Sports and Exercise,
Luke Bucci

Nutrition in Exercise and Sport, Second Edition,
Ira Wolinsky and James F. Hickson, Jr.

Nutrition Applied to Injury Rehabilitation and Sports Medicine,
Luke Bucci

Nutrition for the Recreational Athlete,
Catherine G.R. Jackson

NUTRITION in EXERCISE and SPORT

Edited by Ira Wolinsky

Published Titles

Sports Nutrition: Minerals and Electrolytes,
Constance V. Kies and Judy A. Driskell

Nutrition, Physical Activity, and Health in Early Life:
Studies in Preschool Children,
Jana Parizkova

Exercise and Immune Function,
Laurie Hoffman-Goetz

Body Fluid Balance: Exercise and Sport,
E.R. Buskirk and S. Puhl

Nutrition and the Female Athlete,
Jaime S. Ruud

Sports Nutrition: Vitamins and Trace Elements,
Ira Wolinsky and Judy A. Driskell

Amino Acids and Proteins for the Athlete—The Anabolic Edge,
Mauro G. DiPasquale

Nutrition in Exercise and Sport, Third Edition,
Ira Wolinsky

Published Titles Continued

Gender Differences in Metabolism: Practical and Nutritional Implications, Mark Tarnopolsky

Macroelements, Water, and Electrolytes in Sports Nutrition, Judy A. Driskell and Ira Wolinsky

Sports Nutrition, Judy A. Driskell

Energy-Yielding Macronutrients and Energy Metabolism in Sports Nutrition, Judy A. Driskell and Ira Wolinsky

Nutrition and Exercise Immunology, David C. Nieman and Bente Klarlund Pedersen

Sports Drinks: Basic Science and Practical Aspects, Ronald Maughan and Robert Murry

Nutritional Applications in Exercise and Sport, Ira Wolinsky and Judy Driskell

NUTRITION in EXERCISE and SPORT

Edited by Ira Wolinsky

Forthcoming Titles

High Performance Nutrition: Diets and Supplements for the Competitive Athlete, Mauro DiPasquale

Nutrition and the Strength Athlete, Catherine R. Jackson

Nutrients as Ergogenic Aids for Sports and Exercise, Second Edition, Luke R. Bucci

SPORTS DRINKS

Basic Science and Practical Aspects

Ronald J. Maughan • Robert Murray

CRC Press
Boca Raton London New York Washington, D.C.

Library of Congress Cataloging-in-Publication Data

Maughan, Ron J., 1951–
  Sports Drinks : basic science and practical aspects / Ronald J. Maughan, Robert Murray.
      p. cm. (Nutrition in exercise and sport)
  Includes bibliographical references and index.
  ISBN 0-8493-7008-6 (alk. paper)
  1. Athletes--Nutrition. 2. Physical fitness--Nutritional aspects. 3. Beverages. I.
Murray, Robert, 1949-II. Title. III. Series
TX361.A8 M375 2000
613.2′088′796—dc21   00-034307
                                                                        CIP

Visit the CRC Press Web site at www.crcpress.com

© 2001 by CRC Press LLC

No claim to original U.S. Government works
International Standard Book Number 0-8493-7008-6
Library of Congress Card Number 00-034307
Printed in the United States of America 2 3 4 5 6 7 8 9 0
Printed on acid-free paper

Series Preface

The CRC series Nutrition in Exercise and Sport provides a setting for in-depth exploration of the many and varied aspects of nutrition and exercise, including sports. The topic of exercise and sports nutrition has been a focus of research among scientists since the 1960s, and the healthful benefits of good nutrition and exercise have been appreciated. As our knowledge expands, it will be necessary to remember that there must be a range of diets and exercise regimes that will support excellent physical condition and performance. There is no single diet–exercise treatment that can be the common denominator, or the one formula for health, or a panacea for performance.

This series is dedicated to providing a stage upon which to explore these issues. Each volume provides a detailed and scholarly examination of some aspect of the topic. Contributors from bona fide areas of nutrition and physical activity, including sports and the controversial, are welcome.

We welcome the contribution *Sports Drinks: Basic Science and Practical Aspects*, edited by R. Maughan and R. Murray. They have assembled an expert roster to prepare this book. It is a valuable addition to the series.

Ira Wolinsky, Ph.D.
University of Houston
Series Editor

Preface

It is quite legitimate to ask, "Why a book on the science of sports drinks?" Such a narrow topic seemingly does not deserve the energy and attention required of writing, editing, and publishing a text. The answer is that, in sporting, scientific, and financial terms, sports drinks have generated considerable interest. The ability of a well-formulated sports drink to benefit physiological function and exercise performance is, considering the relative simplicity of its formulation, somewhat remarkable. While there remains much to learn about the physiological, metabolic, hormonal, performance, and sensory responses to fluid, carbohydrate, and electrolyte ingestion during and following physical activity, there is a wealth of information currently available. *Sports Drinks: Basic Science and Practical Aspects* provides a comprehensive review of the current knowledge based on issues related to the formulation of sports drinks and the physiological responses to their ingestion during physical activity. It also looks at the role that sports drinks play in optimizing performance in sports and exercise for the elite athlete and for the recreational exerciser. In a very real sense, this book is not so much a review of the science of sports drinks as it is an example of how scientific knowledge can be used to both create and evaluate the efficacy of products that have benefited millions of people.

Writing and editing a book is not always a lot of fun, especially when the effort to do so is crammed between countless other professional and personal activities, more than a few of which must be put on hold until the task is accomplished. However, the happy outcome of the late nights, missed deadlines, and work-filled weekends is a book in which we can all take pride. We hope you find it to be a valuable and often-used part of your professional library.

About the Editors

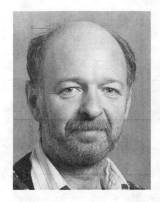

Ronald J. Maughan, Ph.D., FACSM, is currently professor of human physiology at the University Medical School, Aberdeen, Scotland. He obtained his B.Sc. in physiology and Ph.D. from the University of Aberdeen and held a lecturing position in Liverpool before returning to Aberdeen, where he is now based in the Department of Biomedical Sciences. His research interests are in the physiology, biochemistry, and nutrition of exercise performance, with an interest in both the basic science of exercise and the applied aspects that relate to health and to performance in sport. He has published extensively in the scientific literature and is on the editorial board of several international journals.

Dr. Maughan is a Fellow of the American College of Sports Medicine and a member of many scientific organizations, including the Physiological Society, the Nutrition Society, the Biochemical Society, the Medical Research Society, and the New York Academy of Sciences. He chairs the Human and Exercise Physiology group of the Physiological Society. He also chairs the Nutrition Steering Group of the British Olympic Association and played a leading role in the production of the acclimatization strategy that was employed by the British and other competitors preparing for the 1996 Olympic Games held in Atlanta, Georgia. A former runner, he now leads a more sedentary life.

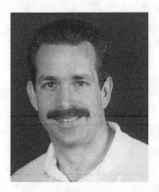

Robert Murray, Ph.D., FACSM, is an exercise physiologist who specializes in sports nutrition, with an emphasis on the physiological and performance effects of hydration and carbohydrate feeding during exercise. He has been director of the Gatorade Sports Science Institute and the Gatorade Exercise Physiology Laboratory since its inception in 1985. As director of the Gatorade lab, Dr. Murray oversees scientific research in a variety of areas in exercise science and sports nutrition, including fluid balance during and after exercise; the effects of fluid, carbohydrate, and electrolyte ingestion during exercise; and the gastric emptying and intestinal absorption of fluid.

A native of Pittsburgh, Dr. Murray earned his B.S. and M.S. degrees in physical education at Slippery Rock State College. He served as assistant professor of physical education and head swimming coach at Oswego State University of New York from 1974–1977 before returning to graduate school to receive his Ph.D. in exercise physiology from Ohio State University. He then served as associate professor of physical education at Boise State University until joining The Quaker Oats Company in Barrington, Illinois to head the Gatorade Exercise Physiology Laboratory.

The author of numerous articles in scientific journals, Dr. Murray is a Fellow of the American College of Sports Medicine.

Acknowledgments

A scientific consensus on any subject does not come quickly or easily and this book is evidence of that fact. As you page through this text, pay particular attention to the lengthy bibliographies for each chapter and you will quickly realize that a book such as this is made possible only as a result of the efforts of a mind-boggling number of scientists. We are as indebted to those scientists as we are to our colleagues and fellow authors, whose expert contributions made this book everything it should be.

Contributors

Luis F. Aragón-Vargas, Ph.D., FACSM
University of Costa Rica
San Jose, Costa Rica

Craig A. Horswill, Ph.D.
Gatorade Sports Science Institute
Barrington, Illinois

John B. Leiper, Ph.D.
University Medical School
Aberdeen, Scotland

Ronald J. Maughan, Ph.D., FACSM
University Medical School
Aberdeen, Scotland

Robert Murray, Ph.D., FACSM
Gatorade Sports Science Institute
Barrington, Illinois

Dennis H. Passe, Ph.D.
The Quaker Oats Company
Barrington, Illinois

Susan M. Shirreffs, Ph.D.
University Medical School
Aberdeen, Scotland

John R. Stofan, M.S.
Gatorade Sports Science Institute
Barrington, Illinois

Contents

1 Fundamentals of Sports Nutrition: Application to Sports Drinks

Ronald. J. Maughan

CONTENTS

1.1 INTRODUCTION

The excitement of sport — for participant and competitor alike — lies in the uncertainty of the outcome. No athlete, and no team competing at a high level, can be sure of winning every competition in which they take part. When evenly matched competitors are involved, the margin between victory and defeat is small, and the serious athlete looks for every advantage that might sway the result. Talent

— whatever that is — is the key factor in setting the potential of the individual, but everyone can improve with training and practice. Performance can continue to improve over many years with sustained intensive training, provided the athlete remains free from serious illness and injury. Psychological factors, including motivation and determination, and tactical awareness are also key elements. Good training facilities and the best available equipment can also help. When all of these things are equal, however, the athlete must search for something else.

1.2   DIETARY SUPPORT FOR TRAINING AND COMPETITION

In all sports, diet can influence performance, yet athletes are slow to appreciate the extent to which their performance is affected by what they eat and are even slower to develop eating strategies that will allow them to optimize their performance. Where athletes do consider nutrition, the focus is generally on eating and drinking in the hours prior to competition or during the event itself. However, as well as affecting performance in competition, an adequate diet is necessary to support the athlete's daily training load. Improvements in performance in competition come from consistent hard training, and the nutrient demands of training must be met if injury and illness are to be avoided. Attention to the training diet may therefore be more important than manipulation of the pre-competition meal.

1.3   NUTRITIONAL TARGETS AND EATING STRATEGIES

There are several barriers to implementation of good dietary practices among sportsmen and -women. The first is a limited awareness of the impact that diet can have on performance. Athletes who are unaware that there is a need to change their eating habits are unlikely to do so, but if they can be convinced of the performance benefits that can accrue, then change will be welcomed. The first step then is to identify the nutritional goals that will allow each athlete to achieve the best possible performance. This requires assessment of the limiting factors in training and in competition and an assessment of each athlete's nutritional needs.

The second barrier to implementation of a successful nutritional program is set by the athlete's nutritional knowledge. Many athletes, for example, know that they should increase their dietary carbohydrate intake, but such awareness is not useful without a knowledge of the carbohydrate content of different foods. Each athlete's nutritional goals must therefore be translated into an eating strategy that will identify the types and amounts of foods that will provide the necessary nutrients. This process must take account not only of the nutritional goals, but also of the athlete's lifestyle and training schedule, cooking skills, and personal likes and dislikes.

The level of nutritional knowledge in the general population is low, and athletes often know little about the composition of foods. Wootton (1986) used a simple multiple-choice questionnaire to assess nutrition knowledge and beliefs among various groups of athletes and coaches. He found that recreational runners, on average, succeeded in answering only about half of the questions correctly, but they scored higher than qualified track-and-field coaches, international-standard swimmers, or professional soccer players. It might be thought that the situation would have improved in recent years, but Sossin et al. (1997) also found a limited nutritional knowledge among American high-school wrestling coaches, even though most (82%) considered themselves to be very knowledgeable about nutrition. Wiita and Stombaugh (1996) also showed limited nutritional knowledge among adolescent female runners; somewhat alarmingly, they also showed that the level of knowledge did not change over the 3-year period during which their subjects were followed.

A knowledge of nutrition and nutritional goals is only the first stage in developing appropriate eating strategies, and a change in attitude to eating may also be necessary. Changing dietary habits is therefore a slow and difficult process, and in many cases, athletes will require professional help to steer them in the right direction.

1.4   NUTRITION IN TRAINING

1.4.1   ENERGY BALANCE

The diet of the athlete in training must meet the additional nutrient requirement imposed by the training load. Failure to meet the energy demand results in a falling body mass, a loss of active tissue, chronic fatigue, and an inability to adapt to the training program. An inadequate intake of individual nutrients can also have catastrophic consequences. If the diet does not supply sufficient carbohydrate, recovery between training sessions will be incomplete and the training load must be reduced. Many athletes, especially those living and training in hot climates, are likely to face difficulties in meeting fluid needs because of their high sweat losses. Chronic dehydration will also restrict exercise capacity. Protein, vitamins, and minerals must also be supplied by the diet in amounts sufficient to meet the body's needs, and the requirement for many dietary components will be increased by hard training.

Because sport is so varied, and the characteristics of athletes are often at the extremes of the normal distribution, generalizations do not apply to all sports and to all individuals. The demands on the 120-kg basketball player, who may participate in more than 100 games in a year, are very different from those faced by the swimmer or cyclist, who may devote several hours per day to training, or from those on the gymnast with a body mass of 35 kg. Even where the duration of competition may be short, as in sprinting or weightlifting, training may occupy several hours per day for a substantial part of the year. In technical events such as gymnastics, the energy demand of training may be modest, even though the total duration of each day's training sessions may be long. In training for endurance sports, the metabolic rate during training may be 15–20 times the resting rate, and such levels of activity may be sustained for several hours per day. The metabolic rate may remain elevated for at least 12 hours after exercise if the exercise is prolonged and the intensity is high, and this will further increase the energy cost of training for the endurance athlete (Bahr, 1992). If body mass and performance levels are to be maintained, the high rate of energy expenditure must be matched by an equally high energy intake.

Table 1.1 shows reported values from a variety of sources for the energy intake of athletes competing in different sports. Several points need to be borne in mind when considering this information. First, it must be remembered that the body mass of successful performers varies greatly between sports: an American football player with a body mass of 120 kg who has a low training load may still have an energy expenditure that is much greater than that of a 45-kg female marathon runner training at the limit of what she can sustain, and he should therefore have a greater energy intake. It is also the case that not all of the published information is absolutely reliable. There are several potential errors involved in the assessment of energy intake. Dietary recall or weighed-intake methods are subject to reporting errors and there is also an inherent variability due to discrepancies in the energy values in food composition tables. Some subjects will also — whether consciously or not — fail to record all food items consumed, others may alter their diet because of the inconvenience of weighing and recording foods, and others may deliberately conceal information.

TABLE 1.1
Reported Values for Energy Intake of Male and Female Athletes During Training for a Variety of Different Sports

| | Daily Energy Intake | | | | |
| | Males | | Females | | |
	MJ/d	kcal/d	MJ/d	kcal/d	Reference
Triathlon	19.1	4584			van Erp-Baart et al. (1989)
Cycle tour	24.7	5928			Saris et al. (1989)
Rowing	14.6	3504	13.0	3120	van Erp-Baart (1989)
Soccer	16.5	3952			Rico-Sanz et al. (1998)
Soccer	12.8	3072			Maughan (1997)
Offshore sailing	18.5	4440			Bigard et al. (1998)
Track and field	13.1	3141	10.5	2508	Sugiura et al. (1999)
Rhythmic gymnastics			7.1	1703	Sundgot-Borgen (1996)

Note: Values are means for groups of athletes from each sport. This is not a comprehensive list, but rather a selection from the large number of published studies, and is designed to show the wide variability in values. These data, of course, should be interpreted in the context of the training load at the time of the measurement, the body mass of the individuals, and the level of competition.

In one study of runners who were in steady state with regard to training and body mass, and who therefore were presumably in energy balance, a good relationship was found to exist between the energy expended in training and the energy intake as estimated by 7-day weighed intake (Figure 1.1; Maughan et al., 1989). This result is hardly surprising, as a failure to meet the energy demand would result in a progressive loss of body mass, chronic fatigue, and impaired exercise capacity. It seems safe to assume that most athletes with a high training load have a high food intake, but the possibility of short-term severe food restriction remains.

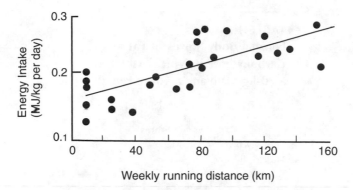

FIGURE 1.1 Energy intake, expressed per unit of body mass, of runners and sedentary controls expressed in relation to the average distance covered per week in training.

Where energy demands are extremely high, there are clearly practical problems in consuming the large amounts of food necessary. This is accentuated by the athlete's reluctance to eat — particularly to eat bulky high-fiber foods — in the pre-exercise period because of a fear of gastrointestinal problems during training and because of a suppression of appetite in the post-exercise period. One solution is to take a significant amount of energy in liquid form, a strategy that is often adopted by athletes with especially high energy intakes (8–10,000 kcal/d or 32–40 MJ/d), such as cyclists competing in multistage races (Westerterp et al., 1986).

1.4.2 CARBOHYDRATE REQUIREMENTS

The energy requirements of training are largely met by oxidation of fat and carbohydrate, with only a small contribution (about 5%) from the breakdown of protein. The higher the intensity of exercise, the greater the total energy demand, and the greater the reliance on carbohydrate as a fuel: at an exercise intensity corresponding to about 50% of maximum oxygen uptake (VO_{2max}), approximately two-thirds of the total energy requirement is met by fat oxidation, with carbohydrate oxidation supplying about one-third. At about 75% of VO_{2max}, the total energy expenditure is increased, and carbohydrate is now the major fuel. If carbohydrate is not available, or is available in only a limited amount, the intensity of the exercise must be reduced to a level where the greater part of the energy requirement can be met by fat oxidation. If carbohydrate is not available, the ability to train at high intensities is reduced and recovery after training is slowed.

Considering that a marathon runner may break down carbohydrate at a rate of 3–4 g/min during training, or that a middle-distance runner can convert 100 g of muscle glycogen to lactate in less than 2 min of hard running, the body stores of carbohydrate are extremely small (Table 1.2). A single training session for each of these athletes will result in a substantial depletion of the muscle glycogen stores. When the muscle glycogen availability is reduced, high-intensity exercise is not possible. More importantly, perhaps, the brain, the red blood cells, and, to a lesser extent, the kidneys, rely exclusively on carbohydrate as a fuel. An inadequate availability of carbohydrate has serious implications for brain function. There is no

TABLE 1.2
Normal Body Stores of Fat and
Carbohydrate in Typical Athletes,
a 70-Kg Male and a 60-Kg Female

	Male	Female
Carbohydrate Stores		
Liver glycogen	90 g	70 g
Muscle glycogen	400 g	300 g
Fat Stores		
Intramuscular	500 g	500 g
Adipose tissue	7–10 kg	12–20 kg

Note: The body fat content can vary greatly, from as little as perhaps 3% of body weight in very lean individuals to 50% or more in the obese.

mechanism to convert the large amount of fatty acids stored in adipose tissue to carbohydrate.

During each strenuous training session, depletion of the glycogen stores in the exercising muscles and the liver takes place. If this carbohydrate reserve is not replenished before the next exercise bout, training intensity must be reduced, leading to corresponding decrements in the training response. Any athlete training hard on a daily basis can readily observe this; if a low-carbohydrate diet, consisting mostly of fat and protein, is consumed after a day's training, it will be difficult to repeat the same training load on the following day. Recovery of the muscle and liver glycogen stores after exercise is a rather slow process, and will normally require at least 24 to 48 hours for complete recovery. The rate of glycogen resynthesis after exercise is determined largely by the amount of carbohydrate supplied by the diet (Ivy, 1998), and the amount of carbohydrate consumed is of far greater importance for this process than the type of carbohydrate.

The training diet, therefore, should be high in carbohydrate; depending on the total energy intake, this may mean that 60% or more of total energy intake comes from carbohydrate. This suggestion conforms to various expert committees' recommendations that carbohydrates provide more than 50% of dietary energy intake. A high-carbohydrate diet (70% of energy intake as carbohydrate) can enable athletes training for 2 hours per day to maintain muscle glycogen levels, whereas if the carbohydrate content is only 40%, a progressive fall in muscle glycogen content is likely to occur. It may be more useful to think of an absolute daily requirement for carbohydrate, rather than relating the need to total energy intake. A daily dietary carbohydrate intake of 500 to 600 g may be necessary to ensure adequate glycogen resynthesis during periods of intensive training, and, for some athletes, the amount of carbohydrate that must be consumed on a daily basis is even greater (Coyle,

1992). The carbohydrate requirement is determined primarily by training volume and intensity, but is also influenced by body size, and a daily requirement of about 6 to 10 g/kg body mass is likely in periods of hard training. These high levels of intake are difficult to achieve without consuming large amounts of simple sugars and other compact forms of carbohydrate, or by increasing the frequency of meals and snacks, which would lead to a "grazing" pattern of eating. Athletes may find that sugar, jam, honey, and high-sugar foods such as confectionery, as well as carbohydrate-containing drinks, such as soft drinks, fruit juices, and sports drinks, can provide a low-bulk, convenient addition of carbohydrate to the nutritious food base (Clark, 1994). There is no evidence that this pattern of eating is in any way harmful, although attention to dental hygiene should, of course, be emphasized.

For the athlete who trains at least once and perhaps two or three times per day, and who also has to work or study, practical difficulties arise in meeting the demand for energy and carbohydrate. Although cyclists may consume a significant part of the day's energy requirement during training, many athletes, particularly runners, find it difficult to train hard until at least 3 hours after food intake. The appetite is also generally suppressed for a time after hard exercise. In this situation, it is particularly important to focus on ensuring a rapid recovery of the glycogen stores between training sessions. This is best achieved when carbohydrate is consumed as soon as possible after training, as the rate of glycogen synthesis if most rapid at this time. At least 50 to 100 g of carbohydrate should be consumed in the first hour and a high-carbohydrate intake continued thereafter. There is clearly a maximum rate at which muscle glycogen resynthesis can occur, and there appears to be no benefit in increasing the carbohydrate intake to levels in excess of 100 g every 2 hours. The type of carbohydrate is less crucial than the amount consumed, but there may be some benefit from ingesting high-glycaemic-index foods at this time to ensure a rapid elevation of the blood glucose level.

1.4.3 PROTEIN REQUIREMENTS

The requirement for vitamins, minerals, protein, and other nutrients is, in some cases, increased by exercise, but to a smaller degree than the energy requirement. In general, it can be said that a varied diet in amounts adequate to meet the energy demand will normally supply these nutrients in adequate amounts. It must be recognized, however, that not all athletes have a high energy intake and that not all eat a varied diet. The latter point may be especially important: a regular routine is a characteristic of the training program of most athletes, and this often includes a regular and monotonous pattern of eating with limited food choices.

Most of the energy requirements of training are met by oxidation of fat and carbohydrate, with only a small contribution from protein. Exercise, whether it is long-distance running, aerobics or weight training, will cause some increase in the rate of protein oxidation relative to the resting state (Lemon, 1991). In a normal 24-hour period, the protein ingested in the diet will be metabolized and nitrogen balance will be maintained. This means that, over the whole day, protein oxidation must account for about 12–15% of total energy expenditure, this being the normal fraction of protein in the diet. The relative contribution of protein oxidation to energy production during the exercise period may decrease to about 5% of the total energy requirement, but the absolute rate of protein degradation is increased during exercise. Hard exercise therefore leads to an increase in the minimum daily protein require- ment, and an intake of 1.2–1.7 g/kg/d is recommended for athletes (Lemon, 1991). This is 50 to 100% in excess of the current recommended intake of about 0.6 to 0.8 g/kg/d for sedentary individuals, but even this increased amount will normally be met if a varied diet adequate to meet the increased energy expenditure is consumed. A diet supplying 3000 kcal, with 12 to 15% of total energy as protein, will give 90 to 112 g of protein; for a 70-kg athlete, this represents 1.3 to 1.6 g/kg (Table 1.3). In spite of the lack of evidence to suggest that athletes' diets are generally deficient in protein or that a further increase in dietary protein intake is in any way beneficial, many athletes ingest large quantities of high-protein foods and expensive protein supplements. Daily protein intakes of up to 400 grams are not unknown in some athletes. Disposal of the excess nitrogen is theoretically a problem if renal function is compromised, but there does not appear to be any evidence that excessive protein intake among athletes is in any way damaging to health, nor is it beneficial to performance.

TABLE 1.3
Protein Intake (in g/kg/d) at Various Levels of Energy Intake for Athletes with Different Body Mass Eating a Diet Giving 15% of Total Energy Intake as Protein

Energy intake (kcal/d)	Body Mass (kg)					
	50 kg	60 kg	70 kg	80 kg	90 kg	100 kg
2000	1.5	1.2	1.1	0.9	0.8	0.7
3000	2.2	1.9	1.6	1.4	1.2	1.1
4000	3.0	2.5	2.1	1.9	1.7	1.5
5000	3.7	3.1	2.7	2.3	2.1	1.9
6000	4.5	3.7	3.2	2.8	2.5	2.2

Note: Values above the recommended intake of 1.2 g/kg body mass are shown in bold.

1.4.4 VITAMINS

There is no good evidence that athletes who eat well-chosen diets with adequate energy are prone to deficiencies of vitamins, but it is also the case that there have been few good studies of vitamin balance in athletes. In many published studies, a comparison of some measure of intake (usually based on a subjective recall method) with the recommended daily intake is used as evidence that vitamin deficiencies are common. This is not so, and the methodology used in these studies is flawed. It is clear from the available limited information on vitamin status of athletes that defi- ciencies are remarkably rare. Nonetheless, several factors may contribute to marginal vitamin status. Lack of imagination or motivation in the preparation of meals, poor cooking skills, and financial constraints all contribute to a limited range of foods being eaten by some athletes and may compromise micronutrient intake.

There is no good evidence that supplementation with any vitamins has a beneficial effect on exercise performance, except when a preexisting deficiency has been corrected. Studies that have shown beneficial effects on performance have usually lacked an appropriate control group, and a placebo effect is being observed. Use of multivitamin supplements in the recommended doses is not harmful, and these are used by many athletes. There have been suggestions that fortification of sports drinks with vitamins, especially those B vitamins involved in carbohydrate metabolism, may be beneficial. This will be discussed in more detail in Chapter 9.

There has been much interest in recent years in the possible role of the antioxidant vitamins in preventing or at least reducing the muscle damage that is associated with hard exercise. There are some suggestions that this damage is the result of free radical formation and that ingestion of large doses of Vitamins C and E can reduce this response (Clarkson, 1995). Many athletes already take supplements containing these vitamins, but the evidence at present is not strong· enough to support the suggestion that athletes should take these as a matter of routine. Furthermore, megadoses of some vitamins may cause adverse effects.

1.4.5   MINERALS

A number of minerals play important roles in the regulation of cellular metabolism, and an adequate intake — sufficient to meet the losses from the body — is essential for maintenance of health. Zinc, copper, magnesium, manganese, chromium, selenium, iodine, and a number of other elements fall into this category. The requirement for some minerals (especially sodium) is increased by hard exercise, in large part because of increased losses in sweat. Many other minerals, including potassium, magnesium, iron, and zinc are also lost in sweat, giving rise to the idea that mineral supplementation may be necessary when sweat losses are high. This also suggests an argument for the addition of these components to drinks intended for consumption during or after exercise. In general, however, the additional losses incurred as a result of exercise are small relative to the total daily requirement. The scope for the addition of minerals to sports drinks is discussed in Chapter 8.

At present, there is no evidence to suggest that mineral deficiencies are common among athletes. Surveys showing an inadequate intake among different athletic groups must be treated with caution, for several reasons. Intake of all of these elements is difficult to assess, particularly because of the problem of obtaining an accurate record of habitual food intake. In addition, food-composition tables are unreliable, so unrealistic values may be obtained even when food intake is measured reliably. The assessment of adequacy of intake also requires a measure of the requirement, and this has not been established with any degree of certainty for many of the micronutrients. Failure to meet a recommended intake may give cause to look closely at the diet, but is certainly not a useful index of adequacy of the intake. Despite apparently low intakes, few athletes show clinical signs of deficiency.

Athletes who are most at risk of inadequate micronutrient intake are those who restrict their food variety and/or total energy intake.

1.4.6 WATER AND ELECTROLYTE REQUIREMENTS IN TRAINING

The discussion above focused on depletion of the glycogen reserve in the exercising muscles as the major cause of fatigue during prolonged exercise. However, problems associated with thermoregulation and fluid balance are much more likely to cause problems for athletes training in warm weather. Even modest levels of dehydration will impair exercise capacity and prevent the athlete from achieving optimum performance. In practice, this means a reduction in the quality of training sessions and a corresponding reduction in the degree of adaptive response. Severe dehydration is potentially fatal, as exercise in the dehydrated state leads to a rapid elevation of body temperature and the onset of heat illness. There is consequently a real need to ensure adequate fluid intake before, during, and after every training session. The idea that the body adapts to dehydration or that the trained individual is more resistant to the negative effects of dehydration is completely wrong.

Heat is evolved as a by-product of all muscular activity and the rate of heat production is set by the rate of energy turnover. At rest, the typical 70-kg human body uses about 300 ml of oxygen per minute and produces heat at a rate of about 70 W. Heat loss from the body surface occurs at the same rate, allowing a constant body temperature to be maintained. The elite cyclist or distance runner can sustain a rate of heat production in excess of 1 kW for prolonged periods. This would cause an intolerable rise in body temperature if the rate of heat loss were not also increased. At high ambient temperatures, the only mechanism by which heat can be lost from the body is evaporation. Evaporation of 1 l of water from the skin will remove 2.4 MJ (580 kcal) of heat from the body. This can be illustrated by the example of a marathon runner with a body weight of 70 kg who completes a race at a steady pace and finishes in a time of 2 hours 30 min. Assuming a flat course and no wind, the average rate of heat production will be about 1 kW. This rate of metabolic heat production can be exactly balanced by evaporative loss alone if sweat can be evaporated from the skin at a rate of about 1.6 l/h. Some sweat will simply drip from the skin without being evaporated and will not contribute to cooling, so a higher sweat rate of about 2 l/h is necessary. This is possible, but would result in the loss of 5 l of body water over the course of the race, corresponding to a loss of more than 7% of body weight (and about 12% of total body water) for a 70-kg runner. For slower runners, the total sweat loss is similar to that of the faster runners: the running time is longer and the sweat rate is lower, but the total loss is similar (Maughan, 1985).

For the typical sedentary young man or woman, daily water intake precisely matches the water losses that occur from the body. Water losses usually amount to about 2–3 l of water per day for individuals living in temperate climates, with about 50% of the total loss in the form of urine (Table 1.4). During hard exercise in a warm environment, however, this amount of fluid may be lost in 1 hour, although sweat rates are typically less than this for most individuals. Sweat losses in training will vary greatly among individuals, even when fitness levels, exercise intensity, and

TABLE 1.4
Approximate Average Values for Water Loss for Sedentary Adult Men and Women Living in a Temperate Climate

	Water losses (ml per day)	
	Men	Women
Urine	1400	1000
Expired air	400	300
Transcutaneous loss	530	280
Sweat loss	650	420
Faecal water	100	90
Total (approximately)	3000	2100

environmental conditions are similar. Many studies have estimated sweat losses during training in groups of athletes from different sports. Typical values are in the range of about 0.8–1.4 l/h, with extremes for the group means of about 0.4–2.6 l/h (Rehrer and Burke, 1996). It should be noted, however, that these mean values conceal the wide variations that occur between individuals.

These measurements are usually based on changes in body mass during training and ignore other losses during the remainder of the day. Advances in the application of isotopic tracer methodology have recently permitted the non-invasive measurement of water turnover, using deuterium as a tracer for body water. The principle of the measurement and the practicalities are both relatively straightforward. Body water is labeled with deuterium, and the water turnover is measured over a period of a few days from the rate of decrease in the tracer concentration in body water. The measurement can be made conveniently on blood or urine samples. Collection of 24-hour urine output allows non-renal losses (consisting mainly of sweat and transcutaneous losses, respiratory water loss, and faecal loss) to be calculated by the difference.

Application of this method to the measurement of water turnover is discussed in detail in Chapter 2 and is mentioned only briefly here. In two studies, it was shown that active individuals had a higher water turnover rate than sedentary control subjects (Leiper et al., 1996; Leiper et al., 1995). In one study, the higher water turnover of a group of runners could be accounted for by a greater urine loss, with no difference in sweat losses (Leiper et al., 1996). It may be that these moderately active runners drank more than their needs because of the emphasis on rehydration in many publications aimed at runners. In contrast, in cyclists with a higher daily traning load, the greater water turnover was accounted for by a greater non-renal water loss (Leiper et al., 1995). In both studies, there was a large inter-individual variability in water turnover, even when the climatic conditions and training load were similar.

Along with water, electrolytes are lost in varying amounts, the major constituents of sweat being those of the extracellular space, i.e., sodium and chloride. Sweat is invariably hypotonic and water is lost in excess of solute. Where sweat losses are large, the electrolyte loss in sweat may become significant, and maintenance of electrolyte balance may require an increased intake, particularly of sodium. Electrolyte balance is important for a number of reasons. The main electrolytes (sodium, potassium, magnesium) play key roles in function of muscle and nerve, but they also help to regulate body water content and the distribution of water among the various body water compartments. The daily intake of electrolytes is subject to wide variation among individuals, with strong trends for differences among different geographical regions. Daily dietary sodium chloride intakes for 95% of the young male UK population fall between 3.8 and 14.3 g with a mean of 8.4 g; the corresponding values for young women are 2.8–9.4 g, with a mean value of 6.0 g (Gregory et al., 1990). For the same population, mean urinary sodium losses were reported to account for about 175 mmol/d (Gregory et al., 1990), which is equivalent to about 10.2 g of sodium chloride. The discrepancy illustrates some of the difficulties with the collection of this type of information.

There are also large differences between countries in the recommended intake of salt: the British advice is for a maximum of 6 g per day, but in Germany, a maximum of 10 g/d is recommended. In contrast, Sweden recommends a maximum of 2 g/d, and Poland recommends a minimum of 1.4 g/d. These differences in the recommendations by different expert committees reflect, in part, different interpretations of the evidence linking salt intake and health, but also reflect regional consumption patterns. Because of the need to excrete excess solute in the urine, the daily salt intake will have implications for an individual's water requirements.

The composition of drinks to be taken before, during, and after exercise will be influenced by the relative importance of the need to supply fuel and water and to replace electrolyte losses. This in turn depends on the intensity and duration of the exercise task, on the ambient temperature and humidity, and on the physiological and biochemical characteristics of the individual. Electrolyte replacement is not normally a priority, but addition of sodium to glucose-containing drinks will promote absorption of glucose and water in the small intestine: this is crucial when rapid replacement is essential, as is the case during exercise (Maughan and Greenhaff, 1991). Electrolyte replacement is also important for fluid volume restoration in the post-exercise period (see Chapter 7)

1.5   NUTRITION FOR COMPETITION

In competition, the aim of nutritional strategies is to target the factors that cause fatigue and impair performance. These include:

- Hyperthermia
- Dehydration
- Hypoglycemia
- Muscle glycogen depletion
- Electrolyte imbalances
- Gastrointestinal distress

All of these factors may, in some situations, contribute to fatigue and limit performance. Nutritional strategies aimed at improving performance should therefore employ interventions that can influence these processes.

1.5.1 HYPERTHERMIA

Except in poorly clad individuals exercising in extreme cold, an increase in body temperature is a normal response to exercise. Core temperature rises from the normal resting level of about 37°C at a rate that is proportional to the ambient temperature, the work rate, and the body mass of the individual (Greenhaff, 1989). The importance of ambient temperature, which plays a major role in determining the rate of rise of core temperature, is well demonstrated by the reduction in exercise performance in warm weather. Even at moderate temperatures (about 20°C), performance of prolonged exercise is already impaired relative to that in cooler (about 10°C) conditions (Figure 1.2). At higher temperatures, performance is dramatically reduced.

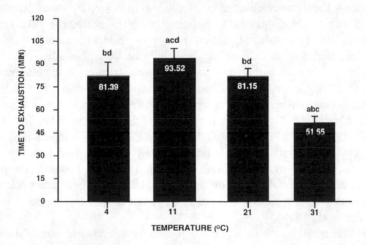

FIGURE 1.2 Endurance performance in moderate-intensity cycling exercise is reduced when the ambient temperature is high, and some impairment is already present at a temperature of only 21°C. The optimum temperature for exercise intensity in these non-acclimated subjects seems to be about 10°C. (Data of Galloway and Maughan, 1997).

There is growing evidence from a number of other sources that body temperature may be a critical factor for the performance of prolonged exercise. Nielsen et al. (1993) reported that subjects performing prolonged exhausting exercise in a hot environment stopped exercising when their core temperature reached a certain critical level (39.7°C with a standard deviation of 0.15°C) and hypothesized that this was related to a reduced motivation or central drive. The improvements in endurance capacity that accompany heat acclimation are not associated with an increased tolerance to an elevated body temperature. Rather, there is a slowing of the rate of rise of temperature due to an increased rate of heat loss resulting from an expanded plasma volume, which allows a greater cardiac output (Nielsen, 1998), an earlier onset of sweating, an increased sweating rate, and a better distribution of sweat secretion over the body surface (Wenger, 1989). There is, however, also some limited evidence from the study of Nielsen et al. (1993) that the rate of change of body temperature is not different after acclimation and that the delay in reaching a critical level is the result of a decrease in the pre-exercise core temperature.

Several studies have also shown that performance of exercise can be enhanced if the core temperature is deliberately reduced prior to exercise in warm or hot environments. Hessermer et al. (1984) exposed subjects to cold air for long enough to reduce mean skin temperature by 4.5°C; in a subsequent 60-min cycling time trial, average power output was increased by 6.8% over a control trial without pre-cooling. Lee and Haymes (1995) pre-cooled runners by exposure to cold air for 30 min before a treadmill run to exhaustion at 82% of VO_{2max} at an ambient temperature of 24°C. The pre-cooling was sufficient to induce a mean decrease of 0.4°C in core temperature, and the running time to fatigue was increased from 22.4 min to 26.2 min. Booth et al. (1997) used 20 min of cold water immersion to induce a fall in core temperature of 0.5°C prior to a maximal 30-min run in hot (32°C), humid (62% rh) conditions. The distance covered in 30 min was increased by about 2% after pre-cooling. More recently, Gonzalez-Alonso et al. (1999) reported the effects of prior immersion in hot, thermoneutral, and cold water on endurance capacity and on the physiological responses to exercise at about 60% of VO_{2max} in a hot (40°C) environment. Mean endurance time was reduced from 46 min in the thermoneutral condition to 28 min after hot water immersion and was increased to 63 min after prior cooling; a clear relationship was reported between the pre-exercise temperature and the time to fatigue. Once again, they reported that subjects voluntarily stopped exercising when the core temperature (in this case esophageal temperature) reached a critical level of 40.1–40.2°C. Brain temperature is hypothesized to be the critical factor, but it cannot be measured directly in man. In the rat, however, the point of cessation of treadmill running with different combinations of heat stress prior to and during running has been shown to occur at a hypothalamic temperature of just over 40°C (Fuller et al., 1998).

These studies all involved relatively prolonged exercise in stressful environments, where the elevation of core temperature might reasonably be considered to be a major factor in fatigue, but Myley et al. (1989) cooled subjects by icing the skin prior to a 6-min all-out rowing test carried out at an ambient temperature of 30°C. Cooling increased the mean power that could be sustained over the 6 min test by 3%. It seems unlikely that core temperature would be sufficiently elevated in 6 min of rowing to reach a critical level, suggesting that other mechanisms may also be involved.

These studies emphasize the importance of strategies to limit the rise in core temperature that occurs in exercise, especially in warm or hot climates. They also call into doubt the benefits of warming up prior to exercise when the ambient temperature is high and where an elevated core temperature may limit performance. Ingestion of fluid during prolonged exercise can help maintain cardiovascular function, attenuate the rise in body temperature that occurs, and improve exercise performance (Coyle and Montain, 1993). The optimum formulation of a drink to achieve this will depend on a number of factors that are described in detail in Chapter 8.

The above description of a possible role for an elevation of body temperature as a factor in the etiology of fatigue does not extend to the inclusion of the various clinical conditions that are referred to as heat illness, heat exhaustion, or heat stroke. These conditions, and the role of fluid replacement in their prevention, have been described by Sutton (1990).

1.5.2 DEHYDRATION

Although the physiological consequences of dehydration due to the sweat loss that occurs during exercise have been the focus of much attention, there has been relatively little scientific interest in the effects of a fluid deficit incurred prior to exercise. Both of these situations, however, are common in sport. Individuals who begin exercise with a fluid deficit will not perform as well as they will when fully hydrated. This has been shown to be true whether the fluid deficit is incurred by prolonged exercise in a warm environment, by passive heat exposure, or by diuretic treatment (Nielsen et al., 1981; Armstrong et al., 1985). An impaired performance is observed whether the exercise lasts a few minutes or is more prolonged, although muscular strength appears to be relatively unaffected, and tasks with a large aerobic component are affected to a greater extent than those that rely primarily on anaerobic metabolism (Sawka and Pandolf, 1990).

In exercise tests lasting more than a few minutes, reductions in performance are apparent at modest levels of body water loss amounting to 1–2% of the pre-exercise body mass (Armstrong et al., 1985). For the average young male (most of the subjects in these studies have been male, but the responses of female subjects do not appear to be different), body water accounts for about 60% of total body mass, so these levels of hypohydration amount to about 2–3% of total body water. It was reported by Adolph et al. (1947) that subjects do not report a sensation of thirst until they have incurred a water deficit of about 2% of body mass. This suggests that athletes living and training in the heat may not be aware that they have become dehydrated to a level sufficient to adversely affect performance.

Fluid losses due to sweating are distributed in varying proportions among the body compartments: plasma, extracellular water, and intracellular water. The decrease in plasma volume that accompanies dehydration may be of particular importance in influencing work capacity. Blood flow to the muscles must be maintained at a high level to supply oxygen and substrates, but a high blood flow to the skin is also necessary to convect heat from the active muscles and the body core to the body surface, where it can be dissipated (Nadel, 1980). When the ambient temperature is high and blood volume has been decreased by sweat loss during prolonged exercise, there may be difficulty in meeting the requirement for a high blood flow to both these tissues. In this situation, skin blood flow is likely to be compromised, allowing central venous pressure and muscle blood flow to be maintained but reducing heat loss and causing body temperature to rise (Rowell, 1986). More recent data, however, suggest that dehydration may cause a reduction in the blood flow to exercising muscles as well as to the skin (Gonzalez-Alonso et al., 1998). It may be that a falling cardiac output and an imminent failure to maintain blood pressure is one of the signals responsible for exhaustion when dehydration occurs during prolonged exercise.

These factors have been investigated by Coyle and his colleagues, whose results clearly demonstrate that increases in core temperature and heart rate and the decreases in cardiac stroke volume during prolonged exercise are graded according to the level of hypohydration achieved (Montain and Coyle 1992a). They also showed that the ingestion of fluid during exercise increases skin blood flow, and therefore thermoregulatory capacity, independent of increases in the circulating blood volume (Montain and Coyle, 1992b). Plasma volume expansion using dextran/saline infusion was less effective in preventing a rise in core temperature than was the ingestion of sufficient volumes of a carbohydrate electrolyte drink to maintain plasma volume at a similar level (Montain and Coyle, 1992b). This raises some questions about the mechanism of action of fluid replacement during exercise, but these studies confirm the importance of the ingestion of drink of a suitable composition and in sufficient volume during prolonged exercise in a warm environment.

1.5.3 ELECTROLYTE IMBALANCES

The normal response to prolonged strenuous exercise is an increase in the plasma concentration of sodium and potassium. The sodium concentration increases for two reasons:

1. Movement of water into the active muscle tissues reduces the plasma volume.
2. The sweat sodium concentration is much less than that of plasma.

The plasma potassium concentration rises because of release of potassium from active muscles and from the liver, as well as from red blood cells and other tissues subjected to membrane damage. Alterations in the distribution of ions among tissues have implications for the maintenance of function, but replacement is not generally an issue, as the movements among compartments are generally reversed in the recovery period.

The sweat that is secreted onto the skin contains a wide variety of organic and inorganic solutes, and significant losses of some of these components will occur where large volumes of sweat are produced. The electrolyte composition of sweat is variable, and the concentration of individual electrolytes as well as the total sweat volume will influence the extent of losses. The normal concentration ranges for the main ionic components of sweat are shown in Table 1.5, along with their plasma and intracellular concentrations for comparison. A number of factors contribute to the variability in the composition of sweat, and much of the published information is suspect because of methodological problems in the collection procedure, including evaporative loss, incomplete collection, and contamination with skin cells. There is also a large inter-individual biological variability (Shirreffs and Maughan, 1997).

Although the sweat composition undoubtedly varies among individuals, it can also change within the same individual depending on the rate of secretion, the state of training, and the state of heat acclimation (Leithead and Lind, 1964). There seem

TABLE 1.5
Concentration (mmol/l) of the Major
Electrolytes in Sweat, Plasma, and
Intracellular Water

	Sweat	Plasma	Intracellular
Sodium	20–80	130–155	10
Potassium	4–8	3.2–5.5	150
Calcium	0–1	2.1–2.9	0
Magnesium	<0.2	0.7–1.5	15
Chloride	20–60	96–110	8
Bicarbonate	0–35	23–28	10
Phosphate	0.1–0.2	0.7–1.6	65
Sulphate	0.1–2.0	0.3–0.9	10

Note: These values are taken from a variety of sources
referred to in Maughan and Shirreffs (1998).

also to be some differences among different sites on the body, and care must be taken in extrapolating from measurements made over a small skin area. In response to a standard heat stress, there is an earlier onset of sweating and an increased sweat rate with training and acclimation. The sweat-sodium concentration decreases in response to acclimation in spite of the increased sweat rate, although it would normally be expected to increase with increasing sweat rate (Wenger, 1989). These adaptations allow improved thermoregulation by increasing the evaporative capacity while conserving electrolytes. The conservation of sodium, in particular, may be important in maintaining the plasma volume and thus maintaining the cardiovascular capacity.

The major electrolytes in sweat, as in the extracellular fluid, are sodium and chloride, although the sweat concentrations of these ions are invariably substantially lower than those in plasma, indicating a selective reabsorption process in the sweat duct. Costill (1977) reported an increased sweat-sodium and -chloride content with increased flow, but Verde et al. (1982) found that the sweat concentration of these ions was unrelated to the sweat flow rate. Acclimation studies have shown that elevated sweating rates are accompanied by a decrease in the concentration of sodium and chloride in sweat (Allan and Wilson, 1971). The potassium content of sweat appears to be relatively unaffected by the sweat rate, and the magnesium content is also unchanged or perhaps decreases slightly. These apparently conflicting results demonstrate some of the difficulties in interpreting the lature in this area. Differences among studies may be due to differences in the training status and degree of acclimation of the subjects used, as well as difference in methodology; some studies have used whole-body washdown techniques to collect sweat, whereas others have examined local sweating responses using ventilated capsules or collection bags.

Because sweat is hypotonic with respect to body fluids, the effect of prolonged sweating is to increase the plasma osmolality, which may have a significant effect on the ability to maintain body temperature. A direct relationship between plasma osmolality and body temperature has been demonstrated during exercise (Greenleaf et al., 1974; Harrison et al., 1978). Hyperosmolality of plasma, induced prior to exercise, has been shown to result in a decreased thermoregulatory effector response; the threshold for sweating is elevated and the cutaneous vasodilator response is reduced (Fortney et al., 1984). In short-term (30 min) exercise, however, the cardio-vascular and thermoregulatory response appears to be independent of changes in osmolality induced during the exercise period (Fortney et al., 1988). The changes in the concentration of individual electrolytes are more variable, but an increase in the plasma-sodium and -chloride concentrations is generally observed in response to both running and cycling exercise. Exceptions to this are rare and occur only when excessively large volumes of drinks low in electrolytes are consumed over long time periods; these situations are discussed further below.

The plasma potassium concentration has been reported to remain constant after marathon running (Meytes et al., 1969; Whiting et al., 1984), although others have reported small increases, irrespective of whether drinks containing large amounts of potassium (Kavanagh and Shephard, 1975) or no electrolytes (Costill et al., 1976) were given. Much of the inconsistency in the literature relating to changes in the circulating potassium concentration can be explained by the variable time taken to obtain blood samples after exercise under field conditions; the plasma potassium concentration rapidly returns to normal in the post-exercise period (Stansbie et al., 1982). Laboratory studies where an indwelling catheter can be used to obtain blood samples during exercise commonly show an increase in the circulating potassium concentration in the later stages of prolonged exercise and during high-intensity exercise. The potassium concentration of extracellular fluid (4–5 mmol/l) is small relative to the intracellular concentration (150–160 mmol/l), and release of potassium from liver, muscle, and red blood cells will tend to elevate plasma potassium levels during exercise in spite of the losses in sweat. During exercise, there is a substantial loss of potassium from the active muscles, and the potassium content of the venous blood draining the active muscles increases in proportion to the exercise intensity (Gullestad et al., 1991). The local extracellular potassium concentration within active muscles may reach levels that are high enough to reduce membrane excitability. This possibility has been extensively reviewed by McKenna (1995) and Lindinger and Sjogaard (1991).

The plasma-magnesium concentration is generally unchanged after moderate-intensity exercise, and although a modest fall has been reported after extreme exercise, it seems likely that this reflects a redistribution of the available magnesium among body compartments rather than a net loss from the body (Maughan and Greenhaff, 1991). A redistribution between red blood cells and plasma has also been observed in response to daily walking for 2 h in a hot (40°C) environment over a period of 10 successive days (Stendig-Lindberg et al., 1998), and again a decrease in the serum-magnesium concentration was observed. A larger fall in the serum magnesium concentration has, however, been observed during exercise in the heat compared with neutral temperatures (Beller et al., 1972), supporting the idea that losses in sweat, rather than a simple movement from the extracellular to the intracellular space, may be responsible. Although the concentration of potassium and magnesium in sweat is high relative to that in the plasma, the plasma content of these ions represents only a small fraction of the whole-body stores, as they are both primarily located in the intracellular space (Table 1.5). Costill and Miller (1980) estimated that only about 1% of the body stores of these electrolytes was lost when individuals were dehydrated by 5.8% of body weight. This raises questions as to the value of adding these electrolytes to drinks intended for consumption before, during, or after exercise.

1.5.4 HYPOGLYCEMIA

The blood glucose concentration falls when the rate of removal of glucose from the circulation by the brain, muscles, and other tissues exceeds the rate at which it is added to the bloodstream by the liver. The normal blood glucose concentration is about 4–6 mmol/l, except after a carbohydrate meal, when it will rise to about 8–10 mmol/l. This provides enough glucose to maintain the supply to the cells of the central nervous system, for which it is the primary fuel. If hypoglycemia — normally defined as a blood glucose concentration of less than about 2.5 mmol/l (about 45 mg/100 ml) — occurs, central nervous symptoms may begin to appear.

There is clearly an opportunity for the gut, provided that it is supplied with carbohydrate, to assist the liver in the maintenance of the blood glucose concentration, particularly in the later stages of exercise. Many studies have shown that regular ingestion of even small amounts of carbohydrate during prolonged exercise can prevent a fall in the blood glucose concentration. It is not clear, however, that hypoglycemia is a cause of fatigue, and even when hypoglycemia is prevented by the ingestion of glucose, exercise performance is not necessarily improved (Felig et al., 1982).

A form of reactive hypoglycemia has been reported to occur in some sensitive individuals when large amounts of carbohydrate are ingested in the fasted state shortly before the performance of hard exercise (Costill et al., 1977). Based on these reports, it was suggested that athletes should not eat carbohydrate-containing foods within the last 3 hours before exercise. The logic is persuasive: the carbohydrate causes a sharp rise in the circulating insulin level, which inhibits fat mobilization and promotes carbohydrate metabolism. When exercise begins, there is a reduced availability of fat as a fuel and an increased rate of carbohydrate oxidation. The blood glucose concentration is therefore likely to fall rapidly, and, in one study, this resulted in an earlier onset of fatigue. On the basis of this result, it was recommended that carbohydrate ingestion should be avoided for at least 2 hours before exercise. The well-fed, well-rested athlete with replete stores of glycogen in liver and skeletal muscle may not need extra carbohydrate at this time, but several more-recent studies have shown that most individuals are not disadvantaged and may even benefit from ingesting carbohydrate in the pre-exercise period, especially if they have been fasted overnight (Gleeson et al., 1986). It appears that the metabolic changes caused by eating carbohydrate are generally rapidly reversed once exercise begins (see Coyle (1991) for a review of these studies). There are some athletes who experience an exaggerated effect, and who might perhaps benefit from avoiding carbohydrate at this time, but most athletes should be able to take carbohydrate snacks or drinks within the last hour before exercise.

Maintaining the blood glucose concentration may have thermoregulatory as well as metabolic benefits. High catecholamine levels during prolonged exercise in warm environments contribute to an increased rate of glycogen breakdown in active skeletal muscles (Febbraio et al., 1996) and in the liver (Hargreaves et al., 1996). Infusing glucose at a high rate to maintain hyperglycemia has been shown to limit the rise in plasma catecholamine levels during prolonged exercise in the heat (Mora-Rodriguez et al., 1996). High catecholamine levels also cause constriction of skin blood vessels, limiting heat loss and contributing to hyperthermia. Dehydration will, of course, also impair thermoregulation, so carbohydrate-containing drinks have clear potential for improvement in performance in all situations where these factors contribute to fatigue.

1.5.5 MUSCLE GLYCOGEN DEPLETION

It is well recognized that the ability to perform prolonged exercise can be substantially modified by dietary intake in the pre-exercise period, and this is important for the individual aiming to produce peak performance on a specific day. The pre-exercise period can conveniently be divided into two phases — the few days prior to the exercise task and the day of exercise itself. In tournament situations or in multistage events, the post-competition phase merges with the preparation phase for the next event, and the recovery diet assumes major importance.

Dietary manipulation to increase muscle glycogen content in the days prior to exercise is recommended for all exercise lasting more than about 1 hour. The method first used by marathon runners was based on a series of Scandinavian laboratory studies in the mid 1960s. These studies examined the effects of diet on muscle glycogen storage and on exercise capacity. The picture that emerged was that the glycogen content of the exercising muscles fell progressively during prolonged exercise (Bergstrom and Hultman, 1966); with the point of fatigue being coincident with the depletion of the glycogen stores (Hermansen et al., 1967). Muscle glycogen synthesis was restricted by feeding a low-carbohydrate diet after exercise, and was promoted by feeding a high-carbohydrate diet at this time. Endurance capacity — the time for which a fixed power output could be sustained to the point of fatigue — was closely related to the size of the pre-exercise muscle glycogen store (Ahlborg et al., 1967). On the basis of these findings, it was recommended that athletes should deplete muscle glycogen by prolonged exercise about 1 week prior to competition. Resynthesis of glycogen was then limited by consuming a low-carbohydrate diet while continuing to train for 2 to 3 days before changing to a high-carbohydrate diet for the last 3 days before competition, during which time little or no exercise was performed. This procedure, which has been shown in the laboratory to double the muscle glycogen content, can increase cycling or running performance, and has been used successfully by many athletes, especially marathon runners. There is now a considerable amount of evidence that it is not necessary to include the low-carbohydrate glycogen-depletion phase of the diet for endurance athletes in regular training. The training load should be reduced over the last 5 or 6 days before competition and the carbohydrate intake increased (Costill, 1988). This avoids many of the problems associated with more-extreme forms of the diet.

Although this glycogen loading procedure is generally restricted to use by athletes engaged in endurance events, similar dietary manipulations have also been shown to influence exercise performance where the intensity is high (close to 100% of VO_{2max}) and the duration is correspondingly short (3 to 10 min); an inadequate carbohydrate intake in the days before exercise reduces performance, and a high-carbohydrate diet can increase performance (Maughan and Greenhaff, 1991). A high muscle glycogen content may be particularly important when repeated sprints at near-maximum speed must be made. Consumption of a high-carbohydrate diet in the days prior to competition may therefore also benefit competitors in games such as football, soccer, or hockey, although it appears not to be usual for these players to pay attention to this aspect of their diet. Karlsson and Saltin (1973) showed that players starting a soccer game with low muscle glycogen content did less running, and much less running at high speed, than those players who began the game with a normal muscle glycogen content. It is common for players to have one game in midweek as well as one on the weekend, and it is likely that full restoration of the muscle glycogen content will not occur between games unless a conscious effort is made to achieve a high carbohydrate intake.

Although it is widely accepted that the point of fatigue during prolonged cycling exercise is closely associated with the depletion of glycogen in the exercising muscles, the evidence that this is so in running is less clear (Sherman et al., 1981). Nonetheless, a high-carbohydrate diet in the days before a long (30 km) run can improve performance (Karlsson and Saltin, 1971). A high-carbohydrate intake (10 g per kg body mass in 24 hours) was also more effective in promoting recovery between prolonged, intermittent, high-intensity shuttle running on consecutive days than a "normal" mixed diet with about half of this amount of carbohydrate (Nicholas et al., 1997). These studies all suggest that glycogen availability or some related factor is involved. Fatigue during exercise in the heat, however, is not associated with depletion of muscle glycogen (Parkin et al., 1999), and some other mechanism, probably involving a thermal factor as described above, must be involved.

1.5.6 CARBOHYDRATE REQUIREMENTS FOR COMPETITION

There is scope for nutritional intervention during exercise only when the duration of events is sufficient to allow absorption of drinks or foods ingested and where the rules of the sport permit. The primary aims must be to ingest a source of energy, usually in the form of carbohydrate, and fluid for replacement of water lost as sweat. To limit the rise in body temperature that would otherwise occur, high rates of sweat secretion are necessary during hard exercise. If the exercise is prolonged, this leads to progressive dehydration and loss of electrolytes. Fatigue toward the end of a prolonged event might result as much from the effects of dehydration as from substrate depletion. Drinks consumed during exercise therefore offer the opportunity to limit the extent of dehydration and to supplement carbohydrate.

It is not entirely clear whether carbohydrate ingested during exercise has a major sparing effect on the muscle glycogen stores. Although some studies have shown glycogen sparing, others have not (see Coyle (1991) for a review of these studies). Even where no slowing of the rate of muscle glycogen use is apparent, however, most studies show that the ingestion of carbohydrate improves the performance of prolonged exercise.

The composition of drinks to be taken during exercise should be chosen to suit individual circumstances. During exercise in the cold, fluid replacement may not be necessary, as sweat rates will be low, but there is still a need to supply additional glucose to the exercising muscles. Consumption of a high-carbohydrate diet in the days prior to exercise should reduce the need for carbohydrate ingestion during exercise in events lasting less than about 2 hours, but it is not always possible to achieve this. Competition on successive days, for example, could prevent adequate glycogen replacement between exercise periods. In this situation, concentrated glucose drinks might be more effective in improving performance. These will supply more glucose, thus supplementing the limited glycogen stores in the muscles and liver without overloading the body with fluid. In many sports environments, there is little provision for fluid replacement; participants in games such as football or hockey can lose large amounts of fluid, but significant replacement is possible only at the half-time interval, with limited opportunities for drinks during time-outs.

Recovery after hard competition requires rest, but rest alone, without restoration of the body's carbohydrate stores and correction of any fluid and electrolyte deficit, will not restore exercise capacity. When the competition has to be repeated after only a short interval, as in a multistage cycle race or in a tennis or rugby tournament, glycogen storage can be promoted by ensuring that carbohydrate is ingested as soon as possible after the end of the exercise period. The same guidelines apply as described above for promoting recovery between training sessions. An intake of 50 to 100 grams of carbohydrate is recommended within the first 2 hours after exercise, as carbohydrate ingestion at this time will promote the fastest rate of muscle glycogen resynthesis. Carbohydrates with a high glycemic index may be more effective than low glycemic index foods.

1.5.7 GASTROINTESTINAL DISTRESS

One problem often encountered by some athletes is a disturbance of gastrointestinal function during training or competition. This may take the form of mild discomfort, flatulence, and a sense of fullness, or may be more serious, with vomiting and bloody diarrhea in extreme cases. In surveys of runners competing in marathon and half-marathon races, it has been reported that the prevalence of gastrointestinal problems of varying severity is typically about 30–50% (Keefe et al., 1984; Riddoch and Trinick, 1988). These surveys, however, are prone to considerable sampling errors; return rates for questionnaires are not high and those responding to questions regarding gastrointestinal problems are likely to be those for whom this is a problem. In addition, most of the questionnaires ask "leading" questions that provoke the response that the investigators are seeking.

In spite of the uncertainty over the extent of the problem, the severity of the symptoms experienced by some individuals indicates that the problem is very real. In some cases, there is an underlying pathology that is exacerbated by hard exercise, perhaps because of some degree of local ischemia or because of mechanical factors associated with repeated jarring while running. This latter argument is supported by the common observation that problems are much more common in runners than in cyclists (Brouns, 1991). The severity of symptoms, especially of gastric bleeding, seems in many cases to be related to the use of non-steroidal anti-inflammatory preparations (Robertson et al., 1987). Hard exercise will also affect the local and systemic concentrations of many of the peptide hormones secreted by the gastrointestinal tract and the liver (Brouns, 1991). Many of these hormones, including gastrin, vasoactive intestinal peptide (VIP), and somatostatin, have metabolic effects as well as their local effects on gut function. O'Connor et al. (1995) measured the circulating concentrations of a number of gastrointestinal peptide hormones in 26 runners before and after a marathon race; the plasma levels of all the peptides except insulin increased during the race, but there was no relationship between the direction and magnitude of these changes and the incidence of gastrointestinal distress, which affected eight of the runners. One proposed mechanism by which exercise might influence the function of the gastrointestinal tract is related to the increased circulating catecholamine level and reduced perfusion of the splanchnic vascular bed during strenuous exercise; these effects have been reviewed by Murray (1987). The factors associated with gastrointestinal problems during exercise have recently been reviewed (Peters et al., 1995), but there remains no clear indication as to the cause of the problem nor of the best way to avoid its occurrence.

Availability of nutrients ingested during exercise is limited by the rate at which they are emptied from the stomach and by the rate of subsequent absorption in the intestine. Where there is a need to replace fluids and carbohydrate during exercise, this may be compromised if either of these processes is slowed. High-intensity exercise slows both gastric emptying and intestinal absorption, but these effects are small at the work rates that can be sustained for prolonged periods (Maughan and Shirreffs, 1998). It is generally the case that the exercise duration would be too short to allow a benefit from ingested food or fluids if the intensity were sufficiently high to markedly slow the availability of ingested nutrients. Food and fluids should, however, be chosen to minimize the possibility of adverse gastrointestinal reactions, and these issues will be discussed in more detail in Chapters 4 and 6.

Because the underlying cause of the gastrointestinal problems encountered by some runners is not clear, it is difficult to suggest interventions that will reduce the frequency of severity of the symptoms that are experienced.

1.6 NUTRITIONAL GOALS AND EATING STRATEGIES

The nutritional needs of athletes are many and varied, but this section has told only one part of the story. It has focused on the nutritional demands of training and competition and has largely ignored issues relating to the selection of foods that will meet the athlete's needs. The increased energy demands of the active individual provide an opportunity for an increased quantity and variety of foods to be consumed. Not all athletes, however, take advantage of this opportunity. Limited awareness of their nutritional goals, combined with poor cooking skills, restricted opportunities for eating due to pressures of work or study, combined with training, financial, and other constraints, prevent many athletes from selecting a varied diet. For many athletes, there is also something reassuring about the regular routine of training and eating.

Once the nutritional goals have been established, many options are open to the athlete. Very different food choices can provide a similar mix of nutrients, allowing the athlete who knows something of the composition of foods considerable scope to indulge personal preferences. There are no good foods or bad foods in the athlete's diet, but poor food choices can result in a poor diet. It cannot be assumed that athletes will choose a diet that will meet their needs, but with sound advice, they should be able to select foods that they enjoy with the knowledge that their diets provide not only enjoyment but also support for their training and competition.

1.7 SUMMARY

The athlete in training must be aware of the nutrient demands imposed by the training load. These will generally be proportional to the intensity, duration, and frequency of training sessions, but will also be affected by the physiological and biochemical characteristics of the individual. The main requirement is to meet the additional energy demand of training, to ensure a high intake of carbohydrate to replace the glycogen stores used by the working muscles, and to ensure that sufficient fluid to replace sweat losses is also consumed. Intake of other nutrients (protein, vitamins, minerals, and fat and essential fatty acids) should be adequate to meet the body's needs. When the nutritional goals have been established, these must be translated into eating and drinking strategies that will identify the types and amounts of foods that should be consumed to provide the necessary nutrients.

Special nutritional strategies may be necessary to meet the demands of competition, and these will vary greatly between sports, depending on the nature of the event. Strategies should target the factors that cause fatigue and impair performance. These include hyperthermia, dehydration, hypoglycemia, muscle glycogen depletion, electrolyte imbalances, and gastrointestinal distress. Food and fluid intake before, during, and after exercise can influence all of these factors, with implications for the success or failure of the performer.

REFERENCES

Adolph, E.F., and associates, *Physiology of Man in the Desert*, Interscience, NY, 1947.

Ahlborg, B., Bergstrom, J., Brohult, J., Ekelund, L.G., Hultman, E., and Maschio, G., Human muscle glycogen content and capacity for prolonged exercise after different diets. *Forsvarsmedicin* 3, 85–89, 1967.

Allan, J.R. and Wilson, C.G., Influence of acclimatization on sweat sodium secretion. *J. Appl. Physiol.* 30, 708–712, 1971.

Armstrong, L.E., Costill, D.L., and Fink, W.J. Influence of diuretic-induced dehydration on competitive running performance. *Med. Sci. Sports Exerc.* 17, 456–461, 1985.

Bahr, R., Excess post-exercise oxygen consumption — magnitude, mechanisms and practical implications. *Acta Physiologica Scandinavica* 144 (suppl. 605), 1–70, 1992.

Beller, G.A., Maher, J.T., Hartley, L.H., Bass, D.E., and Wacker, W.E.C., Serum Mg and K concentrations during exercise in thermoneutral and hot conditions. *The Physiologist* 15, 94, 1972.

Bergstrom, J. and Hultman, E., The effect of exercise on muscle glycogen and electrolytes in normals. *Scandin. J. Clinic.Labor. Invest.* 18, 16–20, 1966.

Bigard, A.-X., Guillemot, P.Y., Chauve, J.Y., Duforez, F., Portero, P., and Guezennec, C.-Y., Nutrient intake of elite sailors during a solitary long-distance offshore race. *Int. J. Sport Nutr.* 8, 364–376, 1998.

Booth, J., Marino, F., and Ward, J.J., Improved running performance in hot humid conditions following whole body precooling. *Med. Sci. Sports Exerc.* 29, 943, 1997.

Brouns, F., Gastrointestinal symptoms in athletes: physiological and nutritional aspects. In *Advances in Nutrition and Top Sport.* Brouns, F., Ed., Karger, Basel,1991, pp. 166–199.

Clark, K., Nutritional guidance to soccer players for training and competition. *J. Sports Sci.* 12 (Special Issue), S43–S50, 1994.

Clarkson, P.M., Micronutrients and exercise: Anti-oxidants and minerals. *J. Sports Sci.* 13 (Special Issue), S11–S24, 1995.

Costill, D.L., Sweating: its composition and effects on body fluids. *Ann. NY Acad. Sci.* 301, 160–174, 1977.

Costill, D.L., Carbohydrates for exercise: dietary demands for optimal performance. *Int. J. Sports Med.* 9, 1–18, 1988.

Costill, D.L. and Miller, J.M., Nutrition for endurance sport. *Int. J. Sports Med.* 1, 2–14, 1980.

Costill, D.L., Branam, G., Fink, W., and Nelson, R., Exercise-induced sodium conservation: changes in plasma renin and aldosterone. *Med. Sci. Sports Exerc.* 8, 209–213, 1976.

Costill, D.L., Coyle, E.F., Dalsky, G., Evans, W., Fink, W., and Hoopes, D., Effects of elevated plasma FFA and insulin on muscle glycogen usage during exercise. *J. Appl. Physiol.* 43, 695–699, 1977.

Coyle, E.F., Timing and method of increased carbohydrate intake to cope with heavy training, competition and recovery. In *Foods, Nutrition and Sports Performance.* Williams, C., Devlin, J.T., Eds., E & FN Spon, London, 1992, pp. 35–62.

Coyle, E.F. and Montain, S.J., Thermal and cardiovascular responses to fluid replacement during exercise. In *Perspect. Exerc. Sci. Sports Med. Vol 6.* Gisolfi, C.V., Lamb, D.R. and Nadel, E.R., Eds., WC Brown, Dubuque, 1993, pp.179–223.

Febbraio, M.A., Snow, R.J., Stathis, C.G., Hargreaves, M., and Carey, M.F., Blunting the rise in body temperature reduces muscle glycogenolysis during exercise in humans. *Experiment. Physiol.* 81, 685–693, 1996.

Felig, P., Cherif, A., Minigawa, A. and Wahren, J., Hypoglycemia during prolonged exercise in normal men. *N. Eng. J. Med.* 306: 895–900, 1982.

Fortney, S.M., Wenger, C.B., Bove, J.R. and Nadel, E.R., Effect of hyperosmolality on control of blood flow and sweating. *J. Appl. Physiol.* 57, 1688–1695, 1984.

Fortney, S.M., Vroman, N.B., Beckett, S.W., Permutt, S. and LaFrance, N.D., Effect of exercise hemoconcentration and hyperosmolality on exercise responses. *J. Appl. Physiol.* 65, 519–524, 1988.

Fuller, A., Carter, R.N., and Mitchell, D., Brain and abdominal temperatures at fatigue in rats exercising in the heat. *J. Appl. Physiol.* 84, 877–883, 1998.

Galloway, S.D.R. and Maughan, R.J., Effects of ambient temperature on the capacity to perform prolonged cycle exercise in man. *Med. Sci. Sports and Exerc.* 29, 1240–1249, 1997.

Gleeson, M., Maughan, R.J., and Greenhaff, P.L., Comparison of the effects of pre-exercise feeding of glucose, glycerol and placebo on endurance and fuel homeostasis in man. *Eur. J. Appl. Physiol.* 55, 645–653, 1986.

Gonzalez-Alonso, J., Calbet, J., and Nielsen, B., Muscle blood flow is reduced with dehydration during prolonged exercise in humans. *J. Physiol.* 513, 895–905, 1998.

Gonzalez-Alonso, J., Teller, C., Andersen, S.L., Jensen, F.B., Hyldig, T., and Nielsen, B., Influence of body temperature on the development of fatigue during prolonged exercise in the heat. *J. Appl. Physiol.* 86, 1032–1039, 1999.

Greenhaff, P.L., Cardiovascular fitness and thermoregulation during prolonged exercise in man. *Brit. J. Sports Med.* 23, 109–114, 1989.

Greenleaf, J.E., Castle, B.L., and Card, D.H., Blood electrolytes and temperature regulation during exercise in man. *Acta Physiologica Polonica* 25, 397–410, 1974.

Gregory, J., Foster, K., Tyler, H., and Wiseman, M., The dietary and nutritional survey of British adults. HMSO, London, 1990.

Gullestad, L., Birkeland, K., Nordby, G., Larsen, S., and Kjekshus, J., Effects of selective beta 2-adrenoceptor blockade on serum potassium and exercise performance in normal men. *Brit. J. Clinic. Pharmacol.* 32, 201–207, 1991.

Hargreaves, M., Angus, D., Howlett, K., Conus, N.M., and Febbraio M., Effect of heat stress on glucose kinetics during exercise. *J. Appl. Physiol.* 81, 1594–1597, 1996.

Harrison, M.H., Edwards, R.J., and Fennessy, P.A., Intravascular volume and tonicity as factors in the regulation of body temperature. *J. Appl. Physiol.* 44, 69–75, 1978.

Hermansen, L., Hultman, E., and Saltin, B., Muscle glycogen during prolonged severe exercise. *Acta Physiologica Scandinavica* 71, 129–139, 1967.

Hessermer, V., Langusch, D., Bruck, K., Bodeker, R.H., and Breidenbach, T., Effect of slightly lowered body temperatures on endurance performance in humans. *J. Appl. Physiol.* 57, 1731–1737, 1984.

Ivy, J.L., Glycogen resynthesis after exercise: effect of carbohydrate intake. *Int. J. Sports Med.* 19, S142–S145, 1998.

Karlsson, J. and Saltin, B., Diet, muscle glycogen and endurance performance. *J. Appl. Physiol.* 31, 203–206, 1971.

Kavanagh, T. and Shephard, R.J., Maintenance of hydration in "post-coronary" marathon runners. *Brit. J. Sports Med.* 9, 130–135, 1975.

Keefe, E.B., Lowe, D.K., and Gross, J.R., Gastrointestinal symptoms of marathon runners. *West. Med. J.* 141, 481–484, 1984.

Lee, D.T. and Haymes, E.M., Exercise duration and thermoregulatory responses following whole body precooling. *J. Appl. Physiol.* 79, 1971–1976, 1995.

Leiper, J.B., Pitsiladis, Y.P., and Maughan, R.J., Comparison of water turnover rates in men undertaking prolonged exercise and in sedentary men. *J. Physiol.* 483, 123P, 1995.

Leiper, J.B., Carnie, A., and Maughan, R.J., Water turnover rates in sedentary and exercising middle-aged men. *Brit. J. Sports Med.* 30, 24–26, 1996.

Leithead, C.S. and Lind, A.R., Heat stress and heat disorders. Casell, London, 1964.

Lemon, P.W.R., Effect of exercise on protein requirements. *J. Sports Sci.* 9, 53, 1991.

Lindinger, M.I. and Sjogaard, G., Potassium regulation during exercise and recovery. *Sports Med.* 11, 382–401, 1991.

McKenna, M.J., Effects of training on potassium homeostasis during exercise. *J. Molec. and Cellular Cardiol.* 27, 941–949, 1995.

Maughan, R.J., Thermoregulation and fluid balance in marathon competition at low ambient temperature. *Int. J. Sports Med.* 6, 15–19, 1985.

Maughan, R.J., Physiology and nutrition for middle distance and long distance running. In *Perspectives in Exercise Science and Sports Med., Vol. 7, Physiology and Nutrition in Competitive Sport,* Lamb, D.R., Knuttgen, H.G., and Murray, R., Eds., Cooper, Carmel, pp. 329–371, 1994.

Maughan, R.J. Energy and macronutrient intakes of professional football (soccer) players. *Brit. J. Sports Med.* 31, 45–47, 1997.

Maughan, R.J. and Greenhaff, P.L., High intensity exercise and acid-base balance: the influence of diet and induced metabolic alkalosis on performance. In *Advances in Nutrition and Top Sport.* Brouns, F., Ed., Karger, Basel, 1991, pp.147–165.

Maughan, R.J. and Shirreffs, S.M., Fluid and electrolyte loss and replacement in exercise. In *Oxford Textbook of Sports Med.*, 2nd ed. Harries, M., Williams, C., Stanish, W.D., and Micheli, L.L., Oxford University Press, New York, 1998, pp.97–113.

Maughan, R.J., Robertson, J.D., and Bruce, A.C., Dietary energy and carbohydrate intakes of runners in relation to training load. *Proc. Nutr. Soc.* 48, 170A, 1989.

Meytes, I., Shapiro, Y., Magazanik, A., Meytes, D., and Seligsohn, U., Physiological and biochemical changes during a marathon race. *Int. J. Biometeorol.* 13, 317, 1969.

Montain, S.J. and Coyle, E.F., Influence of graded dehydration on hyperthermia and cardio-vsacular drift during exercise. *J. Appl. Physiol.* 73, 1340–1350, 1992a.

Montain, S.J. and Coyle, E.F., Fluid ingestion during exercise increases skin blood flow independent of increases in blood volume. *J. Appl. Physiol.* 73, 903–910, 1992b.

Mora-Rodriguez, R., Gonzalez-Alonso, J., Below, P.r., and Coyle, E.F., Plasma catecholamines and hyperglycaemia influence thermoregulation in man during prolonged exercise in the heat. *J. Physiol.* 491, 529, 1996.

Murray, R., The effects of consuming carbohydrate-electrolyte beverages on gastric emptying and fluid absorption during and following exercise. *Sports Med.* 4, 322–351, 1987.

Myley, G.R., Hahn, A.G., and Tumilty, D.M., The effect of preliminary skin cooling on performance of rowers in hot conditions. *Excel* 6, 17–21, 1998.

Nadel, E.R., Circulatory and thermal regulations during exercise. *Federation Proc.* 39, 1491–1497, 1989.

Nicholas, C.W., Green, P.A., Hawkins, R.D., and Williams, C., Carbohydrate intake and recovery of intermittent running capacity. *Int. J. Sport Nutr.* 7, 251–260, 1997.

Nielsen, B., Heat acclimation — mechanisms of adaptation to exercise in the heat. *Int. J. Sports Med.* 19, S154–S156, 1998.

Nielsen, B., Kubica, R., Bonnesen, A., Rasmussen, I.B., Stoklosa, J., and Wilk, B., Physical work capacity after dehydration and hyperthermia. *Scandin. J. Sports Sci.* 3, 2–10, 1982.

Nielsen, B., Hales, J.R., Strange, S., Christensen, N.J., Warberg, J., and Saltin, B., Human circulatory and thermoregulatory adaptations with heat acclimation and exercise in a hot, dry environment. *J. Physiol.* 460, 467–485, 1993.

O'Connor, A.M., Johnston, C.F., Buchanan, K.D., Boreham, C., Trinick, T.R., and Riddoch, C.J., Circulating gastrointestinal hormone changes in marathon running. *Int. J. Sports Med.* 16, 283–287, 1995.

Parkin, J.M., Carey, M.F., Zhao, S., and Febbraio, M.A., Effect of ambient temperature on human skeletal muscle metabolism during fatiguing submaximal exercise. *J. Appl. Physiol.* 86, 902–908, 1999.

Peters, H.P.F., Akkermans, L.M.A., Bol, E., and Mosterd, W. L., Gastrointestinal symptoms during exercise. *Sports Med.* 20, 65–76, 1995.

Rehrer, N.J., Burke, L.M., Sweat losses during various sports. *Australian J. Nutr. and Dietetics* 53, S13–S16, 1996.

Rico-Sanz, J., Frontera, W.R., Mole, P.A., Rivera, M.A., Rivera-Brown, A., and Meredith, C.N., Dietary and performance assessment of elite soccer players during a period of intense training. *Int. J. Sport Nutr.* 8, 230–240, 1998.

Riddoch, C. and Trinick, T., Gastrointestinal disturbances in marathon runners. *Brit. J. Sports Med.* 22, 71–74, 1988.

Roberston, J.D., Maughan, r.J., and Davidson, R.J.L. Faecal blood loss in response to exercise, *Br. Med. J.* 295, 303, 1987.

Rowell, L.B. *Human Circulation.* Oxford University Press, NY, 1986.

Saltin, B. and Karlsson, J., Die Ernährung des Sportlers. In, *Zentrale Themen de Sportmedizin, Springer*, Berlin, 1973, pp. 245.

Saris, W.H.M., van-Erp-Baart, M.A., Brouns, F., Westerterp, K.R., and ten Hoor, F., Study on food intake and energy expenditure during extreme sustained exercise: the Tour de France. *Int. J. Sports Med.* 10, S26–S31, 1989.

Sawka, M.N. and Pandolf, K.B., Effects of body water loss on physiological function and exercise performance. In, *Perspectives in Exercise Science and Sports Medicine, Vol 3.*, Gisolfi, C.V. and Lamb, D.R., Eds., Benchmark Press, Indianapolis, 1990, pp.1–38.

Sherman, W.M., Costill, D.L., Fink, W.J., and Miller, J.M., Effect of exercise-diet manipulation on muscle glycogen and its subsequent utilization during performance. *Int. J. Sport Med.* 2, 114–118, 1981.

Shirreffs, S.M. and Maughan, R.J., Whole body sweat collection in man: an improved method with some preliminary data on electrolyte composition. *J. Appl. Physiol.* 82, 336–341, 1998.

Sossin, K., Gisis, F., Marquart, L.F., and Sobal, J., Nutrition beliefs, attitudes and resource use of high school wrestling coaches. *Int. J. Sport Nutr.* 7, 219–228, 1997.

Stansbie, D., Tomlinson, K., Potman, J.M., and Walters, E.G., Hypothermia, hypokalaemia and marathon running. *Lancet* 2, 1336, 1982.

Stendig-Lindberg, G., Moran, D., and Shapiro, Y., How significant is magnesium in thermoregulation? *J. Basic and Clinic. Physiol. and Pharmacol.* 9, 73–85, 1998.

Sugiura, K., Suzuki, I., Kobayashi, K., Nutritional intake of elite Japanese track-and-field athletes. *Int. J. Sport Nutr.* 9, 202–212, 1999.

Sundgot-Borgen, J., Eating disorders, energy intake, training volume, and menstrual function in high-level modern rhythmic gymnastics. *Int. J. Sport Nutr.* 6, 100–109, 1996.

Sutton, J. R., Clinical implications of fluid imbalance. In, *Perspectives in Exercise Science and Sports Medicine, Vol 3. Fluid Homeostasis During Exercise.* Gisolfi, C.V. and Lamb, D.R., Eds., 1990; 425–448.

van Erp-Baart, A.M.J., Saris, W.H.M., Binkhorst, R.A., Vos, J.A., and Elvers, J.W.H., Nationwide survey on nutritional habits in elite athletes. *Int. J. Sports Med.* 10, S3–S10, 1989.

Verde, T., Shephard, R.J., Corey, P., and Moore, R., Sweat composition in exercise and in heat. *J. Appl. Physiol.* 53, 1540–1545, 1982.

Wenger, C.B. Human heat acclimatization. In *Human Performance: Physiological and Environmental Medicine at Terrestrial Extremes*, Pandolf, K.B., Sawka, M.N., and Gonzalez, R.R., Eds., Cooper, Carmel, 1989, pp.153–197.

Westerterp, K.R., Saris, W.H.M., and Van Es, M., Use of the doubly-labeled water technique in humans during heavy sustained exercise. *J. Appl. Physiol.* 61, 2162–2167, 1986.

Whiting, P.H., Maughan, R.J., and Miller, J.D.B., Dehydration and serum biochemical changes in runners. *Eur. J. Appl. Physiol.* 52, 183–187, 1984.

Wiita, B.G. and Stombaugh, I.A., Nutrition knowledge, eating practices, and health of adolescent female runners: a 3-year longitudinal study. *Int. J. Sport Nutr.* 6, 414–425, 1996.

Wootton, S.A., Nutritional beliefs and eating habits of British athletes and coaches. In *Nutrition in Sport.* Shrimpton, D.H. and Berry Ottaway, P., Eds., Shaklee, Milton Keynes, 1986.

2 Water Turnover and Regulation of Fluid Balance

Susan M. Shirreffs and Ronald J. Maughan

CONTENTS

2.1 INTRODUCTION

2.1.1 BODY WATER AND ITS DISTRIBUTION

Water is the largest component of the human body and the total body water content varies from approximately 45–70% of the total body mass,[1] corresponding to about 33 to 53 l for a 75-kg man. Although body water content varies greatly among individuals, the water content of the various tissues is maintained relatively constant. For example, adipose tissue has a low water content and lean tissue such as muscle and bone has a high water content (Table 2.1), so the total fraction of water in the body is determined largely by the total fat content. In other words, a high fat content is related to a lower total water content as a percentage of body mass.

The body water can be divided into two components — the intracellular fluid (ICF) and the extracellular fluid (ECF); the intracellular fluid is the major component and composes approximately two-thirds of total body water. The extracellular fluid can be further divided into the interstitial fluid (that between the cells) and the plasma, with the plasma volume representing approximately one-quarter of the extracellular fluid volume. This is outlined in Table 2.1.

TABLE 2.1A
Water Content of Various Body Tissues for an Average 75-kg Man

Tissue	% Water	% of Body Mass	Water per 75 kg (in Liters)	% of Total Body Water
Skin	72	18	9.7	22
Organs	76	7	4.0	9
Skeleton	22	15	2.5	5
Blood	83	5	3.1	7
Adipose	10	12	0.9	2
Muscle	76	43	24.5	55

TABLE 2.1B
Body Water Distribution Between the Body Fluid Compartments in an Adult Male[1]

	% of Body Mass	% of Lean Body Mass	% of Body Water
Total body water	60	72	100
Extracellular water	20	24	33
Plasma	5	6	8
Interstitium	15	18	25
Intracellular water	40	48	67

2.1.2 COMPOSITION OF BODY FLUIDS

A wide range of electrolytes and solutes are dissolved in varying concentrations within the body fluids. An electrolyte can be defined as a compound that dissociates into ions when in solution. The major cations (positively charged electrolytes) in the body water are sodium, potassium, calcium, and magnesium; the major anions (negatively charged electrolytes) are chloride and bicarbonate. Sodium is the major electrolyte present in the extracellular fluid, while potassium is present in a much lower concentration (Table 2.2). In the intracellular fluid, the situation is reversed,

TABLE 2.2
Ionic Composition (mmol/l) of Body Water Compartments[2,3] Showing Normal Ranges of the Plasma Electrolyte Compartments

Ion	Plasma	Intracellular Fluid
Sodium	140 (135–145)	12
Potassium	4.0 (3.5–4.6)	150
Calcium	2.4 (2.1–2.7)	4.0
Magnesium	0.8 (0.6–1.0)	34
Chloride	104 (98–107)	4
Bicarbonate	29 (21–38)	12
Inorganic phosphate	1.0 (0.7–1.6)	40

and the major electrolyte present is potassium, with sodium found in much lower concentrations. It is critical for the body to maintain this distribution of electrolytes because maintenance of the transmembrane electrical and chemical gradients is of paramount importance for assuring the integrity of cell function and allowing electrical communication throughout the body.

2.2 CONTROL OF FLUID BALANCE

2.2.1 REGULATION OF PLASMA OSMOLALITY

Sodium and its associated chloride and bicarbonate anions form the major part of the osmotically active components of the plasma, with the plasma proteins also making a smaller but important contribution. Cell membranes are freely permeable to water, and exchange between body fluid compartments is rapid. The osmolality of the extracellular and intracellular fluid compartments is therefore very similar, in spite of the differences in the nature of the osmolytes present. Plasma osmolality is normally regulated in the range of 280 to 290 mosm/kg by controlling water and solute loss by the kidneys and by regulating water intake by the thirst mechanism. The regulatory mechanisms are described below.

Free water clearance is the term used to describe the amount of water excreted or reabsorbed by the kidney to regulate plasma osmolality: the kidney will produce, as required, urine that is hypo-osmotic or hyperosmotic relative to plasma. The "*free water*" refers to the volume of pure water that must be added to or removed from the urine to make it isosmotic with plasma.

The plasma ultrafiltrate entering the renal glomerulus has the same osmolality as the plasma. The loss of this fluid from the body as urine without a change in its composition would give no loss or addition of free water because electrolytes have been neither conserved nor lost.

2.2.2 THIRST AND THE CONTROL OF FLUID INTAKE

In man, daily fluid intake in the form of food and drink (plus that formed from substrate oxidation) is usually in excess of the obligatory water loss (transcutaneous, pulmonary, and renal output), with renal excretion being the main mechanism regulating body water content.[4] However, conservation of water or electrolytes by the kidneys can only reduce the rate of loss; it cannot restore a deficit. The sensation of thirst, which underpins drinking behavior, indicates the need to drink and hence is critical in the control of fluid intake and water balance. While thirst appears to be a poor indicator of acute hydration status in man, the overall stability of the total water volume of an individual indicates that the desire to drink is a powerful regulatory factor over the long term.[5]

The act of drinking may not be directly involved with a physiological need for water intake, but can be initiated by habit, ritual, taste, or desire for nutrients, stimulants, or a warming or cooling effect.[6] A number of the sensations associated with thirst are learned, with signals such as dryness of the mouth or throat inducing drinking, while distention of the stomach can stop ingestion before a fluid deficit has been restored. However, the underlying regulation of thirst is controlled separately by the osmotic pressure and volume of the body fluids and as such is regulated by the same mechanisms that affect water and solute reabsorption in the kidneys and control central blood pressure.

2.2.2.1   Regulatory Mechanisms

Areas of the hypothalamus and forebrain that are collectively termed the thirst control centers appear to be central to the regulation of both thirst and diuresis. Receptors in the thirst control centers respond directly to changes in osmolality, volume, and blood pressure, while others are stimulated by the fluid balance hormones that also regulate renal excretion.[7] These regions of the brain also receive afferent input from systemic receptors monitoring osmolality, circulating sodium concentration, and alterations in blood volume and pressure. Changes in the balance of neural activity in the thirst control centers regulated by the different monitoring inputs determine the relative sensations of thirst and satiety and influence the degree of diuresis. Input from the higher centers of the brain, however, can override the basic biological need for water to some extent and cause inappropriate drinking responses. Cases of water intoxication (hyponatremia) during endurance sports events lasting more than 7 h in which the major cause of the illness is due to overhydration as a result of overdrinking have been reported.[8] Another situation where excess fluid intake commonly occurs is during beer drinking, where large volumes of low-sodium fluids may be consumed in a short space of time without the intake of solid food that might provide electrolytes. Flear et al.[9] reported the case of a man who drank 9 l of beer, with a total sodium content of about 13 mmol, in the space of 20 min; his plasma sodium concentration fell from 143 mmol/l to 127 mmol/l.

A rise of between 2% and 3% in circulating osmolality (i.e., about 6 to 8 mosm/kg H_2O) is sufficient to evoke a profound sensation of thirst coupled with an increase in the circulating concentration of antidiuretic hormone (ADH), also known as vasopressin.[10] The mechanisms that respond to changes in intravascular volume and pressure appear to be less sensitive than those that monitor plasma osmolality, with hypovolemic thirst being evident only following a 10% decrease in blood volume.[4] As fairly large variations in blood volume and pressure occur during normal daily activity, primarily in response to postural changes, this lack of sensitivity presumably prevents overactivity of the volume-control mechanisms. Prolonged exercise, especially in the heat, is associated with a decrease in plasma volume and a tendency for an increase in osmolality, but fluid intake during and immediately following exercise is often less than that required to restore normal hydration status.[5] This appears to be due to a premature termination of the drinking response rather than to a lack of initiation of that response.[6] Also, the composition of the beverage consumed has an effect on the volume of fluid ingested, with water prematurely abolishing the osmotic drive to drink, while sodium-containing drinks help maintain the osmotic drive to drink and increase voluntary intake.

When a water deficit is present and free access to fluid is allowed, the drinking response in man usually consists of a period of rapid ingestion, during which more than 50% of the total intake is consumed, followed by intermittent consumption of relatively small volumes of drink over a longer period.[11] The initial alleviation of thirst occurs before significant amounts of the beverage have been absorbed and entered the body water. Therefore, although decreasing osmolality and increasing extracellular volume promote a reduction in the perception of thirst, other pre-absorptive factors also affect the volume of fluid ingested. Receptors in the mouth, esophagus, and stomach are thought to meter the volume of fluid ingested, while distension of the stomach tends to reduce the perception of thirst.[12] These pre-absorptive signals appear to be behavioral learned responses and may be subject to disruption in situations that are novel to the individual. This could partly explain the inappropriate voluntary fluid intake in individuals exposed to an acute increase in environmental temperature or to exercise-induced dehydration.

2.2.3 ANTI-DIURETIC HORMONE SECRETION AND RENAL REGULATION OF WATER EXCRETION

The volume of urine produced in a healthy individual is largely determined by circulating hormone levels, and in particular, by levels of ADH. ADH is a cyclic, nine amino acid peptide. It is released from the posterior pituitary after having been transported there along the axons of neurons whose cell bodies are located in the paraventricular and supraoptic nuclei of the hypothalamus, the site of ADH synthesis.[14] An increase in the circulating levels of ADH results in reduced urine production. ADH acts on the renal distal tubules and collecting ducts to cause an increased permeability to water and, hence, an increased reabsorption of water from the filtrate. Therefore, a hyperosmotic urine can be formed and the excreted solute load can be accommodated in a small volume of water. A decrease in ADH secretion results in an increase in the volume of urine produced by causing a reduction in the permeability of the renal distal tubule and collecting ducts to water. ADH secretion is largely influenced by changes in plasma osmolality. An increase in plasma osmolality results in a increased ADH secretion and vice versa. The ADH is released rapidly in response to the stimuli and begins to act within minutes. When secretion is inhibited, the half-life of clearance from the circulation is approximately 10 min. Therefore, changes in body fluid tonicity are rapidly translated into changes in water excretion by this tightly regulated feedback system.

In addition to the influence of plasma osmolality on ADH secretion, other (non-osmotic) factors such as baroregulation, nausea, and pharyngeal stimuli also affect thirst. A fall in blood pressure or in blood volume will stimulate ADH release; ADH secretion is, however, less sensitive to these changes than to changes in plasma osmolality. Nausea is an extremely potent stimulus to ADH secretion in man; ADH levels can increase 100- to 1000-fold in response to nausea induced by various chemical agents. After a period of water deprivation followed by access to fluids, ADH levels fall before there is any change in plasma tonicity, suggesting activation of neuronal pathways from the oropharynx.

Aldosterone is a steroid hormone released into the circulation after synthesis by the zona glomerulosa cells of the adrenal cortex. Its primary role, in terms of renal function, is to increase renal tubular reabsorption of sodium. This results in an increased excretion of potassium and, in association with antidiuretic hormone, will increase water reabsorption in the distal segments of the nephron. Aldosterone causes this response by increasing the activity of the peritubular sodium/potassium pump and by increasing the permeability of the luminal membrane to both sodium and potassium. The increased luminal permeability allows potassium to move down its concentration gradient from the inside of the membrane cells into the tubule lumen. The majority of the sodium present is reabsorbed into the cell down the concentration gradient. The sodium absorption and potassium excretion are closely correlated in a ratio of 3 sodium for 2 potassium ions. Chloride follows the sodium to maintain the electrical neutrality of the urine. The release of aldosterone is influenced by a number of factors, in particular the renin angiotensin system. A fall in blood or extracellular fluid volume increases renin production by the kidneys and, via angiotensin II, results in an increase in aldosterone secretion.

The presence in the renal filtrate of ions such as bicarbonate and sulphate, which are not reabsorbed, promotes secretion of potassium into the distal tubule of the nephron and will also result in an increased urinary loss of potassium. Despite this, however, the normal daily loss of potassium in the urine is in the region of 2700 mg in comparison with the total body stores of approximately 140 grams.[2]

2.3 DAILY WATER BALANCE AT REST

Over the course of the day, the body's total water content is normally maintained within a narrow range by intake of food and drink to balance the excretion of fluid and minerals in sweat and urine. Hyperhydration is corrected by an increase in urine production and hypohydration by an increase in water intake via food or drink consumption, as initiated by thirst. Large fluctuations in the intake of non-metabolizable solutes, mostly sodium chloride and the nitrogen moiety of proteins, will also markedly influence renal water loss and stimulate intake. Most fluid intake during the day is related to habit rather than thirst, but the thirst mechanism is effective at driving intake after periods of deprivation.[15]

The major textbooks of nutrition and physiology and dietary surveys include data on the various components of water intake and output, although it is sometimes difficult to find the original data on which the various mean values and ranges are based (e.g., [16,17,18]). For example, the Geigy Scientific Tables[2] suggest that the minimum daily water intake for adults is in the order of 1.5 l, but Nikolaidis[19] indicates that minimum intake should be 2 l/day. Regardless of the discrepancies in the lature regarding minimum daily fluid intake, it should be noted that these values do represent *minimum* values; the daily fluid needs of physically active individuals are usually far in excess of these values.

Body size is clearly a factor that has a major influence on water turnover, but total body water content will also be markedly affected by body composition. Water turnover should therefore be more closely related to lean body mass than to body mass itself. It is expected, therefore, that there will be differences between men and women and between adults and children. Unless otherwise specified, the values given in this chapter relate to the average 70-kg male with a moderate (about 12 to 18%) body fat content.

Environmental conditions affect basal water requirement by altering the losses that occur by various routes (i.e., respiration, sweat, urine). Water requirements for sedentary individuals living in the heat may be two- or threefold higher than the requirement when living in a temperate climate, even when not accompanied by pronounced sweating.[5] Transcutaneous and respiratory losses are markedly influenced by the humidity of the ambient air, and this may be a more important factor than the ambient temperature. Respiratory water losses are incurred because of the humidification of the inspired air with fluid from the lungs. These losses are relatively small in the resting individual in a warm, moist environment (amounting to about 200 ml per day), but will be increased approximately twofold in regions of low humidity and may be as high as 1500 ml per day during periods of hard work in the cold, dry air at higher altitude.[20] To these losses must be added insensible water loss through the skin (about 600 ml per day) and urine loss, which will not usually be less than about 800 ml per day.

Variations in the amount and type of food eaten have some effect on water requirements because of the resulting demand for excretion of excess electrolytes and the products of metabolism. An intake of electrolytes in excess of the amounts lost (primarily in sweat and feces) must be corrected by excretion in the urine, with a corresponding increase in the volume and osmolality of urine formed.

A high-protein diet requires a greater urine output to allow for excretion of water-soluble nitrogenous waste;[21] this effect is relatively small compared with other routes of water loss, but becomes meaningful when water availability is limited. The water content of the food ingested will also be influenced greatly by the nature of the diet, and water associated with food may make a major contribution to the total fluid intake in some individuals. Some water is also obtained from the oxidation of nutrients, and the total amount of water produced will depend on the total metabolic rate and is also influenced by the substrate being oxidized. An energy expenditure of 3000 kcal per day (12.6 MJ per day), based upon a diet composed of 50% carbohydrate, 35% fat, and 15% protein, will yield about 400 ml of water per day (Table 2.3). Reducing the daily energy expenditure to 2000 kcal (8.4 MJ), but keeping the same diet composition, will yield about 275 ml of water. The contribution of this water of oxidation to total water requirements is thus appreciable when water turnover is low, but becomes rather insignificant when water losses are high.

TABLE 2.3
Water from Food Oxidation

1500 kcal from CHO	=	400 g CHO	240 g water
1050 kcal from fat	=	117 g fat	125 g water
450 kcal from protein	=	113 g protein	47 g water
Total	=		412 g

Note: These calculations assume a total energy intake of 3000 kcal/d, with 50% of the total energy intake provided by carbohydrate (CHO), 35% by fat, and 15% by protein, and further assume that the fuels oxidized match exactly the dietary intake.

2.4   DAILY WATER BALANCE DURING EXERCISE

Exercise elevates the metabolic rate, and only about 20 to 25% of the energy made available by the metabolic pathways is used to perform external work, with the remainder being dissipated as heat. When the energy demand is high, as occurs during periods of physical activity, high rates of heat production result. For example, the normal resting oxygen consumption is about 4 ml/kg body mass/min: for a 70-kg individual and this gives a resting rate of heat production of about 60 to 70 W. Running a marathon in 2 h and 30 min requires an oxygen consumption of about 4 l/min to be sustained throughout the race for the average runner with a body mass of 70 kg. [22] The accompanying rate of heat production is now about 1100 W, and body temperature begins to rise rapidly. To limit the potentially harmful rise in core temperature, the rate of heat loss must be increased accordingly. Maintenance of a high skin temperature will facilitate heat loss by radiation and convection, but these mechanisms are effective only when the ambient temperature is low and the rate of air movement over the skin is high. [23] At high ambient temperatures (above about 35°C), skin temperature will be below ambient temperature, and the only mechanism by which heat can be lost from the body is evaporation, as discussed in Chapter 1. Water will also be lost by evaporation from the respiratory tract. During hard exercise in a hot dry environment, this can amount to a significant water loss, although it is not generally considered to be a major heat loss mechanism in man.

In most activities, the energy demand varies continuously; average sweat losses for various sporting activities are well categorized,[24] but much less information is available on occupational tasks, in part because of the wide interindividual variability. Even at low ambient temperatures, high sweat rates are sometimes observed when the energy demand is high, so it cannot be concluded that dehydration is a problem only when the ambient temperature and humidity are high. [25] Sweat loss is, however, closely related to environmental conditions, and substantial fluid deficits are much more common in the summer months and in tropical climates. Body mass losses of 6 l or more are reported for marathon runners in warm weather competition. [26] This corresponds to a water deficit of about 8% of body mass, or about 12 to 15% of total body water. In spite of the large variation among individuals, sweating rate was found to be related to running speed in a heterogeneous group of marathon runners; there was, however, no relationship between total sweat loss and running speed. [25]

It is well established that women tend to sweat less than men under standardized conditions, even after a period of acclimatization. [27] It is likely, however, that a large part of the apparent sex difference can be accounted for by differences in training and acclimation status. There is a limited amount of information on the effects of age on the sweating response, and again, levels of fitness and acclimation are confounding factors, but the sweating response to a standardized thermal challenge generally decreases with age. [28] These observations should not, however, be interpreted as suggesting an inability to exercise in the heat, nor should they be taken to indicate a decreased need for women or older individuals to pay attention to fluid intake during exposure to heat stress.

There are some differences between children and adults in the sweating response to exercise and in sweat composition. The sweating capacity of children is low, when expressed per unit surface area, and the sweat electrolyte content is low relative to that of adults, [29] but the need for fluid and electrolyte replacement is no less important than in adults. Indeed, in view of the evidence that core temperature increases to a greater extent in children than in adults at a given level of dehydration, the need for fluid replacement may well be greater in children. [30]

Dehydration is harmful to athletic performance, and both endurance sports and high-intensity events are adversely affected. It is commonly stated that exercise performance is impaired when an individual is dehydrated by as little as 2% of body mass and that losses in excess of 5% of body mass can decrease the capacity for work by about 30%.[31] An examination of the original data (derived from a total of 13 trials involving three subjects) on which this statement was based, however, shows that the conclusion is much less robust than it might appear. That is, there was no good relationship between the extent of dehydration incurred by sauna exposure and the degree of impairment of the capacity to perform a high intensity exercise test lasting about 6 min, [32] and a large variation in response among and within individuals was observed. Nonetheless, there is convincing evidence that prior dehydration will impair the capacity to perform high-intensity exercise as well as endurance activities.[33,34] For example, Nielsen et al. [33] showed that prolonged exercise that resulted in a loss of fluid corresponding to 2.5% of body weight resulted in a 45% fall in the capacity to perform high intensity exercise. There is equally convincing evidence that the prevention of dehydration by administration of fluids can improve exercise performance, and the evidence to support this will be discussed later.

2.4.1 DISTRIBUTION OF BODY WATER LOSSES

Fluid losses are distributed in varying proportions among the plasma, extracellular water, and intracellular water. The decrease in plasma volume that accompanies dehydration may be of particular importance in influencing work capacity; blood flow to the muscles must be maintained at a high level to supply oxygen and substrates, but a high blood flow to the skin is also necessary to convect heat to the body surface where it can be dissipated. [35] When the ambient temperature is high and blood volume has been decreased by sweat loss during prolonged exercise, there may be difficulty in meeting the requirement for a high blood flow to both of these tissues. In this situation, skin blood flow is likely to be compromised, allowing central venous pressure and muscle blood flow to be maintained, but reducing heat loss and causing body temperature to rise.[36]

The preferential loss of water from the extracellular space reflects the relatively high sodium and chloride concentration in sweat. Electrolyte losses in sweat are a function of sweating rate and sweat composition, and both of these vary over time as well as being substantially influenced by exercise intensity, environmental conditions, and the physiology of the individual. Added to this variability is the difficulty in obtaining a reliable estimate of sweat composition,[37] and these methodological problems have contributed at least in part to the diversity of the results reported in the lature. In spite of the variability in the composition of sweat, however, it is always hypotonic with respect to plasma, and the major electrolytes are sodium and chloride, as in the extracellular space. It is usual to present the electrolyte composition of sweat in mmol (or mEq) per l, and the extent of the sodium losses in relation to daily dietary intake in grams, a confusing comparison that obscures the true magnitude of electrolyte loss. Loss of 1 l of sweat with a sodium content of 50 mmol per l represents a loss of 2.9 grams of sodium chloride. The athlete who sweats 5 l in a daily training session will therefore lose almost 15 grams of salt. Even allowing for a reduced sweat sodium concentration and a decreased urinary output when sodium losses in sweat are considerable, this salt loss is large in comparison with normal intake, and it is clear that the salt balance of individuals exercising regularly in the heat is likely to be precarious. The need for supplementary salt intake in these conditions will be discussed below.

2.5 WATER TURNOVER

2.5.1 METHODS OF MEASUREMENT

There are few reliable measurements of water turnover in normal healthy individuals because of the formidable obstacles that tend to confound the results of measurements of the various components of water intake and water loss. Intake is usually estimated from weighed or measured food- and fluid-intake diaries, but the data are complicated by uncertainties in the water content of foodstuffs. In addition, the act of recording intake tends to change behavior—most commonly in the direction of reduced intake—and under-reporting, either deliberate or inadvertent, is also likely. Measurement of the various avenues of water loss is also beset by similar problems.

As discussed in Chapter 1, body water turnover is now assessed using deuterium as a tracer.

2.5.2 INFLUENCE OF EXERCISE

Using the water turnover method on two groups of subjects, one sedentary and one physically active, showed a higher rate of water turnover in the exercising group.[38] The active group were men with sedentary occupations who ran or jogged a mean distance of 103 km (range 68 to 148 km; similar age, height) during the week of the study. Subjects in the sedentary group had a similar height and weight, and were engaged in similar occupations, but undertook no physically demanding activities in their leisure time. Both groups had similar total body water content. The median daily water turnover (averaged over 7 days) in the active group was 4673 ml per day (range 4320–9609 ml), which was higher (P<0.001) than that of the sedentary subjects (3256 ml per day; range 2055–4185 ml). The average daily urine loss was greater (P<0.001) in the exercising group (3021 ml per day; range 2484–4225 ml) than in the sedentary group (1883 ml per day; range 925–2226 ml). It might have been expected that the runners would have a greater daily sweat loss than the sedentary group, and that this would be reflected in a greater total non-renal loss. There was, however, no significant difference between the groups in non-renal water losses (runners = 1746 ml per day; range 1241–5195 ml; sedentary = 1223 ml per day; range 1021–1950 ml), although there was a tendency for a difference (P<0.08). These results seem surprising, but may reflect the relatively low total exercise load of the runners and the temperate climate (mean maximum daytime temperature of 14°C (range 7–21°C) at the time of the study. The results also suggest that the runners were habituated to drinking a volume of fluid in excess of that required to match the sweat loss incurred during exercise.

The same methodology has been applied to another physically active group, in this case cyclists covering an average daily distance of 50 km in training for competition, and another matched sedentary group. [39] Again, the median water turnover rate was higher (P<0.001) in the active group (3.38 l per day; range 2.88–4.89 l) than in the sedentary individuals (2.22 l per day; range 2.06–3.40 l). In this study, however, there was no difference between the groups in the daily urine output (cyclists = 1.96 l per day; range 1.78–2.36; controls = 1.90 l per day; range 1.78–1.96 l), but the non-renal losses were greater (P<0.001) in the cyclists (1.46 l per day; range 1.06–3.04 l) than in the sedentary group (0.53 l per day; range 0.15–1.72 l). It was again rather cool during the measurement period, with maximum daily temperatures of 10°C (range 4–18°C), which might account for the rather low sweat rates in spite of the high physical activity level of the cyclists.

These two studies emphasize the variability in the normal pattern of fluid intake and loss in both sedentary and active individuals. In all cases, body mass remained rather constant throughout the measurement period, which suggests that the subjects were in energy balance and were maintaining normal hydration status. The variation among individuals was large; one subject (one of the more-active members of the running group) had a daily urine output of 5786 ml, with a range of values from 2817–6290 ml. This is markedly different from the values obtained from most of the subjects, but this subject also had the greatest water turnover values, an average of 9606 ml per day (SD = 4328). [38] This emphasizes the degree to which voluntary drive can override the physiological demand; this subject clearly ingested volumes of fluid greatly in excess of those necessary for maintenance of euhydration.

2.5.3 INFLUENCE OF ENVIRONMENTAL TEMPERATURE

The water turnover studies quoted above used deuterium as a tracer for the hydrogen atoms in water. A doubly labeled water method has been widely used in the last 2 decades to assess energy balance. In this method, tracers are used for both the hydrogen atoms (deuterium) and the oxygen atoms (using O^{15}, a stable isotope of oxygen). Because oxygen atoms are lost from the body in carbon dioxide as well as in water, the rate of decay of the oxygen tracer is faster than that for the hydrogen tracer. The difference gives the rate of CO_2 production, from which the oxygen consumption, and hence the energy expenditure, can be calculated.[40] The doubly labeled water method for assessment of energy expenditure does include a calculation of whole-body water turnover, but these data are seldom presented. Singh et al.,[41] however, have published information on daily water turnover of Gambian women during periods of hard agricultural labor. These measurements were made as part of a study of energy balance in these women. A mean (SD) daily water turnover of 5.2 l (1.4) per day was observed for these women, who had a daily total energy expenditure of about 10.4 MJ (about 2500 kcal) per day; water turnover ranged from 3.2 to 9.0 l per day. This value was compared with a mean value of 3.2 (0.8) l per day in sedentary women in Cambridge, England. The ambient temperature during the measurement period in the Gambia was 23–28°C, and in Cambridge it was 11–19°C. The water turnover values for the Gambian women are high, reflecting the strenuous labor carried out in a tropical climate. The Cambridge women had a higher water turnover than the sedentary Aberdeen men, in spite of their smaller total body water content, and this presumably reflects the warmer weather conditions.

Another unpublished investigation provides further information. A study of water turnover in a group of sedentary individuals living in Jakarta, Indonesia assessed whole-body water balance before, during, and after the period of Ramadan, the month-long Islamic religious observance during which food and fluid are avoided during daylight hours. As might perhaps be expected, the whole-body water turnover was lower during Ramadan (median 1.93 l per day; range 0.58–5.08 l) than it was either before (2.24 l per day; range 1.06–4.15 l) or after (2.19 l per day; range 1.18-3.91 l). This difference was accounted for by a decrease in non-renal losses, with urine output remaining rather constant throughout the measurement periods. Surprisingly, though, considering the prevailing weather (daily outdoor temperature was about 30 to 32°C), the water turnover was rather low. This seems to reflect the low level of physical activity of these subjects and the fact that they spent most of the day in an air-conditioned environment, with little exposure to the outdoors. It cannot be assumed, therefore, that all individuals living in tropical regions are subjected to high heat stress; those who are not, and who are not physically active, may have low water requirements. During Ramadan, when access to food and water was restricted, subjects appeared to respond by further reducing their level of physical activity or exposure to the outdoor environment.

2.6 SUMMARY

In healthy individuals, water is the largest single component of the body. Although water balance is regulated around a range of volumes rather than a finite set point, its homeostasis is critical for virtually all physiological functions. To further assure proper regulation of physiological and metabolic functions, the composition of the individual body water compartments must also be regulated.

Humans continually lose water through the renal system, gastrointestinal system, skin, and respiratory tract, and this water must be replaced. Thirst is implicated in our water intake, although behavioral habits also have an important influence on drinking.

When exercise is undertaken or when an individual is exposed to a warm environment, the additional heat load is lost largely due to sweating and this can greatly increase the individual's daily water loss and therefore the amount that must be consumed. Sweat rates on the order of 2 to 3 l per h can be reached and maintained by some individuals for a number of hours, and it is not impossible for total losses to be greater than 10 l in a day. With such extreme losses, effective fluid replacement relies primarily on the ingestion of appropriate beverages throughout the day. Mealtime is a particularly important drinking occasion and athletes should be encouraged to take their time during meals to help assure adequate fluid intake. A variety of drink types and flavors are likely to be favored by individuals who have extreme losses to replace. Sports drinks have an important role in this regard because their flavor profiles encourage fluid consumption and their electrolyte content is crucial for retention of the ingested water.

REFERENCES

1. Sawka, M.N., Body fluid responses and hypohydration during exercise-heat stress. In: *Human Performance Physiology and Environmental Medicine at Terrestrial Extremes*, Pandolf, K.B., Sawka, M.N., and Gonzalez, R.R., Eds., Cooper Publishing Group, Carmel, pp. 227–266, 1990.
2. Lentner, C., Ed. *Geigy Scientific Tables*. 8th ed. Basle: Ciba-Geigy Limited, 1981.
3. Rose, B.D., *Clinical Physiology of Acid-Base and Electrolyte Disorders*. 2nd ed. McGraw-Hill, 1984, New York.
4. Fitzsimons, J.T., Evolution of physiological and behavioral mechanisms in vertebrate body fluid homeostasis. In: *Thirst: Physiological and Psychological Aspects,* Ramsay, D.J. and Booth, D.A., Eds. ILSI Human Nutrition Reviews, Springer-Verlag, London, 1990, pp. 3–22.
5. Adolph, E.D. et al., *Physiology of Man in the Desert*. Interscience, 1947, New York.
6. Hubbard, R.W., Szlyk, P.C., and Armstrong, L.E., Influence of thirst and fluid palatability on fluid ingestion. In: *Perspectives in Exercise Science and Sports Medicine. Vol 3: Fluid homeostasis during exercise,* Gisolfi, C.V. and Lamb, D.R., Eds. Benchmark Press, Indianapolis, pp. 39–95, 1990.
7. Ramsay, D.J., The importance of thirst in the maintenance of fluid balance. In: *Clinical Endocrinology and Metabolism, vol 3, number 2. Water and Salt Homeostasis in Health and Disease,* Bayliss, P.H., Ed. Baillière Tindall, London, 1989, pp.371–391.

8. Noakes, T.D., Goodwin, N., Rayner, B.L., Branken, T., and Taylor R.K.N., Water intoxication: a possible complication during endurance exercise. *Med Sci Sports Exerc*, 17, 370–375, 1985.

9. Flear, C.T.G., Gill, C.V., and Burn, J., Beer drinking and hyponatraemia. *Lancet*, ii, 477, 1981.

10. Phillips, P.A., Rolls, B.J., Ledingham, J.G.G., Forsling, M.L., and Morton, J.J., Osmotic thirst and vasopressin release in humans: a double-blind crossover study. *Am J Physiol*, 248, R645-R650, 1985.

11. Rolls, B.J., Wood, R.J., Rolls, E.T., Lind, W., Ledingham, J.G.G., Thirst following water deprivation in humans. *Am J Physiol* 239, R476-R482, 1980.

12. Verbalis, J.G., Inhibitory controls of drinking: satiation of thirst. In: *Thirst: Physiological and Psychological Aspects,* Ramsay, D.J., Booth, D.A., Eds., ILSI Human Nutrition Reviews, Springer-Verlag, London, 1990, pp.313-334.

13. Vist, G.E. and Maughan, R.J., The effect of osmolality and carbohydrate content on the rate of gastric emptying of liquids in man. *J. Physiol*, 486, 523-531, 1995.

14. Sterns, R.H. and Spital, A., Disorders of water balance. In: *Fluids and Electrolytes*, 2nd edition, Kokko, J.P. and Tannen, R.L., Eds., Philadelphia, 1990, WB Saunders Company, 139-194.

15. Engell, D.B., Maller, O., Sawka, M.N., Francesconi, R.N., Drolet, L. and Young, A.J. Thirst and fluid intake following graded hypohydration levels in humans. *Physiol Behav*, 40, 229-236, 1987.

16. Astrand, P-O., Rodahl, K., *Textbook of Work Physiology.* McGraw-Hill, NY, 1986.

17. Solomons, N.W. and Young, V.R., The major nutrients. In: *Clinical Nutrition.* Paige, D.M., Ed., Mosby, St. Louis. pp.16-35.

18. Gregory, J., Foster, K., Tyler, H. and Wiseman, M., *The Dietary and Nutritional Survey of British Adults.* HMSO, London. 1990.

19. Nicolaidis, S., Physiology of thirst. In: *Hydration Throughout Life.* Arnaud, M.J., Ed. John Libbey Eurotext, pp.3-8.

20. Ladell, W.S.S., Water and salt (sodium chloride) intakes. In: *The Physiology of Human Survival.* Edholm, O. and Bacharach, A., Eds.. Academic Press. New York. pp.235-299, 1965.

21. LeMagnen, J., Tallon, S.A., Les determinants quantitatif de la prise hydratique dans ses relations avec la prise d'aliments chez le rat. *CR Soc Biol*, 161, 1243-1246, 1967.

22. Maughan, R.J., Leiper, J.B., Aerobic capacity and fractional utilisation of aerobic capacity in elite and non-elite male and female marathon runners. *Eur J Appl Physiol* 52, 80-87, 1983.

23. Leithead, C.S. and Lind, A.R., *Heat Stress and Heat Disorders.* Casell, London 1964.

24. Rehrer, N.J. and Burke, L.M., Sweat losses during various sports. *Aust J Nutr Diet*, 53 (Suppl 4) S13-S16, 1996.

25. Maughan, R.J., Thermoregulation and fluid balance in marathon competition at low ambient temperature. *Int J Sports Med*, 6, 15-19, 1985.

26. Costill, D.L., Sweating: its composition and effects on body fluids. *Ann NY Acad Sci*, 301, 160-174, 1977.

27. Wyndham, C.H., Morrison, J.F. and Williams, C.G., Heat reactions of male and female Caucasians. *J Appl Physiol* 20, 357-364, 1965.

28. Kenney, W.L., Body fluid and temperature regulation as a function of age. In: *Perspectives in Exercise Science and Sports Medicine. Vol 8: Exercise in Older Adults.* Gisolfi, C.V., Lamb, D.R. and Nadel, E., Eds., Cooper Publishing. Carmel. pp.305-352, 1995.

29. Meyer, F., Bar-Or, O., MacDougall, D. and Heigenhauser, G.J.F., Sweat electrolyte loss during exercise in the heat: effects of gender and maturation. *Med Sci Sports Exerc*, 24, 776-781, 1992.
30. Bar-Or, O., Temperature regulation during exercise in children and adolescents. In: *Perspectives in Exercise Science and Sports Medicine. Vol 2: Youth, Exercise, and Sport*, Gisolfi, C.V. and Lamb, D.R., Eds., Benchmark Press. Indianapolis, pp.335-362, 1989.
31. Saltin, B., Costill, D.L., Fluid and electrolyte balance during prolonged exercise. In: *Exercise, Nutrition, and Metabolism*, Horton, E.S. and Terjung, R.L., Eds., Macmillan, New York, 1988, 150-158.
32. Saltin, B., Circulatory response to submaximal and maximal exercise after thermal dehydration. *J Appl Physiol*, 19, 1125-1132, 1964.
33. Nielsen, B., Kubica, R., Bonnesen, A., Rasmussen, I.B., Stoklosa, J. and Wilk, B., Physical work capacity after dehydration and hyperthermia. *Scand J Sports Sci*, 3, 2-10, 1981.
34. Armstrong, L.E., Costill, D.L. and Fink, W.J., Influence of diuretic-induced dehydration on competitive running performance. *Med Sci Sports Exerc* 17, 456-461, 1985.
35. Nadel, E.R., Circulatory and thermal regulations during exercise. *Fed Proc*, 39, 1491-1497, 1980.
36. Rowell, L.B., *Human Circulation*. Oxford University Press, New York, 1986.
37. Shirreffs, S.M. and Maughan, R.J., Whole-body sweat collection in man: an improved method with some preliminary data on electrolyte composition. *J Appl Physiol*, 82: 336-341, 1997.
38. Leiper, J.B., Carnie, A., Maughan, R.J., Water turnover rates in sedentary and exercising middle-aged men. *Br J Sports Med*, 30, 24-26, 1996.
39. Leiper, J.B., Pitsiladis, Y.P. and Maughan, R.J., Comparison of water turnover rates in men undertaking prolonged exercise and in sedentary men. *J Physiol*, 483, 123P, 1995.
40. Westerterp, K.R., Saris, W.H.M., van Es, M. and ten Hoor, F., Use of the doubly labeled water technique in humans during heavy sustained exercise. *J Appl Physiol*, 61, 2162-2167, 1986.
41. Singh, J., Prentice, A.M., Diaz, E., Coward, W.A., Ashford, J., Sawyer, M., Whitehead, R.G., Energy expenditure of Gambian women during peak agricultural activity measured by the doubly labelled water method. *Br J Nutr*, 62, 315-329, 1989.

3 Physiological and Psychological Determinants of Fluid Intake

Dennis H. Passe

3.1 INTRODUCTION

Fluid intake became a focus of systematic research in the early part of this century in military investigations of dehydration in soldiers marching or working under hot conditions. Subsequently, the concept of voluntary dehydration was introduced.[4,111] Temperature and flavor were identified as important variables influencing voluntary fluid consumption. Subsequent research has somewhat refined our understanding of these areas and opened the field for much broader investigation of sensory and psychological variables that may be involved. Underlying these sensory and psychological variables is a network of physiological conditions that modulates the sensation of thirst and sets the stage for drinking behavior. This chapter will selectively review key physiological, psychological, and social variables related to thirst that ultimately modulate drinking behavior and affect the individual's level of hydration. The story encompasses a broad range of research endeavors in biology. The focus of this chapter will be to highlight those areas central to explaining the control of drinking, from physiology to social factors, and to try to integrate these topics into a coherent view of voluntary fluid intake. The methods of physiology have steadily advanced, as have those in psychology, allowing for a more precise measurement of the perception of thirst, which, in turn, is making it possible to conduct more powerful experiments relating the experience of thirst to underlying physiological processes.

3.2 PHYSIOLOGICAL DETERMINANTS OF FLUID INTAKE

A variety of physiological influences on thirst have been identified. While not all of the research has specifically investigated causal relationships between physiological substrates and fluid intake, most discussions have focused on thirst. For the purposes of the current discussion, thirst is a central dependent measure in an understanding of fluid intake. In much research, thirst is either a condition inferred from drinking behavior or is treated as a sensory experience, the perception of which is measured using sensory scales. Most studies have directly measured fluid intake, although discussion of drinking has frequently been in terms of thirst as an intervening variable. That is, physiological conditions give rise to thirst, or "the desire to drink,"[51] which, in turn, is viewed as a direct influence on drinking behavior.

Cellular dehydration and hypovolemia (extracellular dehydration) are the two principal physiological causes of thirst and drinking. Of the two, cellular dehydration is the more important. "Minute" decreases in cellular hydration status result in thirst, while even "modest" reductions in plasma volume do not result in thirst.[131] Rolls et al.[107] have reported that approximately 64–85% of drinking following water deprivation is due to cellular dehydration, and that only about 5–27% of drinking is accounted for by hypovolemia. In adult humans, approximately 60% of the body is composed of water, of which two-thirds is intracellular water and one-third is extracellular water. Normally, these two compartments are in osmotic equilibrium. Deviations from equilibrium can occur by extracellular fluid loss or by an increase in the solute content in the extracellular or intracellular spaces. Usually, the solute content of the body is stable and the osmolality of body fluids is determined by changes in total body water. The usual routes of loss of body water are through urine, skin, and lungs. The following discussion focuses on those physiological systems that mediate drinking arising from these two causes. The area has been extensively reviewed. See Fitzsimons,[42,43] Ramsey and Booth,[97] and Star.[123]

Several key physiological substrates have been identified as regulator mechanisms for thirst and subsequent drinking behavior. Prominent among them are hormones or hormone-like substances, encompassing a wide array of biologically active substances either produced by endocrine glands or originating from other cell structures. For purposes of this discussion, the renin angiotensin system (RAS), and the vasopressin system (VS.) will be the primary focus of attention.

3.2.1 HYPOVOLEMIA

If blood volume decreases, whether by bleeding, sodium deficiency, injections of hyperoncotic colloid, or by obstruction of venous return to the heart, the kidney responds with an increase in renin, which results in an increase in the circulating levels of angiotensin II. This ultimately leads to an increase in drinking. The renin-angiotensin hormone system seems to be critically involved in the drinking behavior that is induced by hypovolemia.[43] Angiotensin II, which has been derived from renal renin and is circulating in blood, contributes to hypovolemic thirst, although it is not exclusively responsible for drinking. In thirst due to cellular dehydration, there is no additional angiotensin II of renal origin, suggesting that circulating angiotensin II is not a determinant of thirst under circumstances of increased osmolality. However, angiotensin II of cerebral origin may play a role in thirst due to cellular dehydration. For a recent and comprehensive review of hypovolemia and hormonal involvement in thirst and drinking, see Fitzsimons.[43]

The demonstration by Fitzsimons and Simons[44] and Epstein et al.[35] that injections of angiotensin II into rats caused drinking, provided strong initial support for the role of hormones in controlling thirst. Fitzsimons and Simons[44] observed a sixfold increase in water intake in male albino rats (n = 20) during the 6-h experimental period as a dose-response function of intra-jugular infusion of angiotensin II dissolved in NaCl solution. A 4.6-fold increase in water intake occurred in nephrectomized rats (n = 34). Epstein et al.[35] reported that direct infusion of angiotensin into septal, preoptic, and anterior hypothalamic regions of the brain caused male rats (n = 44) in normal water balance to drink water. The latency to drink ranged from 10 sec to a few min and typically continued for about 15 min. Szczepanska-Sadowska[124] has pointed out that there is now a general recognition that the central dipsogenic effect of angiotensin II is mediated through the central angiotensin II receptors that usually mediate the effect of angiotensin II of brain origin. Angiotensin II has many actions that may affect drinking, including vasoconstriction, diuresis, stimulation of net fluid absorption from the intestine, increased sodium appetite, increased thirst, and others. The RAS apparently stimulates the anterior hypothalamus, POA, the subfornical organ (SFO), and the vasculosum of the lamina terminalis.[51] The stimulatory effect of injecting angiotensin II into sensitive structures in the brain is robust and is dipsogenic in all vertebrate groups tested, but not amphibians and some fish.[43] According to Szczepanska-Sadowska, "The discovery of the brain renin-angiotensin system allowed explanation of the rapid and powerful dipsogenic effects of Ang II, renin, angiotensinogen and angiotensin I applied directly into the brain tissue (p.113)."[124] Although angiotensin II is the most potent angiotensin, angiotensin III also shows some dipsogenic activity.[82]

While intracranial infusion of angiotensin II is very effective in causing drinking behavior, animal studies have shown varying success in engendering drinking with angiotensin II administered by systemic infusion. The conditions of administration may be more exacting than that for intracranial administration. In man, thirst is not increased by systemic infusion of angiotensin II. Fitzsimons[43] has pointed out that there are well-documented cases in which systemic infusion of angiotensin II has failed to cause drinking.

Angiotensin II participates in the genesis of non-osmotically mediated thirst. As levels of angiotensin II increase, osmoreceptors in the hypothalamus become sensitized, resulting in the release of vasopressin from the pituitary, which is instrumental in the control of body water via plasma osmolality-related mechanisms. Angiotensin II stimulates thirst via mechanisms related to renal blood flow and thereby functions as a backup to the vasopressin-mediated thirst, which is related to plasma osmolality. Loss of extracellular fluid volume will cause the kidneys to increase the output of renin, which ultimately results in an increase in angiotensin II. The role of angiotensin II in fluid intake is complex and involves both circulating and centrally mediated changes in angiotensin II levels.[129] In response to a decrease in extracellular fluid volume, there is an activation of the RAS, resulting in an increase in circulating levels of angiotensin II. Thirst and drinking may be influenced by angiotensin II. It is thought that this might occur either by way of circulating angiotensin II, which might exert an influence on the SFO made possible by a deficient blood–brain barrier, or via angiotensin II in CNS pathways.[83] Hypovolemia is detected by vascular stretch receptors located in various parts of the vascular system. As venous return decreases, there is an unloading of atrial receptors. Similarly, as arterial pressure decreases, there is an unloading of baroreceptors in the carotid sinus and arch of the aorta. Since the input from these atrial and arterial receptors is tonically inhibitory to medullary and hypothalamic cardiovascular control centers, the reduced input from these receptors eventually results in a reflex increase in sympathetic outflow and cardiac performance, increased plasma AVP, and increased renin by the kidneys and activation of the RAS.[129]

3.2.2 CELLULAR DEHYDRATION

Increasing plasma osmolality stimulates thirst. If solute molecules such as dissociated sodium chloride or sucrose, which do not readily permeate through the cell membranes, are added to blood, an osmotic gradient results in the movement of water out of the cells and subsequently causes cell dehydration. Other molecules such as urea or glycerol, if added to blood, do not stimulate thirst to nearly the same degree. Urea and glycerol, even if added to blood in hyperosmolar concentrations, quickly pass through cell membranes, diminishing the osmotic gradient and the stimulus for thirst.[74]

Normally, blood osmolality is maintained within a very narrow range, 280–292 mOsm/kg. At plasma osmolalities of 282 mOsm/kg or higher, vasopressin, an antidiuretic hormone, is released, resulting in water retention by the kidneys, with urine becoming more concentrated and osmolality subsequently decreasing. If plasma osmolality rises sufficiently, thirst is experienced. The plasma osmolality set point for thirst is thought to be about 290 mOsm/kg, but there appears to be substantial variation among individuals.[51] At about 290 mOsm/kg or beyond, thirst occurs, resulting in drinking that moves the plasma osmolality back to the normal physiological range. If blood osmolality goes below about 280 mOsm/kg, vasopressin is not detectable and there tends to be diuresis. This implies that thirst rarely occurs when blood osmolality is within normal physiological range (between 280 and 292 mOsm/kg), which is not supported by clinical experience.[51] The sensory measurement of thirst is not easily accomplished in animals and is inferred from drinking behavior. In humans, however, sensory scales (visual analogue line scales) have been developed that allow a more sensitive assessment of perceived thirst, independent of the measurement of drinking.[73] The sensitivity of these measurements has been great enough to reveal that thirst actually begins much closer to the threshold for vasopressin release than previously thought (Figure 3.1).[73] The termination of drinking, which occurs well before significant changes in plasma osmolality, also occurs coincident with the reduction in vasopressin. McKenna and Thompson[73] have suggested that thirst occurs when vasopressin is released and remains mild until increases in plasma osmolality and subsequent increases in vasopressin result in greater thirst, which promotes larger fluid intakes to meet more-severe fluid deficits. The findings of McKenna and Thompson[73] are consistent with the hypothesis that oropharyngeal and stomach inputs to the hypothalamus cause a cessation of the experience of thirst via regulation of vasopressin. While plasma osmolality is the primary stimulus for modulation of vasopressin, there are nonosmotic factors that can also affect vasopressin levels, including changes in blood volume and blood pressure, catecholamines, angiotensin II, prostaglandins, and atrial natriuretic factor (see Toto[131] for a discussion). Vasopressin is very sensitive to changes in plasma osmolality; a change in plasma osmolality of only 1–2% will produce a change in plasma vasopressin. However, a change in blood volume of 7–10% is required to produce a change in plasma vasopressin (see Star[123] for a discussion). "Plasma osmolality is the most important physiological determinant of vasopressin secretion."[73]

Animal research has indicated that administration of vasopressin does not always result in enhanced thirst (fluid intake) but there does seem to be a lowering of the thirst threshold in dehydrated animals.[9] Effects are observed at moderate doses (0.1 ug/kg) but not higher doses (0.5 ug/kg). High blood levels of vasopressin are associated with reductions of osmotic thirst. A primary action of vasopressin appears to be the lowering of the osmotic thirst threshold. As in the case of angiotensin II, the mode and location of infusion may affect the magnitude of the dipsogenic effect. However, the available evidence seems to indicate that vasopressin may be important for the expression of thirst under physiological conditions and may be a determinant of osmosensitivity.[124] Vasopressin and thirst are central to the control of water balance and thereby are key regulatory mechanisms for the control of plasma osmolality.

Osmoreceptors, cells sensitive to small changes in blood osmolality, are located in the CVO in the anterior hypothalamus, and are thought to have direct access to plasma via gaps in the blood–brain barrier in this region. As plasma osmolality increases, signals from the osmoreceptors are sent to the posterior pituitary, where vasopressin is secreted into the circulation. There are also osmoreceptors located in the splanchnohepatic region with connections to the nucleus tractus solitarius (NTS) and ventral medulla with subsequent input to a number of other regions important in the control of drinking behavior. It seems reasonable to assume that peripheral osmoreceptors may also play some role in thirst, although the precise nature of this role remains uncertain. (See Bourque et al.[15] for a discussion of peripheral osmore-

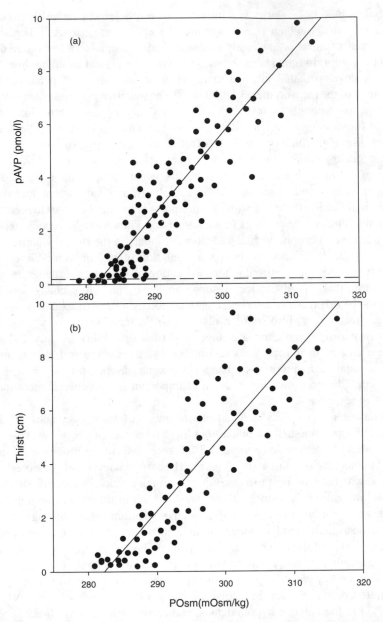

FIGURE 3.1 Results of measurement of (a) plasma vasopressin (pAVP) and (b) thirst in response to hypertonic saline infusion in ten healthy volunteers. ----- assay limit of detection for vasopressin (0.3 pmol/l). _____ regression lines. From McKenna, K. and Thompson, C.,Osmoregulation in clinical disorders of thirst appreciation, *Clin.Endocrin.*, 49, 139–152, 1998. With permission.

ceptors.) Vasopressin is a neuropeptide synthesized principally in the supraoptic nucleus but also in the paraventricular nucleus (PVN), the suprachiasmatic nucleus, and other hypothalamic neurons. As an antidiuretic hormone, it helps regulate water excretion from the kidneys and the sensation of thirst. It is transported via neurons to the posterior pituitary, where it is stored until released into the circulation. (See McKenna and Thompson,[73] Szczepanska-Sadowska,[124] and Toto[131] for discussions of the effect of vasopressin on thirst.)

Szczepanska-Sadowska[125] has discussed the possible interaction of angiotensin II and vasopressin in the control of water intake and concluded that there is not strong evidence for synergistic or interactive effects of these hormones on thirst or fluid intake, at least in the rat. This is a topic remaining to be adequately investigated. Somewhat more-positive information has been generated regarding the interaction of angiotensin II and vasopressin relative to cardiovascular control.[79,125] Species differences in this interaction probably reflect differences in the relative distribution and nature of vasopressin and angiotensin II receptors.[125]

3.2.3 CENTRAL NERVOUS SYSTEM (CNS) CONTROL OF FLUID INTAKE

Cardiovascular and body fluid homeostasis, thirst, and voluntary fluid intake are maintained at a physiological level as a result of the integration of neural and chemical input to the brain.[60] Information is emerging about the integration of neuropharmacological and neuroanatomical elements in the maintenance of body fluid homeostasis. Signals arising from volume receptors reach the CNS via the NTS. Hormonal signals from circulating blood reach the brain through neural sites in the SCVO, which lack a complete blood–brain barrier. Information arising from both neural and blood-borne avenues is projected to an extensive neural network that is responsible for coordinating the effector mechanisms controlling fluid homeostasis. While a complete understanding of homeostatic physiology would require the integration of information from the molecular, cellular, and systems levels, the scope of this section is to elucidate the relationships among neuronal and hormonal inputs and key CNS anatomical sites, especially as they relate to thirst and its expression in voluntary fluid intake. The role of CNS structures in fluid homeostasis has been reviewed by Fitzsimons,[43] Johnson et al.,[60] Johnson and Edwards,[61] and Johnson.[58]

Before considering the functional interrelationships among CNS structures in the control of drinking behavior, it is useful to clarify some fundamental anatomical relationships and terminology.[75] The lamina terminalis, occupying the anterior wall of the third ventricle, consists of three structures: the SFO and the organum vasculosum of the lamina terminalis (OVLT), both of which lack a blood–brain barrier, and the median preoptic nucleus (MnPO). Anatomically, the SFO protrudes into the third ventricle and has extensive reciprocal connections with the MnPO and the OVLT in the anteroventral third ventricle (AV3V) region. The AV3V consists of the OVLT, the ventral MnPO, ventral lamina terminalis, anteroventral PVN, and the anterior paraventricular preoptic nucleus. The CVO consist of the SFO, the OVLT, and the area postrema (AP). The AV3V and lateral terminalis have the OVLT and MnPO in common (see Oldfield[83]).

Strong evidence implicating the SFO in fluid balance was forthcoming in studies by Simpson and Routtenberg[120] and Simpson et al.[119] They found that blood-borne angiotensin II acts on the SFO to induce fluid intake in rats. In addition, circulating angiotensin II stimulates vasopressin release in the SFO. The evidence for the role of the SFO relative to the dipsogenic effects of circulating angiotensin II is strong in the rat, but in the sheep, SFO lesions have little effect on drinking induced by injected blood-borne angiotensin II. This suggests that in this species there may be another site, perhaps the OVLT, more sensitive to circulating angiotensin II.[75] The dog, on the other hand, seems to have the SFO as a key angiotensin II-related dipsogenic center. The species differences that have been observed suggest that species may vary in the relative importance of the CVO structure mediating the dipsogenic effects of circulating angiotensin II.[75] Destruction of the SFO results in loss of drinking in response to intravenous injection of angiotensin II in most species. Since angiotensin II is a powerful dipsogen when injected directly into the brain, it is therefore thought to be important in circulating blood as a stimulus to drinking. There are angiotensin II-sensitive neurons in various parts of the brain, many found in highly vascularized structures with deficient blood–brain barrier properties. Angiotensin II receptors in the SFO and OVLT are primarily responsible for drinking in response to circulating angiotensin II, although the AP may also be involved.

Central injection and lesion work[17,59] has also implicated the OVLT and MnPO sites in body fluid regulation. Lesions destroying the paraventricular nuclei surrounding the AV3V, including the OVLT and ventral MnPO, produced acute adipsia and chronic impaired drinking. Lesions to both the SFO and AV3V areas impaired angiotensin-related responses.

While circulating angiotensin II does not get to the MnPO, signals from the SFO to the MnPO presumably play an important role in angiotensin II-mediated thirst and drinking behavior since severing efferents from the SFO to the MnPO disrupts drinking induced by intravenous angiotensin II.[75] Other angiotensin-sensitive brain structures lie inside the blood–brain barrier and are not directly affected by circulating angiotensin II, including the MnPO, the PVN, the POA, and the central gray area of the midbrain to which the POA projects. It is possible, however, that these structures may be stimulated by angiotensin generated in the brain.

Johnson et al.[60] proposed that circulating angiotensin II acts on the SFO to activate a descending angiotensinergic pathway that terminates in the ventral MnPO. Not all descending fibers from the SFO terminate in the MnPO; some continue to other forebrain structures such as the major hypothalamic and limbic nuclei. Johnson et al.[60] have also proposed that there is a selective action of noradrenaline in the ventral lamina terminalis on angiotensin-induced drinking and that noradrenaline amplifies the effects of angiotensinergic innervation. Cathecholaminergic cell groups clustered in the hindbrain give rise to the noradrenergic innervation of the MnPO. Changes in blood pressure and blood volume affect the activity of these cell groups, including noradrenaline turnover during hypovolemia.

The CVO appears to be an important interface between circulating blood and the brain, allowing the brain to monitor body fluids in the periphery while protecting the integrity of the blood–brain barrier against harmful substances and major homeostatic imbalances. These structures are richly vascularized with many angiotensin II receptors, allowing them to monitor blood chemistry. Considerable evidence indicates that three of them (SFO, OVLT, and AP) play roles in the control of drinking behavior, renal function, and blood pressure.[43] The SFO in particular may be important in the control of drinking behavior relative to blood-borne angiotensin II. It is thought to be the principal site mediating circulating angiotensin II-induced drinking behavior.[43] The OVLT, also very well vascularized, lies in the lamina terminalis, in tissue surrounding the AV3V region. While it is clear that the AV3V region is involved in angiotensin II-induced drinking, the specific role played by the OVLT is less clear. It seems likely that the OVLT serves several functions and responds to more than one stimulus. The OVLT is also a major site for osmoreceptors, as is the SFO. It is possible that the CVO responds to both circulating angiotensin II and plasma hyperosmolality.[43] The AP is located near the fourth ventricle and central canal of the spinal cord and projects into the NTS. A highly vascularized area, the AP has been implicated in drinking behavior and the sense of taste. It appears that the AP and NTS areas monitor extracellular fluid volume on the basis of vascular stretch receptor input and circulating angiotensin II levels. Signals are then sent from the AP and NTS to the MnPO, AV3V areas, SFO, PVN, supraoptic nucleus (SON), and the amygdala via ascending noradrenergic and other pathways.

In summary, the CVO, MnPO, and AV3V regions play a critical role in thirst and drinking, especially relative to angiotensin II stimulation. The SFO, OVLT, and AP areas are sensitive to blood-borne angiotensin II and are chiefly responsible for drinking behavior as well as other elements of fluid homeostasis. The projections of the SFO and OVLT to other brain regions such as MnPO, the POA, the anterior hypothalamic area, and limbic area serve to initiate drinking behavior.[43] In addition to its role in organizing and mediating responses to hypovolemia, the CNS plays a critical role in mediating thirst and drinking behavior due to intracellular dehydration. A growing body of research is suggesting that there may be CNS structures outside the blood–brain barrier that are sensitive to increased osmolality of extracellular fluid.[15] Attention has focused on the SFO and OVLT. Destroying either site interferes with neurohypophysical hormone responses to systemic hypertonicity as well as causing a deficit in osmotically evoked drinking.[15] Anatomically, the SFO and OVLT have direct connections to the magnocellular neurosecretory cells (MNCs) of the supraoptic and PVN, which in turn project axon terminals to the posterior pituitary, where vasopressin and oxytocin are synthesized. As indicated above, the SFO and OVLT have projections to the MnPO. The MnPO has projections to hypothalamic MNCs. It would appear that the SFO and OVLT function as primary receptors in the osmotic control of drinking behavior.[15]

In humans, the effectiveness of rehydration is frequently not complete, with sizable fluid deficits remaining after voluntary drinking has ceased.[3,111] Rothstein et al.[111] called this "voluntary dehydration" and pointed out the value of temperature and flavor in enhancing fluid intake. The thirst mechanism in humans is not as precise as in other species studied, with thirst subsiding before rehydration is complete. In the dog[1] and burro,[3] the amount of fluid required to replace lost water is consumed immediately. Rothstein et al.[111] suggested that voluntary dehydration is related to an inhibition of water intake and the thirst sensations that go with it, pointing out that thirst is not necessarily an effective indicator of water balance in man. The following sections go beyond the physiological substrates of thirst and fluid intake to touch on the psychological factors that may affect drinking behavior.

3.3 PSYCHOLOGICAL DETERMINANTS OF FLUID INTAKE

3.3.1 THIRST PERCEPTION AND VOLUNTARY FLUID INTAKE

There is a biological continuum of integrated control of voluntary fluid intake. The neuro-hormonal, sensory, psychological, social, and cultural elements that compose the milieu in which we find ourselves conspire to generate the mix of beverage choices and levels of fluid intake that occur during rest and exercise. As discussed above, the physiological substrates of thirst set the occasion for drinking behavior. Thirst may be thought of as motivation to drink. However, we will also consider socially driven occasions when the level of thirst actually experienced during drinking may be low or nonexistent, or even in the direction of satiation. Because of the complexity and interplay of the factors contributing to fluid intake in humans, we do not always consume sufficient quantities to completely rehydrate. This lack of completeness of rehydration observed in humans appears to be an exception in the animal world. Interestingly, humans also hyperhydrate during social occasions. This aspect of fluid intake is relatively unexplored from the physiological perspective but has received more attention from psychology.

The general issue of adequate hydration has been framed by Eichna et al.,[31] who observed inadequate levels of voluntary intake in men working in simulated jungle conditions (32.2–32.8°C/90–91°F, relative humidity of 94%–96%). "No man drank enough water voluntarily to replace the water lost in the sweat during work in humid heat. Thirst did not appear until considerable water deficits had developed. Since it lags behind the water needs, thirst constitutes an insensitive guide to the water requirement (p. 45)." Recently, attention has been given to fluid replacement strategies of athletes performing under severe temperature and humidity conditions.[69] Sporting events held in hot and humid environments have placed extraordinary demands on athletes, sometimes even putting them at substantial physical risk. An important element of reducing the risk of serious heat illness and maintaining peak physiological function and performance is an effective rehydration strategy. An effective strategy includes not only the amount and timing of beverage ingestion, but also beverage composition.

The idea of palatability relative to voluntary fluid intake is a pervasive one. However, it remains an ill-defined concept, used both as a dependent measure and as an explanation for voluntary fluid intake. It is variously measured using scaling techniques (e.g., a 9-point hedonic scale[90]), inferred from differences in voluntary fluid intake (e.g., the beverage consumed in the greatest quantity is, by definition, the most palatable one), and used as an explanation for voluntary fluid intake (e.g., the beverage consumed in the greatest quantity was so consumed because it is more palatable). The reason for this confusion appears to arise from a shifting focus on palatability among researchers. Palatability can refer to an invariant attribute of the beverage (e.g., flavor quality) or it can refer to the pleasantness or hedonic experience of consuming the beverage. Evidence for such a distinction among subjects comes from Yeomans and Symes,[140] who asked subjects to rate the "palatability" and "pleasantness" of two isoenergetic meals differing in blandness, before and following *ad libitum* intake. In this study of 50 male adult university staff and student volunteers, two distinct sub-populations emerged. While essentially all of the subjects rated the pleasantness of eating the food as decreasing as they approached satiety, one sub-group rated the palatability as also decreasing while the other sub-group indicated that the palatability of the food did not change, even though the pleasantness of eating it was decreasing. This suggests that the second sub-group interpreted "palatability" as an invariant attribute of the food, separating it from the hedonic experience of eating it. Clearly, the wording of the questionnaire and how and whether terms are defined for the subjects are critical in determining the conclusions that we draw about the perception of beverages and the hedonic experience of drinking.

3.3.2 TEMPERATURE

Early research on fluid intake in soldiers quickly identified the importance of the temperature of available fluids in voluntary intake of water.[111] In one experiment, Rothstein et al.[111] compared two groups of men (n = 7 for each group) walking for 2 h under 39°C (103°F) ambient conditions. Following this, the men had access to cooled water (13°C, 55°F) or warm water (28°C, 82°F). The group that was given the cooled water replaced 87% of lost body water compared with 75% for the group given the warm water (significance level not reported). In another field study of soldiers marching in the desert, Sohar et al.[121] conducted experiments on 19 heat-acclimatized men (18–21 y) marching 617 km (370 miles) over a 24-day period. On 7 days the men had access to either cooled water (10–15°C/50–59°F) warm water (20–30°C/68–86°F). On 6 of the 7 days there was a preference for the cooled water, with the exception occurring on a day when access to the cooled water was made more difficult by other activities. Hubbard et al.,[56] taking a more controlled look at the impact of temperature on fluid intake, marched 29 males (23 ± 3 y) on a treadmill for 14.5 km (8.7 miles) under environmental conditions of 40°C (104°F) and 32% RH. Subjects received either water or a flavored beverage at two different temperatures: 15°C (59°F) or 40°C (104°F). The temperature effect was substantial, with an increase in fluid intake of 87% for the cooled beverage over the warm one. Szlyk et al.[126,127], in another study of men (n = 14, 21–33 y) marching under simulated desert conditions (6 h of intermittent marching, 40°C/104°F, 42% RH), also found substantial effects of temperature on voluntary fluid intake. Intakes of the cooled water averaged 88% higher than the warm water. Using a similar protocol of 6 h of intermittent marching under similar environmental conditions, Armstrong et al.[7] investigated voluntary fluid intake in 12 healthy men (23 ± 2 y) using a dose-response approach. In a between-groups design, subjects were randomly assigned to one of three beverage-temperature treatment groups (6, 22, 46°C). Subjects participated in non-chlorinated water and chlorinated water segments for each of the treatment conditions. Although there was no significant difference in intake between the 6°C (43°F) and 22°C (72°F) treatments, both were consumed in significantly greater quantities than 46°C (115°F) water at all points over the course of the 6-h exercise protocol. In another dose-response approach to the impact of temperature on fluid intake, Boulze et al.[14] examined the effects of water ranging in temperature from 0–50°C (32–122°F) on fluid intake of mountain patrol guards (n = 140) who had first dehydrated by mountain climbing for a half day without food or water, and on fluid intake of patients (n = 260) who had first dehydrated by sitting in a warm spa-like environment (cave at Luchon, France with interior dry- and wet-bulb temperatures of 40°C/104°F). Subjects were assigned to groups of n = 20 in a between groups design. Water temperatures were 0–50°C in 5-degree increments (32–122°F in 9-degree increments). In both populations of subjects, fluid intake was maximized at 15°C (59°F). In a follow-up experiment with the patients, subjects were allowed to mix water from hot and cold reservoirs to identify the most acceptable temperature. Water of this temperature was then consumed ad lib after dehydration. The result of this experiment closely replicated the previous findings. The mean temperature of the self-mixed water was 15°C (59°F) and was consumed in volumes not significantly different from those consumed by the mountain guards or the other patient subjects. Hedonic measures revealed that although 15°C (59°F) was the preferred temperature in terms of intake, water down to 0°C (32°F) also maintained a high level of rated palatability. Boulze et al.[14] speculated that drinking dropped off at the higher temperatures because the fluid became less palatable, and that it dropped off at the coldest temperatures because cold water was more satiating, thereby more effectively diminishing the drive to drink. Unfortunately, this explanation is encumbered by the fact that palatability was measured only with a sip-and-spit technique. No hedonic measures were taken during *ad libitum* fluid intake periods, thereby precluding measurement of any reductions in liking that may have occurred to the coldest temperatures due to possible sinus discomfort associated with consumption of the very cold water. An assessment of the impact of drink temperature on subsequent level of thirst was made by Rolls et al.[104] In their study they fed vegetable juice at 1°C or 60–62°C (34°F or 140–144°F) to males and females (n = 15 each sex, 18-35 y) and measured thirst 2 min later. Relative to a no-drink control condition, males showed a significant reduction in thirst following the cold drink but not the hot drink. This effect, however, was not seen in the females.

In an unpublished study conducted in our laboratory, we examined the impact of beverage temperature on fluid intake following exercise at moderate intensity (70–85% of age-predicted maximum heart rate[5,40] for 30 min in an exercise circuit. The drink was a citrus-flavored 6% CHO-electrolyte sports beverage at four temperatures (2, 7, 15, 22°C/36, 45, 59, 72°F) consumed ad lib immediately after exercise. In a repeated-measures design, 58 subjects (laboratory personnel volunteers) were exposed to all four treatments. Fluid intake and liking of beverage temperature were measured after drinking had voluntarily ceased (usually within 10 min). Results are shown in Figure 3.2. Although no significant differences in fluid intake were observed among the temperature conditions in this study, the numerical maximum at 15°C (59°F) is consistent with the results of Boulze et al.[14] Also consistent with Boulze et al. was a trend for palatability to increase with decreasing temperature. Cardello and Maller,[20] while not assessing the impact of temperature on intake, did examine an array of beverages along a continuum of serving temper-

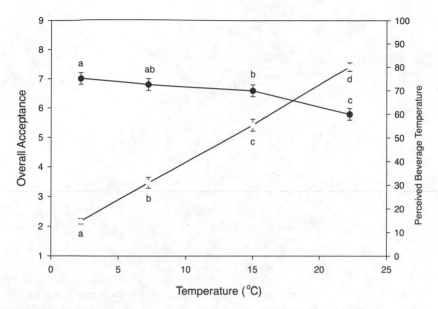

FIGURE 3.2 Impact of beverage temperature on overall acceptance. Closed circles (●) show overall acceptance (9-point scale) of beverage as a function of beverage serving temperature. Open circles (○) show perceived beverage temperature (100-point scale) as a function of beverage serving temperature. Within each curve, points not sharing a common letter are significantly different from each other ($p < 0.05$).

atures and related temperature to palatability in a sedentary setting. Utilizing laboratory personnel volunteers (n = 36), the investigators presented fruit-flavored noncarbonated beverages, lemonade, milk, tea, and coffee at temperatures ranging from 3°C to 57°C (38–135°F). Palatability was measured by a 9-point category scale (like extremely = 9 to dislike extremely = 1). They observed a strong trend for drinks normally served cold to be preferred cold. For most such drinks there was a monotonically increasing function of palatability with decreasing temperature. Significant temperature, beverage, and interaction effects were observed. It is interesting to note that water had one of the steepest gradients, that is, showed the most sensitivity of palatability to temperature. Water at a warmer temperature was disliked to a greater extent than are many of the flavored and carbohydrate-containing beverage alternatives at comparable temperatures. This interaction of beverage and temperature is of considerable importance when attempting to maximize voluntary fluid intake. In an unpublished study conducted in our laboratory, we directly compared a 6% carbohydrate electrolyte sports beverage (formulated with an optimized lemon-lime flavor system) with commercially available bottled water. Laboratory personnel volunteers (n = 57) exercised for 30 min at 70–85% of age-predicted maximum heart rate, after which they had *ad libitum* access to one of the beverages, in a crossover design. Both beverages were served at 32°C (90°F). Fluid intake, liking of beverage temperature, and overall beverage palatability were measured. Results are presented in Figure 3.3. Beverage temperature was disliked for both beverages, but even more so for the water ($p < 0.04$). Overall acceptance of the flavor-optimized

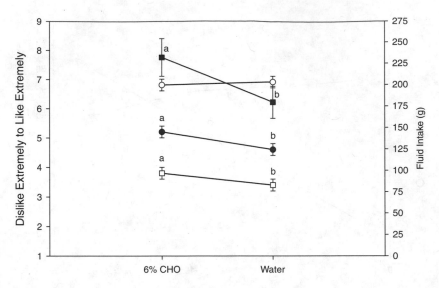

FIGURE 3.3   Liking of beverage temperature, overall beverage acceptance, and fluid intake for a 6% CHO-electrolyte sports beverage and water. Closed circle (●) shows overall acceptance (9-point scale) of warm beverage. Open circle (○) shows overall acceptance (9-point scale) of chilled beverage. Closed square (■) shows fluid intake of warm beverage (g). Open square (□) shows liking of warm temperature (9-point scale). Within each curve, points not sharing a common letter are significantly different from each other (p < 0.05).

sports beverage was significantly greater than water (p < 0.01), and significantly more of the sports beverage than water was consumed (p < 0.001). These results are consistent with the interaction between beverage and temperature observed by Cardello and Maller.[20] The negative impact of elevated serving temperature is not equal across all beverages. Water appears to suffer more than most beverages tested to date in this regard. The critical impact of flavor optimization on voluntary fluid intake is discussed in greater detail below.

While it is important to understand the relationship between beverage temperature and fluid intake, the reciprocal impact of exercise state on liking of beverage temperature as well as perception of temperature may also be important. Sandick et al.[115] investigated these relationships in a study in which subjects rated perception of water temperature and liking of water temperature before and after exercise. The temperatures of the water were 5, 16, 22, and 38°C (41, 61, 72, 100°F). Subjects (18 military personnel volunteers) participated in both control and experimental sessions in a counterbalanced fashion. Subjects rated the perceived temperature of water before and after control and exercise sessions using a 12-category "temperature wheel" devised for this purpose. They also rated the palatability of the water before and after control and exercise sessions using a 9-point hedonic scale. Subjects were allowed *ad libitum* access to all of the water samples following the control and exercise periods. Sandick et al.[115] found significant interactions between exercise condition and water temperature for fluid intake and palatability. The amounts consumed for the two coldest temperatures were significantly greater on exercise than control days. There were no significant differences in intake between exercise and control sessions for the two warmer samples. A significant interaction was also found between exercise state and water temperature for water palatability, suggesting at least a directional shift for greater palatability for the cooler beverage temperatures following exercise. Palatability of the 16.0°C (60.8°F) sample was greater on exercise days than control days. Although there appeared to be a shift in liking of temperature, there were no significant differences between control and exercise conditions in the perception of water temperature. That is, exercise condition did not affect ability to perceive beverage temperature, but only liking of beverage temperature. Consistent with the results of Boulze et al.,[14] Sandick et al.[115] showed a steady increase in palatability with decreasing temperature both in sedentary conditions and immediately following exercise. Cardello and Maller[20] also reported a similar monotonic increase for three of the five beverages examined in their study, although there appeared to be a downward inflection in acceptability rating for the coldest temperature for two of the beverages (water and lemon-lime drink). The greatest intake in the study of Sandick et al.[115] was for the coldest beverage (5°C) rather than for the 16°C beverage, as might have been predicted from previous research.[14] A major difference between these two studies was that Boulze et al.[14] allowed only a short time to drink (10–15 seconds), while Sandick et al.[115] allowed 15 min to drink, possibly avoiding sinus discomfort caused by the cold temperature of the water. Hubbard et al.[57] have pointed out that, as a general rule, increasing water temperature dramatically decreases fluid intake.

An additional dimension to the hedonic impact of temperature already discussed is the role of temperature expectation. Zellner et al.[142] have pointed out that many beverages have culturally mediated temperature-appropriate expectations attached to them. For instance, coffee is to be served hot, and white wine or beer should be served chilled. According to these authors, the sensory impact of temperature occurs in combination with the cognitive element of "appropriateness" or "expectation." In their first experiment, (with 22 university student and staff volunteers), subjects rated (no tasting was involved) how much they thought they would like various beverages if served hot, at room temperature, or cold. Clear differences in temperature appropriateness were observed for all of the beverages. In a second experiment with 13 university student and staff volunteers, subjects tasted a subset of the beverages from Experiment 1, served hot, at room temperature, and cold. Overall results suggested that tasting the beverage at an inappropriate temperature lowered the hedonic rating (consistent in direction and trend with Experiment 1). However, at least for some beverage–temperature combinations, tasting them at an inappropriate temperature did not result in as large a hedonic decrement as might have been predicted from Experiment 1. In Experiment 3, with two groups of 12 undergraduate volunteers, subjects were given novel tropical fruit juices (guanabana and tamarind) and were either told nothing about the appropriate temperature at which these drinks were typically consumed or were told that they were typically consumed at room temperature. Samples were served cold and at room temperature. The group that was told that the appropriate serving temperature was room temperature scored these drinks significantly higher at room temperature than did the subjects not given any information on appropriate serving temperature, suggesting that temperature expectation can have an impact on beverage liking.

In the case of sweetened beverages, temperature may exert an impact on palatability through modifying perceived sweetness intensity. Calvino[19] generated psychophysical sweetness-intensity curves at beverage temperatures of 7°C, 37°C, and 50°C (45°F, 99°F, 122°F). Solutions at 37°C (99°F) and 50°C (122°F) were perceived as being sweeter than when tasted at 7°C (45°F). In addition, the slopes of their functions were lower than at 7°C (45°F); that is, the sweetness function was steeper at 7°C (45°F) than at the warmer temperatures.

Boulze et al.[14] and Engell and Hirsch[32] have pointed out that the trend seen in humans for chilled beverages to be preferred over warm ones is opposite to that seen in animals. In animals, intake is maximized when the water is tepid (30°C/86°F) or even warm (36–37°C/97–99°F).

Rolls et al.[104] investigated the impact of temperature of a beverage on subsequent ratings of thirst in the context of a follow-up meal. Thirty subjects (15 males and 15 females, 18–35 y) reported to the laboratory at their usual lunch time. They received a vegetable juice, either cold (1°C, 34°F) or warm (60–62°C, 140–144°F), or a no-drink control condition followed by a lunch. Ratings of thirst were obtained before and 2 min following consumption of the beverage. Relative to the no-drink condition, males showed a reduction in thirst following the cold drink but not the warm drink condition. For males, the reduction in thirst for the cold drink condition was also greater than for the warm drink condition. Females showed a reduction in thirst relative to the no-drink condition for both the cold and warm drink conditions, with no significant difference between the cold and warm drink conditions. These results suggest, at least for males, that temperature may have a direct impact on thirst, and that a cool beverage may have greater thirst-quenching properties than a warm one.

3.3.3 FLAVOR

In addition to beverage temperature, flavor is an important element in encouraging voluntary fluid intake. Rothstein et al.[111] observed that, in addition to the impact of temperature on voluntary fluid intake, providing some flavoring enhanced palatability. Anecdotal reports from soldiers indicated that they preferred some flavoring to mask the taste of salt added to their water. In controlled studies of men marching in the desert, Sohar et al.[121] compared the palatability of an array of beverages including tea, sweetened citrus drink, juice, milk, soda water, carbonated cola, beer, and water. They found that the preponderance of choices was for chilled citrus-flavored drinks. Conversely, the least popular drinks were those containing carbonation. When asked to rate the beverages, 17 of 19 participants stated a preference for citrus-flavored beverages. Others have also found positive effects for flavor. In a study of 77 steelworkers in a naturalistic setting, Spioch and Nowara[122] investigated the impact of an herb tea with electrolytes vs. water (water, soda water, and mineral water) on voluntary dehydration. In a between-groups design, workers had *ad libitum* access to either tea (n = 30) or a water (n = 47) on their shift for 17 days. Total sweat loss between the two groups did not differ. However, significantly more of the flavored electrolyte tea than water was consumed, resulting in significantly less voluntary dehydration for that group. The tea group was also reported to have experienced less fatigue and better subjective feelings. Szlyk et al.[126,127] reported that, in reluctant drinkers, flavoring warm water (raspberry flavor) increased voluntary fluid intake by 79%. Engell and Hirsch[32] reported an increase in fluid intake in soldiers when the water was sweetened and cherry flavored. Hubbard et al.[56] investigated the impact of flavored beverage on palatability and fluid intake in 29 young men (23 ± 3 y) under simulated desert marching conditions (14.5 km/9.1 mile walk in the heat over a 6-h period). They showed fluid intake increases of approximately 40% for flavored iodinated water over unflavored iodinated water under both warm and chilled conditions. The relative impact of temperature vs. flavor was also disclosed in studies reported by Hubbard et al.[56] They reported an increase of voluntary fluid intake of about 50% when the water was chilled, 40% when the water was flavored, and an increase of about 80% when water was both chilled and flavored. Rose et al.[110] investigated the impact of 2.5% carbohydrate electrolyte solutions varying in magnesium, potassium, and phosphate content on voluntary fluid intake in soldiers working in the heat. Subjects also had access to other beverages such as soft drinks and juice throughout the test period. When data were partitioned according to flavored beverages (combining all sources) vs. water, the investigators found that up to 10 times as much flavored beverage was consumed as water ($p < 0.001$). In research conducted in our laboratory (unpublished), the interaction between temperature and flavor can be seen in comparisons between a commercially available sports beverage formulation (6% carbohydrate electrolyte beverage) and water (commercially available) when served chilled (4.4°C, 39.9°F) and at desert temperature (32.2°C, 90.0°F.). In Experiment 1, 51 adults (25 males and 26 females) exercised at moderate intensity (70–85% of maximum age-predicted HR) for 30 min, after which either a lemon-lime-flavored 6% carbohydrate electrolyte sports beverage or water was evaluated for overall acceptance. Beverage temperature was 4.4°C (39.9°F). In Experiment 2, 56 adults (25 males and 31 females) participated in a protocol essentially identical to that of Experiment 1, except that the beverages were served at 32.2°C (90.0°F). In Experiment 1, both the sports beverage and the bottled water scored essentially the same (6.8 ± 0.2 and 6.9 ± 0.2, respectively). When both beverages were served at 32.2°C (90.0°F, approximately desert ambient temperature), the overall palatability of both beverages decreased ($p < 0.01$), with water scoring significantly lower than the sports beverage (5.2 ± 0.2 and 4.6 ± 0.2, respectively; $p < 0.01$). In both studies, care was taken to obtain a high-quality water containing no off notes from purification chemicals.

As a result of extensive investigation of the relationship between flavor and drinking in animals and humans, Rolls[103] has concluded: "The taste of the available drinks is a major determinant of the amount consumed (p. XIII–5)." Basic research in rats has identified the importance of sweetness-mediated palatability. Adding saccharin[36,107,109] or nutritive sweeteners such as sucrose or glucose[102] to water greatly increased the level of fluid intake, resulting in positive fluid balance. Extending this finding to the presence of essences added to the water, Rolls and colleagues[105,107] observed that when an odor essence was added to the water of nondeprived rats for an hour, fluid intake increased by 88% ($p < 0.001$). When variety was enhanced by presenting four different essences in succession over the same time period, fluid intake increased by 182% over plain water (p < 0.001). In a similar paradigm with humans (Rolls et al.[107]), 18 nondeprived subjects consumed three low-energy drinks successively over a 30-minute period in three 10-minute bouts. Drinks were either the same or three different flavors (orange, lemon, or lime). Twelve of the subjects were also tested in a water control condition. Fluid intake was increased by 99% over the water condition by the addition of one flavor. Adding three flavors increased voluntary fluid intake over water by 143%. In subsequent research on the effect of various beverages on food intake, Beridot-Therond et al.[10] reported that sweetened beverages served prior to a meal were consumed in significantly greater quantities than unsweetened beverages, resulting in significantly greater total energy intake for the day. Although outside the scope of this chapter, the post-ingestive effects of foods, prior exposure to specific foods, preloading, and sensory-specific satiety have been discussed as possible factors contributing to the hedonic value of foods.[18,101,102,104,106]

Maughan and Shirreffs.[71] investigated a variety of factors influencing the restoration of fluid and electrolyte balance after exercise. Addressing palatability, Maughan et al.[70] examined the impact of four drinks (a glucose-electrolyte beverage, aerated water, a commercial sports beverage, and a juice mixture) on voluntary fluid intake. More of the sports drink and juice mixtures were consumed, and they were also reported as being more pleasant tasting. Although hedonic measurements were not reported, their general findings are consistent with the preponderance of evidence in this area. In a study comparing some commonly available beverage alternatives, Passe et al.[85] examined water (Evian®), diluted fruit juice (Minute Maid® premium pulp-free orange juice diluted 50%) a homemade 6% CHO-electrolyte beverage,[21] and a commercially available 6% CHO-electrolyte sports beverage (Gatorade®). All of the drinks except water were of orange flavor. Fifty triathletes and runners exercised for 75 min at 80–85% of age-predicted heart rate. To simulate conditions in which athletes have limited time to drink, they were allowed *ad libitum* access to a beverage for 1 minute after 30 and after 60 min of exercise. Results showed that the commercial sports beverage scored significantly higher than all of the other beverages in overall acceptance (p < 0.05) at both measurement times. Acceptance scores were combined across times and are graphed in Figure 3.4a. The commercial sports beverage was also consumed in significantly greater quantities than all of the other beverages (p < 0.05, Figure 3.4b), resulting in significantly lower dehydration (p < 0.05, Figure 3.4c) than all of the other beverages. This suggests that the actual delivery of flavor quality may not be optimum with a homemade sports beverage, diluted orange juice or water, and that the avidity of consumption may be reduced relative to an optimized commercial flavor system.

While most of the research investigating fluid intake has been with adults, the scope of investigation has been expanded to include children. Differences in sweat electrolyte composition, as well as other possible differences between children and adults in thermoregulatory responses, make this population an important focus of rehydration research.[37,77] Bar-Or et al.[8] established that boys (10–12 y) do not voluntarily consume sufficient water during intermittent exercise in the heat. This

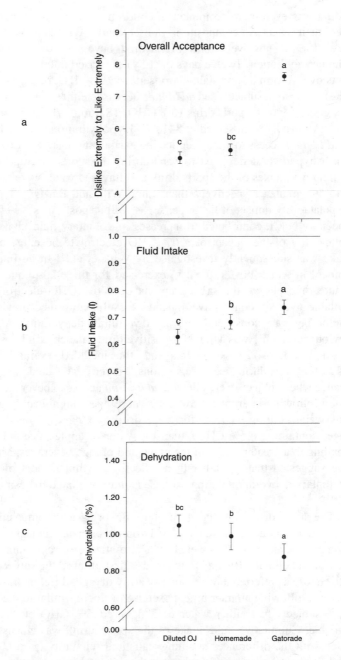

FIGURE 3.4 a, overall acceptance (9-point scale); b, fluid intake (g); and c, % dehydration. Values not sharing a common letter are significantly different from each other ($p < 0.05$).

finding was even more prominent in children with cystic fibrosis, a condition that alters their sweat Na composition. Subsequently, Wilk and Bar-Or[136] reported evidence for the positive impact of flavored beverages over water in maintaining voluntary hydration. Twelve boys (9–12 y) exercised intermittently (four 20-minute bouts over 3 h) in a warm laboratory setting (35 $\pm$ 1°C, rh 40–45%). In a repeated-measures design, subjects had *ad libitum* access to either water, grape-flavored water, or a grape-flavored sports drink (6% CHO, 18.0 mmol/l NaCl, commercially available). All drinks were served at 8–10°C. Hypohydration occurred under conditions of *ad libitum* access to water, replicating earlier findings.[8] However, subjects significantly hyperhydrated relative to water during the sports beverage phase of the study. Cumulative intakes of the sports drink and flavored water were approximately 90% and 45% greater, respectively, than water. Wilk and Bar-Or[136] have suggested that the palatability impact of flavor per se, as well as post-ingestive effects of CHO and especially NaCl, contributed to increases in voluntary fluid intake over water. The replicability of the impact of a 6% CHO electrolyte beverage on voluntary fluid intake was subsequently investigated by Wilk et al.[137] In an intermittent exercise protocol in which boys (10–12 y) exercised for three 20-minute bouts over a 70-minute time period, the same grape-flavored 6% CHO electrolyte beverage was available over six consecutive sessions. Results confirmed previous research[136] in that this beverage consistently prevented voluntary dehydration. Also consistent with previous research[136] was a trend for positive fluid balance. Mild positive fluid balance occurred in 67 of 72 sessions. In a study that included several different drink types and CHO levels during exercise sessions, Meyer et al.[78] demonstrated positive fluid balance when subjects were allowed *ad libitum* access to beverage during a recovery period following intermittent exercise. There was a significantly greater increase in body weight during recovery for grape drink (13.9% CHO) and orange sport beverage (containing 6.5% CHO), than for water or apple juice (11.2% CHO) corresponding to a greater intake of the grape and orange beverages. Meyer and Bar-Or[77] have suggested that "…rather than reflecting an impairment of thirst perception, involuntary dehydration during exercise is mainly related to desirability of the drink (p. 9)."

The study of the impact of beverage flavoring and composition has also been extended to heat-acclimatized boys in a tropical climate. Subjects in this study, unlike those in Wilk and Bar-Or,[136] were heat acclimatized, exercise trained, and indigenous to a tropical climate. Rivera-Brown et al.[99] first allowed the subjects (12 boys 11–14 y) to choose a preferred flavor among an array of eight different flavors. In subsequent sessions, following an intermittent exercise protocol similar to that of Wilk and Bar-Or,[136] subjects had either water or a flavored 6% CHO electrolyte drink freely available. Cumulative fluid intake of the sports drink was consistently higher than water, with the differences attaining statistical reliability (p < 0.05) after 110 min. Total fluid intake was 32% higher for the sports drink over water. Similarly, there was a progressive pattern of hypohydration with water, which also reached statistical reliability after 110 min. These findings, which are consistent with the results of Wilk and Bar-Or,[136] suggest that unflavored water is not sufficient to maintain euhydration in young boys under these conditions. These results are also consistent with previous findings in heat-acclimatized boys[116] in whom voluntary intake of water, under a similar protocol of intermittent exercise in the heat, resulted in voluntary dehydration.

In an investigation of two different commercial sports beverages (6% CHO and 8% CHO, also differing in electrolyte composition, carbonation, and other formulation parameters) and water, Wilmore et al.[138] observed that both commercial sports beverages were consumed in greater quantities than water during a 90-minute rest period following 90 min of running at 60% VO_{2max}. Sensory measurements at the end of the rest period were taken to identify liking of the beverages. Significantly more of the more-liked sports beverage than water was consumed during exercise, suggesting an important role for hedonics in voluntary fluid intake. In experiments that have taken a more systematic look at the role of flavor palatability and voluntary fluid intake, Passe et al.[84] investigated palatability as an independent variable, an approach not taken before. Forty-nine triathletes and runners (33 males, 16 females) first participated in a sedentary sensory evaluation of an array of 10 different flavors of sports beverage (all 6% CHO electrolyte beverages differing only in the flavor component of the formula) to determine palatability. The most acceptable flavor for each subject, the least acceptable flavor for each subject, and water were subsequently made available *ad libitum*, during 3 h of aerobic exercise (65-75% of maximum age-predicted heart rate). Each subject participated in three exercise sessions and received each treatment. Chilled beverage was replenished every 15 min to help maintain its temperature and to facilitate measurement of voluntary fluid intake. Sensory measurements were taken after 90 min and 180 min of exercise. Cumulative fluid intakes are presented in Figure 3.5 (Passe et al.[86]). The most acceptable flavor was consumed in greater quantities than both the least acceptable flavor and water throughout the first 75 min, and was consumed in greater quantities than water throughout the entire exercise period. Of particular interest is the finding that total consumption of the least acceptable flavor of the sports beverage was also greater than water. This is consistent with the hedonic measurements taken at 90 min and 180 min, which are shown in Figure 3.6. In sedentary testing the most acceptable flavor scored higher than water (p < 0.01), which scored higher than the least acceptable flavor (p < 0.01). However, during exercise, the palatability of the least acceptable flavor increased and exceeded that of water at both 90 min and 180 min (p < 0.01). In a replication experiment with the same flavors and a similar aerobic exercise protocol, the most acceptable flavor and the least acceptable flavor of the sports beverage for each individual subject were paired with water in a two-choice (two-bottle) test. Subjects reported to the laboratory for two exercise sessions and received the two treatments (most acceptable flavor vs. water, or least acceptable vs. water) in counterbalanced fashion. Consistent with the first study, the flavored sports beverage, whether originally identified as most acceptable or least acceptable, was consumed in significantly greater quantities than water, even after only 15 min of exercise. These findings highlight the importance of flavor in contributing to voluntary fluid intake, and suggest that a powerful interaction exists between flavor palatability and exercise state. This interaction is consistent with the findings of Horio and Kawamura,[55] who have reported that a shift in the hedonic value of a beverage can occur as a function of exercise.

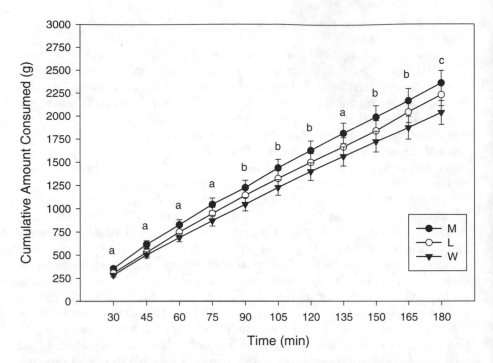

FIGURE 3.5 Cumulative fluid intake (g) for the most acceptable flavor (M), the least acceptable flavor (L), and water (W). Statistical annotation: a: M > L and W (p < 0.05), b: M > W (p < 0.05), c: M > W (P < 0.01), L > W (p < 0.05). From Passe, D., Horn, M., and Murray, R.M., The effects of beverage carbonation on sensory responses and voluntary fluid intake following exercise, *Appetite,* in press. With permission.

While most of the published research on the topic of flavor and voluntary intake has examined the positive impact of palatable flavors, less attention has been given to how to optimize flavors for voluntary intake. To date, there have been few, if any, published reports of systematic investigations of flavor components that can increase or decrease palatability of beverages during exercise. In a series of unpublished experiments in our laboratory, we investigated the dose-response relationships between key flavor components (sweetness, saltiness, tartness, flavor strength), and palatability measured immediately following exercise. Healthy adult males and females (n = 42–52, ages = 23–58 y) exercised for 30 min (aerobic training circuit) at moderate intensity (75–85% of maximum heart rate based on age-predicted maximum rates[5,40] after which they had *ad libitum* access to a beverage which they evaluated using hedonic (9-point) and descriptive (100-point) sensory scales. Subjects returned to the laboratory to complete a series of sessions in which they were exposed to all treatment conditions, administered in a Latin square arrangement. Palatability ratings and perceived intensity, as functions of stimulus intensity for sweetness, tartness, saltiness, and overall flavor strength, are presented in Figures 3.7–3.10. Each figure represents a separate experiment. The impact of CHO level (6%, 8%, 10%) on perceived sweetness and palatability is shown in Figure 3.7. Perceived sweetness of 10% CHO was significantly greater than 8% CHO (p < 0.05),

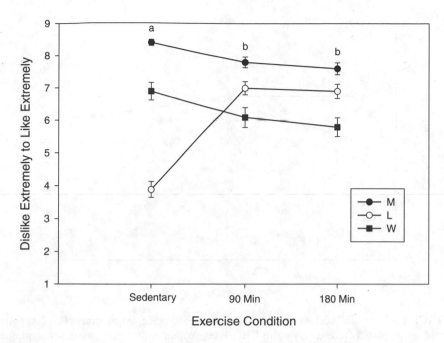

FIGURE 3.6 Overall acceptance of the most acceptable flavor (M), least acceptable flavor (L), and water (W) under sedentary and exercise conditions. Statistical annotation: a: M > W (p < 0.01), W > L (p < 0.01), b: M > L (p < 0.05), L > W (p < 0.01). From Passe, D., Horn, M., and Murray, R.M., The effects of beverage carbonation on sensory responses and voluntary fluid intake following exercise, *Appetite*, in press. With permission.

which was significantly sweeter than 6% CHO (p < 0.05). The overall acceptance of the 10% CHO was significantly lower than both the 6% and 8% CHO beverages, indicating that, in this study, a hedonic optimum had been reached, beyond which palatability of the beverage decreased. The impact of varying citric acid level on subsequent measures of tartness and overall acceptance is shown in Figure 3.8. As citric acid level increased (0.2%, 0.28%, 0.40%, 0.50%), so did perception of tartness (p < 0.05 for all mean differences). The palatability of the 0.5% citric acid beverage was significantly lower (p < 0.05) than all of the other levels of citric acid, as measured by overall acceptance. The palatability of 0.4% citric was significantly lower than the 0.2% and 0.28% citric acid beverages, again pointing to the existence of a hedonic optimum. Figure 3.9 shows the effect of sodium level (0, 20, 40, 60 mmol/l) on perceived saltiness and palatability. As sodium concentration was increased beyond 20 mmol/l, perceived saltiness increased. 60 mmol/l was perceived as being saltier than 40 mmol/l (p < 0.05), which was perceived as saltier than the 20-mmol/l and 6-mmol/l beverages (p < 0.05). There was not a significant difference in perceived saltiness between the 20-mmol/l and 6-mmol/l beverages. The 60-mmol/l beverage was liked significantly less (p < 0.05) than the 6-, 20-, or 40-mmol/l beverages, among which there were no significant differences. The impact of flavor concentration on perceived flavor strength and overall acceptance was investigated by combining commercially available dry-mix powder of a lemon-lime-flavored

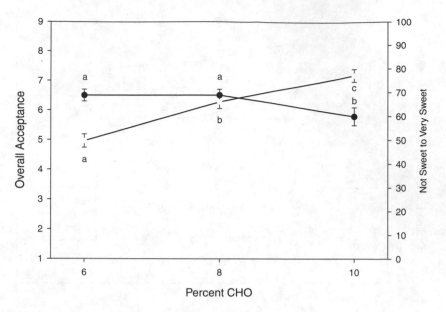

FIGURE 3.7   Overall acceptance (●, 9-point scale) and perceived sweetness (○, 100-point scale) of a sports beverage varying in CHO level. Within each curve, points not sharing a common letter are significantly different from each other ($p < 0.05$).

sports beverage with water to create a range of concentrations (10%, 25%, 50%, 75%, 100%, and 150% of recommended mixing instructions). As can be seen in Figure 3.10, perception of flavor strength increased monotonically as a function of beverage concentration. From concentrations of 25% to 100%, overall acceptance increased as a function of concentration with the highest level of acceptability measured at 100% concentration. There appeared to be an inflection beyond 100% suggesting a tapering off or reduction in palatability at the highest concentration, although this difference was not statistically significant. Together, these studies suggest, at least for major flavor components of a sports beverage, that there are optima that must be achieved to fully enhance beverage flavor quality and that deviation from optimum with either higher or lower concentrations reduces palatability. The sodium palatability results are consistent with those of Wemple et al.[135] who investigated the impact of sodium at two levels (25 and 50 mmol/l) in flavored 6% CHO drinks on voluntary fluid intake following dehydration. Subjects were given 3 h to rehydrate, with *ad libitum* access to the sodium-containing beverage or flavored water control. Results indicated that fluid intake was significantly enhanced for the 25 mmol/l beverage over water but not for the 50 mmol/l beverage. Leshem et al.[65] have reported an increase in salt preference in soup following exercise. Subjects (21 male students, 24 ± 1 y) engaged in "routine exercise" for 1 h, after which they were allowed to self-adjust the salt level in tomato soup. Relative to baseline measurements and a control group that did not exercise, subjects increased the level of salt in the soup by about 50% (from approximately 1.3% NaCl, to approximately 2% NaCl, weight/weight percentage).

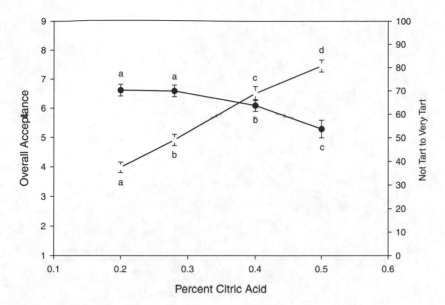

FIGURE 3.8 Overall acceptance (●, 9-point scale) and perceived tartness (○, 100-point scale) of a sports beverage varying in citric acid level. Within each curve, points not sharing a common letter are significantly different from each other (p < 0.05).

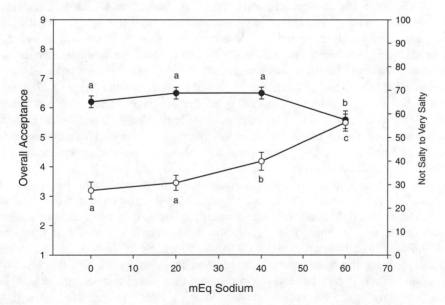

FIGURE 3.9 Overall acceptance (●, 9-point scale) and perceived saltiness (○, 100-point scale) of a sports beverage varying in sodium level. Within each curve, points not sharing a common letter are significantly different from each other (p < 0.05).

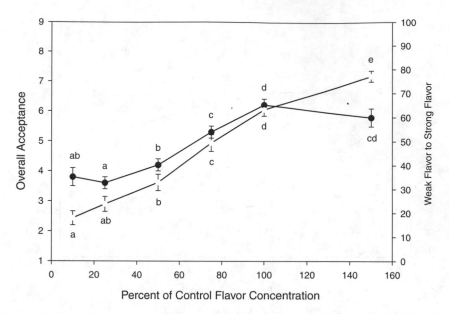

FIGURE 3.10   Overall acceptance ($\bullet$, 9-point scale) and perceived flavor strength ($\bigcirc$, 100-point scale) of a sports beverage varying in flavor concentration. Within each curve, points not sharing a common letter are significantly different from each other (p < 0.05).

Carbonation has also been investigated for its impact on beverage palatability in exercising subjects. The impact of beverage carbonation (0, 1.1, 2.3, 3.0 vol CO_2) on palatability was investigated in a dose-response study by Passe et al.[87] with 52 subjects who exercised for 30 min at 75%–85% of their maximum age-predicted heart rate. A single beverage was consumed following exercise in a repeated-measures design in which all subjects were exposed to all treatments. Figure 3.11 shows that at 2.3 and 3.0 vol CO_2, palatability of the beverage decreased significantly (P < 0.01). This reduction in palatability also corresponded with significantly lower voluntary fluid intake levels immediately following exercise. These carbonation levels (2.3 and 3.0 vol CO_2) correspond to "medium" levels of beverage carbonation,[133] with some soft drinks containing 3.5 vol CO_2 or higher. Figure 3.11 shows a relatively steep slope of perceived carbonation intensity vs. stimulus intensity (vol CO_2). This is consistent with the steep psychophysical function for carbonation observed by Yau & McDaniel,[139] who wrote: "…a small CO_2 concentration change could cause a large change in carbonation perception in a carbonated beverage system (p. 126)." The exponents of the power functions for carbonation are much higher than for the basic tastes.[139] In addition to gustatory stimuli, this level of discrimination may be related to gastrointestinal feedback. Ploutz-Snyder et al.,[92] in the first study to use magnetic resonance imaging (MRI) to quantify gastric gas, investigated fluid and gas emptying, and perception of gastric distress over a 1 h period following ingestion of 800 ml of water, a commercially available non-carbonated 6% carbohydrate electrolyte sports beverage, a commercially available lightly carbonated (1.15-vol CO_2) 8% carbohydrate electrolyte sports beverage, and

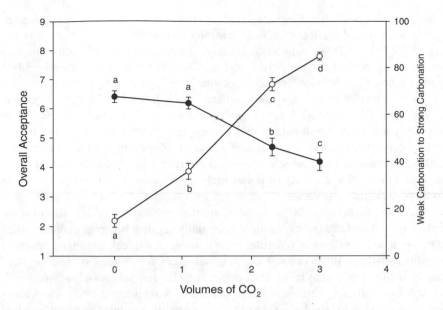

FIGURE 3.11   Overall acceptance (●, 9-point scale) and perceived carbonation (○, 100-point scale) of a sports beverage varying in volumes of CO_2. Within each curve, points not sharing a common letter are significantly different from each other ($p < 0.05$).

a commercially available carbonated 10% carbohydrate (3.2 vol CO_2) cola. The lightly carbonated carbohydrate electrolyte beverage (1.15 vol CO_2) and the soft drink (3.2 vol CO_2) had significantly slower gastric emptying times than water or the non-carbonated carbohydrate electrolyte beverage. Additionally, gastric distress for the carbonated soft drink was significantly greater than all of the other beverages at all of the time-points at which it was measured (10, 20, 45 min post-consumption). This appears to be due to the combined large total gastric volume (liquid + gas) that may enhance the perception of carbonation in a beverage.

While the impact of flavor and beverage temperature may be a key driver of voluntary fluid intake during exercise, there appears to be a reciprocal relationship between exercise and hedonic experience. That is, exercise state may impact the hedonic experience of the flavor being tasted. Lluch et al.[66] demonstrated that the pleasantness of a low-fat meal increased after exercise (50 min of cycling at 70% VO_{2max}) relative to the same meal consumed after rest. Subjects were lean, dietary-restrained women who were regular exercisers. A similar finding was reported by King et al.[63] for women but not for men.[62] Lluch et al.[66] observed that the increase in the hedonic value of foods following exercise occurred predominantly for the high-carbohydrate (low-fat) items in the menu, consistent with the need for carbohydrate related to glycogen use during exercise.

In addition to the positive impact that the correct combination of beverage characteristics can have on hedonics and voluntary fluid intake, there is also the dark side of beverage formulation with its negative effects. Failure to eliminate or at least to minimize negative beverage characteristics may produce potent negative reactions, as has been observed when water is tainted by off-flavors,[111,126,127] when the beverage type is mismatched for the exercise occasion,[121] or when the temperature is too warm.[7,14,56,115,126,127] In an unpublished study in our laboratory, 49 adult subjects consumed a variety of beverages (lemon-lime-flavored 6% carbohydrate electrolyte sports beverage, apple juice, mixed-vegetable juice, bottled water, and a cola) *ad libitum* in a repeated-measures Latin square design following 30 min of aerobic activity at 65–75% of maximum heart rate. At the end of the study, subjects were asked to complete a questionnaire that probed how "annoyed" they would be if certain beverage characteristics existed. The questionnaire consisted of 18 questions (100-point analogue line scales anchored on either end by "not annoyed" to "very annoyed") directed to a variety of issues including nausea, mouthfeel (sensation in mouth of stickiness or dryness), beverage texture (thickness), sweetness, undesirable flavors, flavor strength, saltiness, tartness, aftertaste, color and others. Results (see Table 3.1) indicated that the most salient potentially negative beverage characteristics related to nausea, feelings of bloating, objectionable mouthfeel, perceived beverage viscosity, off-flavor (objectionable flavor), and excessive sweetness. The negative characteristics identified as being least important were low saltiness, low sweetness, low tartness, and high artificial color appearance. A replication study was subsequently conducted in which 43 subjects participated in a similar protocol and had *ad libitum* access to a lemon-lime-flavored 6% carbohydrate electrolyte sports beverage, iced tea, a carbonated lemon-lime soft drink, orange juice, milk (2% fat), and tap water immediately after exercise. Again, every subject was exposed to all treatment conditions in a Latin square design and at the end of the study was asked to complete the "annoyance" questionnaire. Essentially the same pattern of findings was observed. The correlation between the mean values from these two studies was $r = 0.98$ (df = 16, p < 0.01). While these studies did not directly manipulate the flawed beverage characteristics as independent variables, the questionnaire data do suggest a ranking of annoyance values for potential flaws and suggest directions for future optimization research. Consistent with the above results, Pelchat and Rozin[88] observed in a survey study that nausea was the most potent correlate of acquired dislike of the taste of food. The impact of post-ingestional gastrointestinal distress can be a powerful one and is a central theme in the area of conditioned taste aversion learning. See Garcia et al.[46] and Rozin and Kalat[113] for discussions.

3.3.4 TEXTURE

There appears to be little or no published information on the impact of texture or mouthfeel on voluntary fluid intake. However, it may have a profound impact on the hedonic value placed on the beverage. Beverages that have a syrupy mouthfeel score lower in acceptability (unpublished research). In a series of exercise-sensory studies (unpublished), which were conducted over a 10 y period and which investigated a range of beverages (e.g., sports beverages, juices, soft drinks, waters, milk, beer), those beverages that scored the lowest in overall acceptance were also described by subjects as having a heavy mouthfeel and a syrupy or somewhat viscous texture. Beverages that were rejected for mouthfeel characteristics included juices, soft drinks, and milk. In addition, as reported above (Table 3.1), objectionable

TABLE 3.1
Level of Annoyance with Various Beverage Flaws

Annoyance Question	Study 1	Study 2
Beverage causes nausea	93	91
Beverage leaves mouth sticky and dry	80	78
Beverage is too thick and syrupy	79	76
Beverage is too sweet	77	76
Beverage has off flavor	76	77
Beverage leaves you feeling bloated	72	70
Beverage does not quench thirst	68	65
Beverage is too salty	64	74
Aftertaste is too strong	62	60
Flavor is too strong	57	57
Beverage has artificial flavor	55	56
Beverage is too tart	45	50
Aroma is too strong	43	39
Flavor is too weak	42	46
Beverage is not tart enough	37	37
Beverage appears artificially colored	33	34
Beverage is not sweet enough	25	30
Beverage is not salty enough	20	17

Note: Scale is 100-point analogue line scale, anchored on the left by "Not Annoyed" and on the right by "Very Annoyed."

mouthfeel characteristics ranked high in importance among exercising subjects completing "annoyance" questionnaires.

3.3.5 OROPHARYNGEAL FACTORS, ORAL METERING, AND GASTROINTESTINAL FACTORS

While flavor and beverage temperature may be thought of as oropharyngeal factors, these key drivers of voluntary fluid intake have been addressed in some detail above. The oropharyngeal sensation of thirst, oral metering (from sensory cues arising from the act of swallowing), and gastrointestinal factors such as stomach distension may play important roles in the initiation and termination of drinking. These are critical elements that may exert control before intracellular and extracellular influences fully come into play. Zeigler has described the anatomy and functional morphology of drinking.[141] The important roles played by oropharyngeal factors have been discussed by Fitzsimons,[42] Rolls and Rolls,[105] Rolls et al.,[108] and Rolls et al.[107] Early research in sham-drinking (in which the fluid is prevented from reaching the stomach, usually by means of an esophageal or gastric fistula) demonstrated that relatively large volumes are drunk in rat,[80,81] dog,[2] and monkey.[68]

It has become clear that the oropharyngeal cues associated with drinking can maintain drinking in the absence of gastrointestinal cues, plasma dilution, or expansion of extracellular fluid.[107] In experiments with humans, Rolls et al.[107] investigated the subjective sensations of thirst and the pleasantness ratings of water following an overnight fast. As subjects drank to satiety, their pleasantness ratings of the taste of the water decreased steadily over the 20-minute rehydration time. Subjects who were not allowed to drink *ad libitum*, but who were restricted to small sips for sensory testing purposes, showed less reduction in pleasantness ratings. In a study investigating the relationship among dehydration, oropharyngeal factors, fluid intake, and sensory perception, Rolls et al.[108] fasted five healthy males (24–33 y) for 24 h and measured voluntary fluid intake for 1 h, fluid balance and subjective sensations. A significant fluid deficit was evidenced by significant decreases in extracellular fluid and plasma volume, and increases in plasma osmolality. Drinking was rapid, with 65% of the total fluid intake occurring during the first 2.5 min, well before plasma sodium and osmolality had approached normal values, which did not occur until after 12.5 min. Cellular rehydration does not appear to have accounted for the initial time course and early decrease of drinking. However, sensory measures of thirst, pleasantness of the taste of the water, and mouth dryness showed substantial decreases during the first five min of drinking, establishing a correspondence between these oropharyngeal elements and early drinking. The perception of stomach distention also coincided with the first break in drinking in this study, suggesting a possible feedback role for this sensation.

In subsequent research, investigating *ad libitum* drinking under non-laboratory conditions, Phillips et al.[91] observed that drinking occurred in the absence of significant body fluid changes and was coincident with feelings of thirst, mouth dryness, and a general emptiness in the stomach. Drinking terminated with the cessation of feelings of thirst and mouth dryness and with an increase in perceived fullness in the stomach. Goldman et al.[50] observed a close correspondence between the time course of desire for water and that of vasopressin (AVP) levels. Subjects received an infusion of saline followed by a bolus of water. Within 5–10 min after water ingestion, there was a substantial reduction in desire for water and a parallel reduction in plasma AVP. Plasma osmolality and plasma sodium did not show significant changes until 20 and 25 min after water ingestion, respectively. Figaro and Mack[41] more directly investigated the role of oropharyngeal factors and oral metering on fluid intake in humans in a study employing the use of nasogastric infusion and extraction of fluid from the stomach. In a repeated-measures design, six adults were exposed to mild exercise in the heat for 2 h, resulting in body water loss of about 29 ml/kg. After exercise, subjects were allowed to rehydrate for 75 min via:

1. *ad libitum* drinking (Control)
2. infusion of an amount of water similar to control directly into the stomach for the first 25 min followed by a combination of infusion and *ad libitum* drinking during the remaining 50 min (Infusion)
3. *ad libitum* drinking with simultaneous extraction of the fluid as it entered the stomach (Extraction)

Consistent with the results of Goldman et al.,[50] there was a sharp drop in perceived thirst (although Goldman et al.[50] measured desire to drink and not perceived thirst) and AVP during the first 5 min of rehydration for Control and Extraction conditions but not for the Infusion condition. This suggests an impact of oropharyngeal factors on perceived thirst and circulating AVP. In the Infusion condition, even though all of the water deficit had been infused and plasma osmolality and volume had returned to normal, there were still strong thirst ratings and an urge to drink, with subjects consuming about 20% of their original deficit within 5 min, again pointing to a possible role for oropharyngeal factors in the control of drinking. During the Extraction condition, the volume of water consumed only exceeded the water deficit by about 15%, suggesting an effective form of oral metering in humans. The findings of Goldman et al.[50] and Figaro and Mack[41] on the relationship between oropharyngeal stimulation and AVP confirm previous findings in dogs,[6,130] sheep,[11,12] and humans.[47,128]

A simple model for the integration of oropharyngeal, gastrointestinal, and post-absorptive factors has been suggested by Verbalis[134] (Figure 3.12). This framework is consistent with the conclusions drawn by Rolls et al.,[108] Rolls and Rolls,[105] and Fitzsimons.[42] It is likely that drinking is normally terminated by a combination of oropharyngeal stimulation, gut distension, osmotic effects of water in the gut and hepatic portal system, and systemic dilution and expansion.[108] It has also been suggested that species differences in voluntary fluid intake can be understood in terms of the relative importance of oropharyngeal, gastrointestinal, and postabsorptive factors.[134] For additional discussion integrating the multiple control loci for drinking, see Mack.[67]

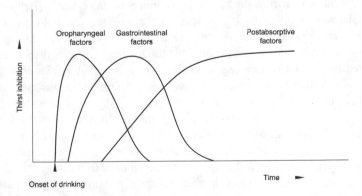

FIGURE 3.12 Schematic diagram depicting the onset and duration of various inhibitory signals to continued fluid ingestion following initiation of drinking in response to body fluid deficits. Although each signal by itself is capable of terminating ingestion (depending upon the species), it is the overlapping nature of these sequentially activated mechanisms that produces and sustains the inhibition of further water ingestion. From Verbalis, J.G., Inhibitory controls of drinking: satiation of thirst, in *Thirst: Physiological and Psychological Aspects,* Ramsey, D.J. and Booth, D., Eds., Springer-Verlag, London, 1991, chap. 19. With permission.

Oral metering may be a key oropharyngeal element for some species. As pointed out by Fitzsimons,[42] "...the advantage to the animal of being able to complete the ingestion of an amount of water appropriate to its needs and in advance of any significant absorption is obvious (p. 88)." The dog[1] seems particularly adept at replacing body water deficit, thereby being able to accurately replace lost fluid in minutes. When an amount of water equal to the deficit was placed directly into the stomach, the dog still drank an amount equal to the deficit, if allowed to begin drinking within 10 min of placement of the stomach load. Drinking did not occur if it was delayed by more than 15 min. The rat, conversely, seems more sensitive to the effects of stomach distention than oral metering, although oropharyngeal factors and oral metering clearly play a role in controlling fluid intake in the rat as well.[42] Direct evidence from Figaro and Mack[41] suggests a role for oral metering in humans also.

3.3.6 ERGONOMIC FACTORS

3.3.6.1 Proximity

The proximity of the beverage to the subject has been found to be an important factor affecting the amount of fluid consumed. Systematic field observations of body weight changes and voluntary fluid intake of basketball, netball, and soccer teams during training and competition in Australia[16] suggested that proximity to water bottles, and individualized water bottles may contribute to fluid intake, although experimental manipulation of bottle proximity was not conducted. Engell et al.,[33] in a between-groups laboratory study with 36 adult males (40 ± 13 y), positioned water on a lunch table, across the room (about 6 m from the table), and out of sight of the table (about 13 m from the table), in a "luncheon taste test." They found that water intake was significantly higher when it was on the table (444 ± 260 g) than when it was 6 m away (197 ± 100 g) or 13 m away (187 ± 155 g). In experiments with soldiers (reviewed by Engell and Hirsch[32]), ease of use of drinking systems contributed to amount of beverage consumed. In a repeated-measures experiment with 10 adult cyclists,[117] a metered drink system was compared with two *ad libitum* drink conditions during a 1 h ride at 50% of VO_{2max}. Subjects were allowed to drink every 15 min from the metered system (which dispensed water in 200 ml aliquots), were given *ad libitum* access to water every 15 min, or were given *ad libitum* access to water throughout the 60 min ride. Significantly more water was consumed during the metered-system trial than during the two *ad libitum* trials, suggesting that this form of portion control enhanced intake. Beverage proximity may be particularly relevant in industrial settings where workers must spend many hours active in a hot environment or in sports settings where the duration of practice or competition is such that continual access to fluid is important to encourage complete hydration.

3.3.6.2 Container

The shape or configuration of the beverage container may affect ease of use, liking of the package, and amount of fluid consumed. In a repeated-measures study comparing six beverage packages (unpublished data), 48 fit adults exercised for 30 min (aerobic training circuit) at moderate intensity (75–85% of maximum heart rate based on age-predicted maximum rates[5,40]), after which they had *ad libitum* access to a flavored 6% CHO electrolyte sports beverage in one of six bottle or package types (16-oz plastic, 16-oz glass, 32-oz glass, 10-oz glass, 12-oz can, 25-ml drink box). Hedonic and descriptive sensory evaluations were made using 9-point and 100-point scales, respectively. Subjects returned to the laboratory to complete a series of sessions in which they were exposed to all treatment conditions, which were administered in a Latin square arrangement. Clear differences were observed in liking of container type (Figure 3.13), with the two 16-oz bottles being liked more than the 250-ml drink box ($p < 0.05$) in this adult sample. Similarly, fluid intakes were higher for the two 16-oz bottles than the 250-ml drink box ($p < 0.05$). Written comments from the subjects suggested that the small size of the drink box and the mandatory use of a straw may have created an annoyance factor that could have brought down the hedonic score and made drinking difficult, especially when the subjects had just finished exercise and may have been eager to drink avidly. This may also help to explain the relatively low hedonic score for the 32-oz glass bottle, which subjects (especially women) reported was somewhat difficult to hold, but from which it was easy to drink. The 32-oz glass bottle had a 53-mm closure size that was larger than the two 16-oz bottles, which had closures of approximately 40 mm, and the 10-oz glass bottle, which had a closure size of 28 mm. Other human-factor elements such as the use of a water bladder, multiple bottles, or plasticity of sport bottle could possibly play a role in encouraging voluntary fluid intake.

3.3.7 SOCIAL, CULTURAL, AND PSYCHOLOGICAL FACTORS

An important element in the continuum of factors controlling fluid intake is the social/cultural/psychological one. Fitzsimons[42] has acknowledged that there clearly are reasons other than thirst that contribute to *ad libitum* drinking in the normal course of homeostasis. Cognitive factors, including learning mechanisms, play a role in the control of voluntary fluid intake.[134] Holland[53] has described in some detail several psychological mechanisms including stimulus control properties arising from Pavlovian and operant conditioning, and the contribution of associative and non-associative learning, and drive-reduction theory. Ramirez et al.[93–96] have demonstrated in rats that gastric infusions of carbohydrate solution, given when rats drank a flavored solution (saccharin, NaCl, cherry flavor, oligosaccharide), increased fluid intake of the flavored solution. Perez et al.[89] have also demonstrated robust post-ingestional effects on flavor preference in rats preexposed to a varied diet. Ramirez[96] has suggested that these results, and those of others investigating post-ingestive effects on preference,[76,96,118] point to a form of Pavlovian conditioning. Schedule-induced polydipsia is a condition in which drinking occurs as a function of the temporal distribution of non-contingent reinforcers, or reinforcers contingent on behaviors other than drinking. It has been extensively investigated in animals and has been suggested as a possible basis for excessive behavior in humans,[38,39,48] although the extent to which schedule-induced polydipsia occurs in everyday life is uncertain.[49] In laboratory experiments with humans, Doyle and Sampson[29,30] demonstrated that the non-contingent delivery of monetary rewards in a video slot

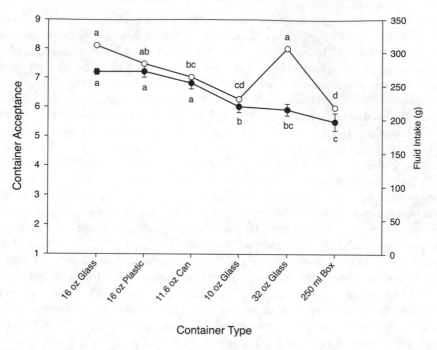

FIGURE 3.13 Beverage-package acceptance (●, 9-point scale) and fluid intake (○, g). Within each curve, points not sharing a common letter are significantly different from each other (p < 0.05).

machine at intervals of 130 seconds and 190 seconds could engender significant increases in intake of water and beer at the 190-second interval. Rogers et al.[100] examined the post-ingestive effects of caffeine on preference for a novel flavored drink in moderate-caffeine and low-caffeine users. Subjects first ranked an array of seven novel beverages. The beverage of middle rank for each subject was then presented immediately after breakfast for 10 d, with or without caffeine, in a between-groups design. Subjects had only water to drink for 24 h prior to testing. Moderate-caffeine users developed an increase in relative preference for the caffeine-containing beverage and a relative dislike for the non-caffeine version. Low-caffeine users, however, developed an increase in relative preference for the non-caffeine beverage and showed no significant change in liking of the caffeine-containing beverage. In addition, mood in the moderate-caffeine users who received the non-caffeine beverage was lower than in the group of moderate-caffeine users who received the caffeine-containing beverage. Mood in the low-caffeine users was largely unaffected by caffeine. It appears that the moderate-caffeine users developed an aversion to the non-caffeine beverage because it was associated with the negative consequences of caffeine abstinence. It is this alleviation of the adverse effects of abstinence (negative reinforcement, Honig[54]) that may be maintaining caffeine-beverage use in some individuals. De Castro[23] has also emphasized the importance of non-homeostatic mechanisms for a complete understanding of the control of fluid intake, contending that social context and food intake are more important than homeostatic fluid balance status in predicting voluntary fluid intake. While focused on eating as well as fluid intake, De Castro[25] has provided a comprehensive framework in which to view the social factors involved in the regulation of intake. Complex social situations including immediate social as well as enduring cultural influences are relevant. A key method employed in this research is the complete dietary self-report method,[24] which involves creating a detailed 7-d log of all food and beverage consumed, including time, amount, method of preparation, social situation, and environmental context. (This method, which requires subjects to carry the dietary log, is to be distinguished from diet-recall methods in which subjects attempt to remember dietary practice at the end of a day or other fixed period of time.) The subjective state and social situation (especially number of people present) may have a profound effect on amount eaten. Significant positive correlations between food intake and measures of elation and anxiety have been reported.[28] Meals eaten in the presence of other people were 44% larger than meals eaten alone. The more people present, up to an average of approximately 13 people, the greater the amount of food eaten.[27] A power function describes the size of the meal relative to the number of people present: Meal size = 485 $N^{0.23}$.[131] More research needs to be done in this area for beverage intake. Through manipulating the number of other people present, social facilitation has been shown to be a causal influence on food intake.[98] An analysis of self-reported fluid intakes of 36 adults[22] indicated that the regulation of fluid intake under *ad libitum* conditions is secondary to the regulation of food intake. In regression analyses, the amount of food consumed accounted for over 50% of the variation in voluntary fluid intake. For a more complete discussion of the effects of eating on drinking, see Kraly.[64] De Castro[23] concludes: "... something other than the levels of fluids in the intracellular and extracellular compartments at the time of a bout would appear to be responsible for regulating the amount and timing of fluid intake (p.352)." McCarty[72] has reported that the amount of beverage consumed in bars increases as the number of people present increases. The role of advertising and marketing on beverage choice and volume consumed has been briefly considered by Gilbert.[49] Marketing efforts are directed at changing trends in coffee, soft drink, and alcohol purchase frequency as well as amount consumed via increasing serving size. The role of advertising and marketing in shaping cultural influences on fluid intake are largely unexplored. The role of social and cultural influences has been broadly considered by Booth[13] and Tuorila.[132] In many social contexts, the offer of a drink from one person to another may not be related to any underlying body water deficit, but may relate to cultural factors, learning, and peer pressure. Within the U.S., there are ethnic differences related to the appropriateness of beverage choice.[132] The differences observed among countries in consumption of various categories of beverages also illustrate enduring cultural influences.[132] In a cross-cultural survey with 1281 subjects from Belgium, France, Japan, and the U.S., Rozin et al.[112] have focused on the psychology of food in terms of "negative" (worry, fear regarding health implications of food choice) and "positive" (pleasure, anticipation of eating) views of food, the importance of food in life, and how people view food relative to diet and health. Substantial cultural differences were observed with significant main effects for country ($p < 0.001$) for most categories. For instance, Americans seem to worry more than all of the other countries about the health implications of diet and to modify their diets to support health more than any other country, yet are the least likely to view themselves as being healthy eaters. Gender effects were also seen, but with a lower frequency of statistical reliability. Age effects tended to be small and not statistically reliable. While this study did not directly address fluid intake, the insight that can emerge from these types of investigations may contribute to a more complete understanding of factors controlling food (and fluid) intake. Rozin and Millman[114] have suggested that environmental influences (family environment) are of greater importance than genetic ones in accounting for food preferences. See Galef[45] for a discussion of social influences on fluid intake in the rat and non-human primate.

3.4 SUMMARY

Clearly, there is an array of control loci for drinking, ranging from homeostatic mechanisms to cultural and social influences. This chapter has attempted to highlight some of the prominent elements in that array. See Ramsey and Booth[97] and Rolls and Rolls[105] for additional discussions of a wide range of controlling factors for drinking behavior. There is a need for closer integration of the physiological and psychosocial elements that have been identified as influences on fluid intake. An excellent framework for discussing such an integration has been provided by Greenleaf,[51] who took a multiple-regression approach to better understand the relative contribution of 22 metabolic variables. The analysis[52] revealed that six elements were relatively important and accounted for 62% of the variation in water intake. Engell et al.[34] took a similar statistical approach and created an equation that accounted for 65% of the variation in water intake. Both investigators found that plasma osmolality was important. However, this approach could be expanded to include those other factors since identified as being important determinants of fluid intake. Beverage palatability, temperature, negative attributes, social context, and mood, or psychological status, in addition to metabolic variables, could all be included in a model, thereby providing a single context for evaluating the relative importance of all of the potential controlling factors. While individual studies have each identified robust effects for many of the homeostatic, oropharyngeal, sensory, social, and psychological variables that have been tested, expanding the model suggested by Greenleaf[51] and Engell et al.[34] could provide the basis for a much more integrated analysis.

REFERENCES

1. Adolph, E.F., Measurements of water drinking in dogs, *Am.J.Physiol.*, 125, 75-86, 1939.
2. Adolph, E.F., Thirst and its inhibition in the stomach, *Am.J.Physiol.*, 161, 374-386, 1950.
3. Adolph, E.F. and Dill, D.B., Observations on water metabolism in the desert, *Am.J.Physiol.*, 123, 369-378, 1938.

4. Adolph, E.F. and Wills, J.H., Thirst, in *Physiology of Man in the Desert,* Adolf, E.F., Ed., Interscience Publishers, NY, 1947, chap. 15.

5. American College of Sports Medicine. ACSM's Guidelines for Exercise Testing and Prescription, Balado, D. Ed., Baltimore, Williams & Wilkins 5, 274, 1995.

6. Appelgren, B.H., Thrasher, T.N., Keil, L.C., and Ramsey, D.J., Mechanism of drinking-induced inhibition of vasopressin secretion in dehydrated dogs, *Am.J.Physiol.,* 261, R1226-R1233, 1991.

7. Armstrong, L.E., Hubbard, R.W., Szlyk, P.C., Matthew, W.T., and Sils, I.V., Voluntary dehydration and electrolyte losses during prolonged exercise in the heat, *Aviat.Space Environ.Med.,* 56, 765-770, 1985.

8. Bar-Or, O., Dotan, R., Inbar, O., Rothstein, A., and Zonder, H., Voluntary hypohydration in 10- and 12-year-old boys, *J.Appl.Physiol.: Respirat.Environ.Exercise Physiol.,* 48, [1], 104-108, 1980.

9. Barker, J.P., Adolf, E.F., and Keller, A.D., Thirst tests in dogs and modifications of thirst with experimental lesions of the neurohypophysis, *Am.J.Physiol.,* 173, 233-245, 1953.

10. Beridot-Therond, M.E., Arts, I., Fantino, M., and De La Gueronniere, V., Short-term effects of the flavour of drinks on ingestive behaviours in man, *Appetite,* 31, 67-81, 1998.

11. Blair-West, J.R., Gibson, A.P., Sheather, S.J., Woods, R.L., and Brook, A.H., Vasopressin release in sheep following various degrees of rehydration, *Am.J.Physiol.,* 253, R640-R645, 1987.

12. Blair-West, J.R., Gibson, A.P., Woods, R.L., and Brook, A.H., Acute reduction of plasma vasopressin levels by rehydration in sheep, *Am.J.Physiol.,* 248, R68-R71, 1985.

13. Booth, D.A., Influences on human fluid consumption, in *Thirst: Physiological and Psychological Aspects,* Ramsey, D.J. and Booth, D., Eds., Springer-Verlag, London, 1991, chap. 4.

14. Boulze, D., Montastruc, P., and Cabanac, M., Water intake, pleasure and water temperature in humans, *Physiol.Behav.,* 30, [1], 97-102, 1983.

15. Bourque, C.W., Oliet, S.H.R., and Richard, D., Osmoreceptors, osmoreception, and osmoregulation, *Front.Neurendocrinol.,* 15, 231-274, 1994.

16. Broad, E.M., Burke, L.M., Cox, G.R., Heeley, P., and Riley, M., Body weight changes and voluntary fluid intakes during training and competition sessions in team sports, *Int.J.Sport Nutr.,* 6, 307-320, 1996.

17. Buggy, J. and Johnson, A.K., Preoptic-hypothalamic periventricular lesions: thirst deficits and hypernatremia, *Am.J.Physiol.,* 233, [1], R44-52, 1977.

18. Cabanac, M., Physiological role of pleasure, *Science,* 173, 1103-1107, 1971.

19. Calvino, A.M., Perception of sweetness: the effects of concentration and temperature, *Physiol.Behav.,* 36, [6], 1021-1028, 1986.

20. Cardello, A.V. and Maller, O., Relationships between food preferences and food acceptance ratings, *J.Food Sci.,* 47, 1553-1561, 1982.

21. Clark, N. *The New York City Marathon Cookbook*, Rutledge Hill Press, Nashville, 1994, 219.

22. De Castro, J.M., A microregulatory analysis of spontaneous fluid intake by humans: evidence that the amount of liquid ingested and its timing is mainly governed by feeding, *Physiol.Behav.,* 43, 705-714, 1988.

23. De Castro, J.M., Bout pattern analysis of *ad libitum* fluid intake, in *Thirst: Physiological and Psychological Aspects,* Ramsey, D.J. and Booth, D., Eds., Springer-Verlag, London, 1991, chap. 21.

24. De Castro, J.M., Methodology, correlational analysis, and interpretation of diet diary records of the food and fluid intake of free-living humans, *Appetite,* 23, 179-192, 1994.

25. De Castro, J.M., How can eating behavior be regulated in the complex environments of free-living humans? *Neurosci.Biobehav.Rev.,* 20, [1], 119-131, 1996.

26. De Castro, J.M. and Brewer, E.M., The amount eaten in meals by humans is a power function of the number of people present, *Physiol.Behav.,* 51, [1], 121-125, 1992.

27. De Castro, J.M. and De Castro, E.S., Spontaneous meal patterns of humans: influence of the presence of other people, *Am.J.Clin.Nutr.,* 50, [2], 237-247, 1989.

28. De Castro, J.M. and Elmore, D.K., Subjective hunger relationships with meal patterns in the spontaneous feeding behavior of humans: evidence for a causal connection, *Physiol.Behav.,* 43, 159-165, 1988.

29. Doyle, T.F. and Samson, H.H., Schedule-induced drinking in humans: a potential factor in excessive alcohol use, *Alcohol Depend.,* 16, 117-132, 1985.

30. Doyle, T.F. and Samson, H.H., Adjunctive alcohol drinking in humans, *Physiol.Behav.,* 44, 775-779, 1988.

31. Eichna, L.W., Bean, W.B., Ashe, W.F., and Nelson, N., Performance in relation to environmental temperature, *Bull.Johns Hopkins Hosp.,* 76, 25-58, 1945.

32. Engell, D. and Hirsch, E., Environmental and sensory modulation of fluid intake in humans, in *Thirst: Physiological and Psychological Aspects,* Ramsey, D.J. and Booth, D., Eds., Springer-Verlag, N.Y., 1991.

33. Engell, D., Kramer, M., Malafi, T., Salomon, M., and Lesher, L., Effects of effort and social modeling on drinking in humans, *Appetite,* 26, 129-138, 1996.

34. Engell, D.B., Maller, O., Sawka, M.N., Francesconi, R.P., Drolet, L., and Young, A.J., Thirst and fluid intake following graded hypohydration levels in humans, *Physiol.Behav.,* 40, [2], 229-236, 1987.

35. Epstein, A.N., Fitzsimons, J.T., and Rolls, B.J., Drinking induced by injection of angiotensin into the brain of the rat, *J.Physiol.,* 210, 457-474, 1970.

36. Ernits, T. and Corbit, J.D., Taste as a dipsogenic stimulus, *J.Comp.Physiol.Psychol.,* 83, [1], 27-31, 1973.

37. Falk, B., Bar-Or, O., and MacDougall, J.D., Thermoregulatory responses of pre-, and mid-, and late-pubertal boys to exercise in dry heat, *Med.Sci.Sports Exerc.,* 24, [6], 688-694, 1992.

38. Falk, J.L., The environmental generation of excessive behavior, in *Behavior in Excess: An Examination of the Volitional Disorders,* Mule, S.J. Ed., Free Press, New York, 1981.

39. Falk, J.L. and Tang, M., Schedule induction and overindulgence, *Alcohol Clin.Exp.Res.,* 4, [3], 266-270, 1980.

40. Fardy, P.S., Yanowitz, F.G., and Wilson, P.K., *Cardiac Rehabilitation, Adult Fitness, and Exercise Testing,* Lea & Febiger, Philadelphia, 1988, 171.

41. Figaro, M.K. and Mack, G.W., Regulation of fluid intake in dehydrated humans: role of oropharyngeal stimulation, *Am.J.Physiol.,* 272, R1740-R1746, 1997.

42. Fitzsimons, J.T. *The Physiology of Thirst and Sodium Appetite,* Cambridge, University Press, 1979.

43. Fitzsimons, J.T., Angiotensin, thirst, and sodium appetite, *Physiol.Rev.,* 78, [3], 583-686, 1998.

44. Fitzsimons, J.T. and Simons, B.J., The effect on drinking in the rat of intravenous infusion of antiotensin, given alone or in combination with other stimuli of thirst, *J.Physiol.,* 203, 45-57, 1969.

45. Galef, B.G., Social influences on fluid intake: Laboratory experiments with rats, field observations of primates, in *Thirst: Physiological and Psychological Aspects,* Ramsey, D.J. and Booth, D., Eds., Springer-Verlag, London, 1991, chap. 20.

46. Garcia, J., Hankins, W.G., and Rusiniak, K.W., Behavioral regulation of the milieu interne in man and rat, *Science,* 185, 824-831, 1974.

47. Geelen, G., Keil, L.C., Kravik, S.E., Wade, C.E., Thrasher, T.N., Barnes, P.R., Pyka, G., Nesvig, C., and Greenleaf, J.E., Inhibition of plasma vasopressin after drinking in dehydrated humans, *Am.J.Physiol.,* 247, R968-R971, 1954.

48. Gilbert, R.M., Drug abuse as excessive behaviour, *Can.Psychol.Rev.,* 17, 231-240, 1976.

49. Gilbert, R.M., Alcohol- and caffeine-beverage consumption: causes other than water deficit, in *Thirst:Physiological and Psychological Aspects,* Ramsey, D.J. and Booth, D., Eds., Springer-Verlag, London, 1991, chap. 23.

50. Goldman, M.B., Robertson, G.L., and Hedeker, D., Oropharyngeal regulation of water balance in polydipsic schizophrenics, *Clin.Endocrin.,* 44, 31-37, 1996.

51. Greenleaf, J.E., Problem: thirst, drinking behavior, and involuntary dehydration, *Med.Sci.Sports Exer.,* 24, [6], 645-656, 1992.

52. Greenleaf, J.E., Averkin, E.G., and Sargent II, F., Water consumption by man in a warm environment: a statistical analysis, *J.Appl.Physiol.,* 21, [1], 93-98, 1966.

53. Holland, P.C., Learning, thirst and drinking, in *Thirst: Physiological and Psychological Aspects,* Ramsey, D.J. and Booth, D., Eds., Springer-Verlag, London, 1991, chap. 17.

54. Honig, W.K. *Operant Behavior: Areas of Research and Application*, Appleton-Century-Crofts, New York, 1966.

55. Horio, T. and Kawamura, Y., Influence of physical exercise on human preferences for various taste solutions, *Chemical Senses,* 23, 417-421, 1998.

56. Hubbard, R.W., Sandick, B.L., Matthew, R.P., Francesconi, R.P., Sampson, J.B., Durkot, M.J., Maller, O., and Engell, D.B., Voluntary dehydration and alliesthesia for water, *J.Appl.Physiol.,* 57, 868-873, 1984.

57. Hubbard, R.W., Szlyk, P.C., and Armstrong, L.E., Influence of thirst and fluid palatability on fluid ingestion during exercise, in *Perspectives in Exercise Science and Sports Medicine Volume 3: Fluid Homeostasis During Exercise,* Gisolfi, C.V. and Lamb, D.R., Eds., Brown & Benchmark, Carmel, IN, 1990.

58. Johnson, A.K., Brain mechanisms in the control of body fluid homeostasis, in *Perspectives in Exercise Science,* Gisolfi, C.V. and Lamb, D.R., Eds., Brown & Benchmark, Carmel, 1990, chap. 10.

59. Johnson, A.K. and Buggy, J., Periventricular preoptic-hypothalamus is vital for thirst and normal water economy, *Am.J.Physiol.,* 234, [3], R122-129, 1978.

60. Johnson, A.K., Cunningham, J.T., and Thunhorst, R.L., Integrative role of the lamina terminalis in the regulation of cardiovascular and body fluid homeostasis, *Clin.Exp.Pharmacol.Physiol.,* 23, [2], 183-191, 1996.

61. Johnson, A.K. and Edwards, G.L., Central projections of osmotic and hypovolaemic signals in homeostatic thirst, in *Thirst: Physiological and Psychological Aspects,* Ramsey, D.J. and Booth, D., Eds., Springer-Verlag, London, 1991, chap. 9.

62. King, N.A. and Blundell, J.E., High-fat foods overcome the energy expenditure induced by high-intensity cycling or running, *Eur.J.Clin.Nutr.,* 49, [2], 114-123, 1995.

63. King, N.A., Snell, L., and Blundell, J.E., Effects of short-term exercise on appetite responses in unrestrained females, *Eur J.Clin.Nutr.,* 50, [10], 663-667, 1996.

64. Kraly, F.S., Effects of eating on drinking, in *Thirst: Physiological and Psychological Aspects,* Ramsey, D.J. and Booth, D., Eds., Springer-Verlag, London, 1991, chap. 18.

65. Leshem, M., Abutbul, A., and Eilon, R., Exercise increases the preference for salt in humans, *Appetite,* 32, 251-260, 1999.

66. Lluch, A., King, N.A., and Blundell, J.E., Exercise in dietary restrained women: no effect on energy intake but change in hedonic ratings, *Eur.J.Clin.Nut.,* 52, 300-307, 1998.

67. Mack, G.W., Recovery after exercise in the heat: Factors influencing fluid intake, *Int.J.Sports Med.,* 19, S139-S141, 1998.

68. Maddison, S., Wood, R.J., Rolls, E.T., Rolls, B.J., and Gibbs, J., Drinking in the rhesus monkey: peripheral factors, *J.Comp.Physiol.Psychol.,* 94, [2], 365-374, 1980.

69. Maughan, R., Symposium Proceedings: Dehydration, rehydration, and exercise in the heat, *Can.J.Appl.Physiol.,* 24, [2], 149-151, 1999.

70. Maughan, R.J., Leiper, J.B., and Shirreffs, S.M., Factors influencing the restoration of fluid and electrolyte balance after exercise in the heat, *J.Sports Med.,* 31, 175-182, 1997.

71. Maughan, R.J. and Shirreffs, S.M., Recovery from prolonged exercise: restoration of water and electrolyte balance, *J.Sports Sci.,* 15, 297-303, 1997.

72. McCarty, D., Environmental factors in substance abuse: the micro-setting, in *Determinants of Substance Abuse: Biological, Psychological, and Environmental Factors,* Galizio, M. and Maisto, S.A., Eds., Plenum Press, NY, 1985.

73. McKenna, K. and Thompson, C., Osmoregulation in clinical disorders of thirst appreciation, *Clin.Endocrin.,* 49, 139-152, 1998.

74. McKinley, M.J., Osmoreceptors for thirst, in *Thirst: Physiological and Psychological Aspects,* Ramsey, D.J. and Booth, D., Eds., Springer-Verlag, London, 1991, chap. 5.

75. McKinley, M.J., Pennington, G.L., and Oldfield, B.J., Anteroventral wall of the third ventricle and dorsal lamina terminalis: headquarters for control of body fluid homeostasis? *Clin.Exp.Pharmacol.Physiol.,* 23, [4], 271-281, 1996.

76. Mehiel, R. and Bolles, R.C., Learned flavor preferences based on calories are independent of initial hedonic value, *Anim.Learn.Behav.,* 16, 383-387, 1988.

77. Meyer, F. and Bar-Or, O., Fluid and electrolyte loss during exercise, *Sports Med.,* 18, [1], 4-9, 1994.

78. Meyer, F., Bar-Or, O., Salsberg, A., and Passe, D., Hypohydration during exercise in children: Effect on thirst, drink preferences, and rehydration, *Int.J.Sport Nutr.,* 4, 22-35, 1994.

79. Michelini, L.C., Barnes, K.L., and Ferrario, C.M., Arginine vasopressin modulates the central action of angiotensin II in the dog, *Hypertension,* 5, 94-100, 1999.

80. Mook, D.G., Oral and postingestional determinants of the intake of various solutions in rats with esophageal fistulas, *J.Comp.Physiol.Psychol.,* 56, 645-659, 1963.

81. Mook, D.G., Culberson, R., Gelbart, R.J., and McDonald, K., Oropharyngeal control of ingestion in rats: acquisition of sham-drinking patterns, *Behav.Neurosci.,* 97, [4], 574-584, 1983.

82. Mosimann, R., Imboden, H., and Felix, D., The neuronal role of angiotensin II in thirst, sodium appetite, cognition and memory, *Biol.Rev.,* 71, 545-559, 1999.

83. Oldfield, B.J., Neurochemistry of the circuitry subserving thirst, in *Thirst: Physiological and Psychological Aspects,* Ramsey, D.J. and Booth, D., Eds., Springer-Verlag, London, 1991, chap. 10.

84. Passe, D., Horn, M., and Murray, R. Effect of beverage palatability on voluntary fluid intake during exercise, *Med.Sci.Sports Exerc.,* 30, [5], S156-S156, 1998.

85. Passe, D., Horn, M., and Murray, R. Palatability and voluntary intake of sports beverages, diluted fruit juice, and water during exercise, *Med.Sci.in Sports Exerc.,* 31, [5], S322, 1999.

86. Passe, D., Horn, M., and Murray, R., Impact of beverage acceptability on fluid intake during exercise, *Appetite,* In press., 2000.
87. Passe, D., Horn, M., and Murray, R.M. The effects of beverage carbonation on sensory responses and voluntary fluid intake following exercise, *Int.J.Sport Nutr.,* 7, 286-297, 1997.
88. Pelchat, M.L. and Rozin, P., The special role of nausea in the acquisition of food dislikes by humans, *Appetite,* 3, 341-351, 1998.
89. Perez, L., Fanizza, J., and Sclafani, A., Flavor preferences conditioned by intragastric nutrient infusions in rats fed chow or a cafeteria diet, *Appetite,* 32, 155-170, 1999.
90. Peryam, D.R. and Pilgrim, F.J., Hedonic scale method of measuring food preferences, *Food Technol.,* 11, [9], 9-14, 1957.
91. Phillips, P.A., Rolls, B.J., Ledingham, J.G.G., and Morton, J.J., Body fluid changes, thirst and drinking in man during free access to water, *Physiol.Behav.,* 33, [3], 357-363, 1984.
92. Ploutz-Snyder, L., Foley, J., Ploutz-Snyder, R., Kanaley, J., Sagendorf, K., and Meyer, R., Gastric gas and fluid emptying assessed by magnetic resonance imaging, *Europ.J.Appl.Physiol.,* 79, 212-220, 1999.
93. Ramirez, I., Stimulation of fluid intake by carbohydrates: interaction between taste and calories, *Am.J.Physiol.,* 266, R682-R687, 1994.
94. Ramirez, I., Stimulation of fluid intake by maltodextrins and starch, *Physiol.Behav.,* 57, [4], 687-692, 1995.
95. Ramirez, I., Stimulus specificity in flavor acceptance learning, *Physiol.Behav.,* 60, [2], 595-610, 1996.
96. Ramirez, I., Stimulation of fluid intake by nutrients: oil is less effective than carbohydrate, *Am.J.Physiol.,* 272, [R289], R293, 1997.
97. Ramsey, D.J. and Booth, D.A. *Thirst: Physiological and Psychological Aspects,* Springer-Verlag, London, 1991.
98. Redd, E.M. and De Castro, J.M., Social facilitation of eating: effects of instructions to eat alone or with others, *Physiol.Behav.,* 52, [4], 749-754, 1992.
99. Rivera-Brown, A.M., Gutierrez, R., Gutierrez, J.C., Frontera, W.R., and Bar-Or, O. Drink composition, voluntary drinking, and fluid balance in exercising, trained, heat-acclimatized boys, *J. Appl. Physiol.,* 86, [1], 78-84, 1999.
100. Rogers, P.J., Richardson, N.J., and Elliman, N.A., Overnight caffeine abstinence and negative reinforcement of preference for caffeine-containing drinks, *Psychopharmacology,* 20, 457-462, 1995.
101. Rolls, B.J., Sensory-specific satiety, *Nut.Rev.,* 44, [3], 93-101, 1986.
102. Rolls, B.J., Sweetness and satiety, in *Sweetness,* Dobbing, J.Eds., Springer-Verlag, London, 1987, chap. 11.
103. Rolls, B.J., Palatability and fluid intake, in *Fluid Replacement and Heat Stress,* Marriott, B.M. and Rosemont, C., Eds., National Academy Press, Washington, D.C.: 1991.
104. Rolls, B.J., Fedoroff, I.C., Guthrie, J.F., and Laster, L.J., Effects of temperature and mode of presentation of juice on hunger, thirst and food intake in humans, *Appetite,* 15, 199-208, 1990.
105. Rolls, B.J. and Rolls, E.T., *Thirst,* Cambridge University Press, Cambridge, MA, 1982.
106. Rolls, B.J., Rolls, E.T., Rowe, E.A., and Sweeney, K., Sensory specific satiety in man., *Phys.& Beh.,* 27, 137-142, 1981.
107. Rolls, B.J., Wood, R.J., and Rolls, E.T., Thirst: the initiation, maintenance, and termination of drinking, *Prog.Psychol.Physiol.Psychol.,* 9, 263-321, 1980.

108. Rolls, B.J., Wood, R.J., Rolls, E.T., Lind, H., Lind, W., and Ledingham, J.G.G., Thirst following water deprivation in humans, *Am.J.Physiol.,* 239, R476-R482, 1980.
109. Rolls, B.J., Wood, R.J., and Stevens, R.M., Palatability and body fluid homeostasis, *Physiol.Behav.,* 20, [1], 15-19, 1978.
110. Rose, M.S., Szlyk, P.C., Francesconi, R.P., Lester, L.S., Armstrong, L., Matthew, W., Cardello, A.V., Popper, R.D., Sils, I., Thomas, G., Schilling, D., and Whang, R. Effectiveness and acceptability of nutrient solutions in enhancing fluid intake in the heat, 1-256, 1988. Natick, USARIEM.
111. Rothstein, A., Adolf, E.F., and Wills, J.H., Voluntary dehydration, in *Physiology of Man in the Desert,* Adolf, E.F., Ed., Interscience Publishers, N.Y., 1947, chap. 16.
112. Rozin, P., Fischler, C., Imada, S., Sarubin, A., and Wrzesniewski, A., Attitudes to food and the role of food in life in the USA, Japan, Flemish Belgium and France: possible implications for the diet-health debate, *Appetite,* 33, 163-180, 1999.
113. Rozin, P. and Kalat, J.W., Specific hungers and poison avoidance as adaptive specializations of learning, *Psychol.Rev.,* 78, 459-486, 1971.
114. Rozin, P. and Millman, L., Family environment, not heredity, accounts for family resemblances in food preferences and attitudes: a twin study, *Appetite,* 8, 125-134, 1987.
115. Sandick, B.L., Engell, D.B., and Maller, O., Perception of drinking water temperature and effects for humans after exercise, *Physiol.Behav.,* 32, [5], 851-855, 1984.
116. Santana, J.R.R., Rivera-Brown, A.M., Frontera, W.R., Rivera, M., Mayol, P.M., and Bar-Or, O., Effect of drink pattern and solar radiation on thermoregulation and fluid balance during exercise in chronically heat acclimatized children, *Am.J.Human Biol.,* 7, 643-650, 1995.
117. Schroeder, J.M., Heck, K.L., and Potteiger, J.A., A comparison of three fluid replacement strategies for maintaining euhydration during prolonged exercise, *Can.J.Appl.Physiol.,* 22, [1], 48-57, 1997.
118. Sclafani, A., How food preferences are learned: laboratory animal models, *Proc.Nutr.Soc.,* 54, [2], 419-427, 1995.
119. Simpson, J.B., Epstein, A.N., and Camardo, J.S. Jr., Localization of receptors for the dipsogenic action of antiotensin II in the subfornical organ of rat, *J.Comp.Physiol.Psychol.,* 92, [4], 581-608, 1978.
120. Simpson, J.B. and Routtenberg, A., Subfornical organ: a dipsogenic site of action of angiotensin II, *Science,* 201, [4353], 379-381, 1978.
121. Sohar, E., Kaly, J., and Adar, R., The prevention of voluntary dehydration, in *Symposium on Environmental Physiology and Psychology in Arid Conditions,* United Nations Educational Scientific and Cultural Organization, Paris, 1962.
122. Spioch, F.M. and Nowara, M., Voluntary dehydration in men working in heat, *Int.Arch Occup.Environ.Health,* 46, 233-239, 1980.
123. Star, R.A., Southwestern Internal Medicine Conference: Hyperosmolar States, *Am.J.Med.Sci.,* 300, [6], 402-412, 1990.
124. Szczepanska-Sadowska, E., Hormonal inputs to thirst, in *Thirst: Physiological and Psychological Aspects,* Ramsey, D.J. and Booth, D., Eds., Springer-Verlag, London, 1991.
125. Szczepanska-Sadowska, E., Interaction of vasopressin and angiotensin II in central control of blood pressure and thirst, *Regul.Pept.,* 66, [1-2], 3-11, 1996.
126. Szlyk, P.C., Hubbard, R.W., Matthew, R.P., Armstrong, L.E., and Kerstein, M.D., Mechanisms of voluntary dehydration among troops in the field, *Military Medicine,* 152, [8], 405-407, 1987.

127. Szlyk, P.C., Sils, I.V., Francesconi, R.P., Hubbard, R.W., and Armstrong, L.E., Effects of water temperature and flavoring on voluntary dehydration in men, *Physiology & Behavior,* 45, [3], 639-647, 1989.

128. Thompson, C.J., Burd, J.M., and Baylis, P.H., Acute suppression of plasma vasopressin and thirst after drinking in hypernatremic humans, *Am.J.Physiol.,* 252, R1138-R1142, 1987.

129. Thrasher, T.N., Volume receptors and the stimulation of water intake, in *Thirst: Physiological and Psychological Aspects,* Ramsey, D.J. and Booth, D., Eds., Springer-Verlag, London, 1991, chap. 6.

130. Thrasher, T.N., Keil, L.C., and Ramsey, D.J., Drinking, oropharyngeal signals, and inhibition of vasopressin secretion in dogs, *Am.J.Physiol.,* 253, R509-R515, 1987.

131. Toto, K.H. Regulation of plasma osmolality, *Crit.Care Nurs.Clin.North Am.,* 6, [4], 661-674, 1994.

132. Tuorila, H., Individual and cultural factors in the consumption of beverages, in *Thirst: Physiological and Psychological Aspects,* Ramsey, D.J. and Booth, D., Eds., Springer-Verlag, London, 1991, chap. 22.

133. Varnam, A.H. and Sutherland, J.P., *Beverages: Technology, Chemistry, and Microbiology,* Chapman & Hall, London, 1994.

134. Verbalis, J.G., Inhibitory controls of drinking: satiation of thirst, in *Thirst: Physiological and Psychological Aspects,* Ramsey, D.J. and Booth, D., Eds., Springer-Verlag, London, 1991, chap. 19.

135. Wemple, R.D., Morocco, T.S., and Mack, G.W., Influence of sodium replacement on fluid ingestion following exercise-induced dehydration, *Int.J.Sport Nut.,* 7, 104-116, 1997.

136. Wilk, B. and Bar-Or, O., Effect of drink flavor and NaCl on voluntary drinking and hydration in boys exercising in the heat, *J.Appl.Physiol.,* 80, [4], 1112-1117, 1996.

137. Wilk, B., Kriemler, S., Keller, H., and Bar-Or, O., Consistency in preventing voluntary dehydration in boys who drink a flavored carbohydrate-NaCl beverage during execise in the heat, *Int.J.Sport Nut.,* 8, 1-9, 1998.

138. Wilmore, J.H., Morton, A.R., Gilbey, H.J., and Wood, R.J., Role of taste preference on fluid intake during and after 90 min of running at 60% of VO_{2max} in the heat, *Med.Sci.SportsExerc.,* 30, [4], 587-595, 1998.

139. Yau, N.J.N. and McDaniel, M.R., The power-function of carbonation, *J.Sens.Studies,* 5, 117-128, 1990.

140. Yeomans, M.R. and Symes, T., Individual differences in the use of pleasantness and palatability ratings, *Appetite,* 32, 383-394, 1999.

141. Zeigler, H.P., Drinking in mammals: functional morphology, orosensory modulation and motor control, in *Thirst: Physiological and Psychological Aspects,* Ramsey, D.J. and Booth, D., Eds., Springer-Verlag, London, 1991, chap. 15.

142. Zellner, D.A., Stewart, W.F., Rozin, P., and Brown, J.M., Effect of temperature and expectations on liking for beverages. *Physiol. Behav.,* 44, [1], 61-68, 1988.

4 Gastric Emptying and Intestinal Absorption of Fluids, Carbohydrates, and Electrolytes

John B. Leiper

CONTENTS

0-8493-7008-6/01/$0.00+$.50
© 2001 by CRC Press LLC

4.1 INTRODUCTION

Ingestion of carbohydrate electrolyte drinks before and during exercise has been shown to help delay the fatigue process. Before the body can utilize the constituents of drink they must be absorbed by the small intestine and transported to the appropriate body pools. The role of the gastrointestinal tract in regulating the absorption of a drink and delivering the nutrients to the circulation is therefore crucial in determining the benefits that can be derived from fluid ingestion.

The intestinal tract is a tube approximately 9 meters in length, continuous from the mouth to the anus (Figure 4.1). Highly regulated contractions of the muscular walls produce peristaltic waves that propel the intestinal contents along the length of the intestine. Other rhythmical contractions of the intestinal wall cause mixing of the intestinal contents that promotes digestion and absorption.

The esophagus extends from the back of the mouth (pharynx) and passes through the thorax and diaphragm into the abdomen, where it opens into the stomach. The stomach functions as a reservoir that regulates the rate at which ingested material enters the small intestine, which is a coiled tube about 6.3 meters in length lying in the central and lower region of the abdomen and consisting of the duodenum, the jejunum, and the ileum. The diameter of the small intestine is about 5.0 cm at the start of the duodenum and it progressively tapers along its length until, at the end of the ileum, it has a diameter of approximately 2.5 cm. The duodenum is about 12 cm in length and is roughly crescent shaped. It is the first part of the small intestine

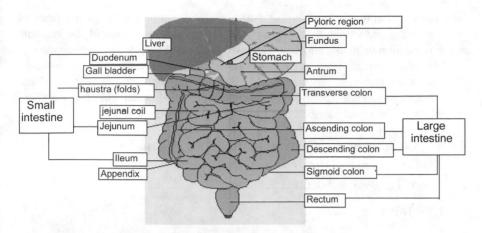

FIGURE 4.1   Schematic diagram of the gastrointestinal tract.

and the biliary and pancreatic secretions, important in facilitating the absorption of fats and the digestion of proteins, respectively, are discharged into this region of intestine. The next region of the small intestine is the jejunum, which is about 2.5 meters long. The jejunum is characterized by the rapid, vigorous, peristaltic waves that sweep along its length, and most of the absorption of the diet occurs in this region. The last region of the small intestine is the ileum, which is approximately 3.6 meters in length. Apart from some specialist absorptive functions, the main purpose of the ileum appears to be to provide reserve absorptive capacity.

The ileum terminates at the ileoceacal valve, where the small intestine ends and the large intestine begins. The large intestine is about 1.6 meters long, and consists of the cecum, appendix, colon, rectum, and anal canal. The cecum is a blind-ended pouch approximately 8 cm in diameter at the proximal end of the large intestine. The main part of the large intestine is the colon, which is not coiled, but consists of three relatively straight regions — the ascending colon, the transverse colon, and the descending colon — and the pelvic or sigmoid colon. The pelvic colon leads to the rectum, which in turn becomes the anal canal. The large intestine receives the liquid by-products of digestion and, by absorption of most of the water and electrolytes, forms the more solid consistency of feces. Apart from just before defecation, peristalsis in the large intestine is slower and less propulsive than that of the small intestine.

The highly sophisticated and complex gastrointestinal tract fulfills a variety of functions that are important for normal living. It is internally and externally innervated, is highly vascularized with a complex network of fine capillaries around the gastric glands and in the villi of the small intestine, and secretes a great variety of hormones and biologically active peptides. While the main role of the small intestine is to digest and absorb food, it also helps regulate the desire for, and the amount of, nutrients and water that are ingested, and it assists in the preservation of water and electrolyte balance. It plays an important role in maintaining the immunological integrity of the body, acts as a major reservoir of blood, and many of the hormones and biologically active peptides secreted by intestinal cells appear to influence organs far removed from their site of release. Although the functions of the gastrointestinal tract are many and varied, this chapter will concentrate on the role of the intestine in the regulation of intake and absorption of drinks and the solutes they contain.

Ingested water and nutrients are not immediately available for use by the body. They must be absorbed into the circulation from whence they can be assimilated into the appropriate body pools. Sports drinks supply both water and energy and are formulated to be rapidly absorbed and utilized in the body.

4.1.1   THE ROLE OF THE GASTROINTESTINAL TRACT IN THE REGULATION OF INTAKE AND ABSORPTION OF FLUIDS AND SOLUTES

4.1.1.1   Thirst

The sensation of thirst is a fundamental mechanism that ensures that the individual will actively seek out fluids and drink adequately before a serious body water deficit occurs. An increase in the osmotic pressure or a decrease in the volume of the body fluids each separately causes an increase in the perception of thirst (Ramsay, 1989). This increase in the thirst response, caused by a decrease in the body water content, is intimately associated with the regulation of the secretion of the fluid-balance hormones that affect water and electrolyte reabsorption in the kidneys and play a role in the control of blood pressure (Ramsay, 1989; Leiper, 1998). This system therefore ensures that while water losses are being restricted, there is an increased desire to drink to restore the water deficit. However, thirst need not be caused by a physiological need for water intake; drinking is more likely to be due to habit or to a craving for some stimulant or pleasurable sensation. Most drinks are normally consumed along with food, and about 70% of daily fluid intake is usually associated with mealtimes. Daily fluid intake in man is normally more than obligatory water losses with the excretion of dilute urine maintaining the total body water content.

Modulation of the thirst response (Figure 4.2) can be caused by sensations in the intestinal tract that need not be related to the content of the body water pools. For example, a dry mouth or throat can stimulate thirst, while a full stomach can inhibit drinking before sufficient fluid has been absorbed. Even when initiated by hypohydration in man, the sensation of thirst diminishes and cessation of drinking usually occurs before recovery of the circulating levels of osmolality, fluid-balance hormones, or blood volume (Verbalis, 1990). There are thought to be various receptors in the mouth and esophagus that respond to different tactile, temperature, chemical, and pressure stimuli that are involved in controlling the sensation of thirst. The act of swallowing and receptors in the oropharyngeal cavity, esophagus, and stomach appear to assist in monitoring the volume of fluid ingested. Gastric distention tends to inhibit the drinking response due to increased activity of the stretch receptors in the stomach, although the sensation of thirst may be unaffected (Verbalis, 1990). After fluid has emptied from the stomach, it is difficult to determine whether the concomitant reduction in the thirst response is caused by the presence of the fluid in the lumen of the small intestine or by the effect that absorbed water has on restoring the body water pools. The integration of the pre- and post-absorptive stimuli modulates the sensation of thirst and the volume of drink consumed.

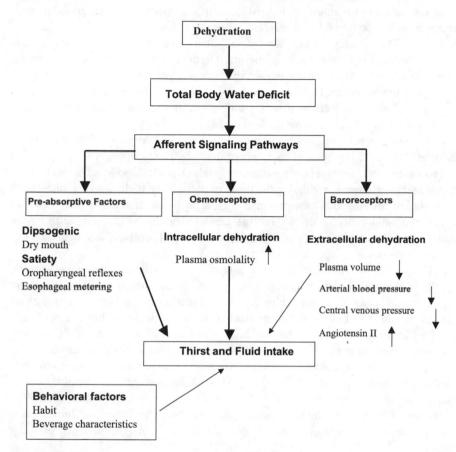

FIGURE 4.2   Control diagram illustrating multiple afferent signaling pathways involved in thirst generation and the stimulation of drinking behavior in humans. (Mack, G.W., Recovery after exercise in the heat factors influencing fluid intake, *Int. J. Sports Med.*, 1998; redrawn with permission.)

4.1.1.2   Influence of Beverage Composition

Fluids can be used as a vehicle to supply a wide variety of different solutes. Beverages can range from distilled water containing only trace amounts of solutes to liquid meals that contain all the macronutrients, micronutrients, vitamins, and minerals required for normal nutrition. While there are various benefits in supplying nutrients in liquids rather than in solid meals, the main advantage lies in the faster absorption of fluids (Leiper, 1997). In normal daily life in industrialized countries, the regulation of energy intake supersedes fluid intake. The factors that modulate daily nutrient intake are more numerous and complex than those controlling water intake and are beyond the scope of this chapter.

Sports drinks were originally developed as solutions with relatively simple formulations of carbohydrates and electrolytes in amounts known to stimulate rapid fluid absorption in the intestine; however, recent variations contain ingredients such as amino acids, proteins, lipids, glycerol, alcohol, caffeine, organic acids, vitamins, and herbs. The efficacy, or lack thereof, of some of these additional ingredients is covered in detail in Chapter 9. It is important to note that the addition of any solute to a sports drink may have an impact on both the palatability and physiological efficacy of the beverage. For example, the presence of sugars in too high a concentration may initiate a feeling of satiety and result in negative organoleptic characteristics such as a thicker, unpalatable mouthfeel.

The development of satiety, and therefore the cessation of drinking that is associated with the ingestion of energy-containing nutrients, appears to be controlled by orosensory and pre- and post-absorptive signals (Blundell and MacDiarmid, 1997) that are similar to those regulating the thirst response. The inclusion of solutes, such as alcohol or caffeine, that have pharmacological properties that make them addictive affects the palatability of drinks, but the greater stimulus would appear to be the desire to satisfy a pharmacologically induced craving. Therefore, the main effect of some solutes occurs after intestinal absorption.

Although man appears to enjoy the taste of sodium chloride, the human appetite for salt is appreciably less than that shown by many animals. In addition, relatively high concentrations of sodium chloride are discerned as being bitter and may cause nausea. Because sodium is the main electrolyte in extracellular fluid, it is closely involved in the homeostatic control of body water and, hence, many of the sensory signals and mechanisms controlling water intake also influence sodium intake. While there may be some receptors that specifically respond to the sodium content of body fluids, it is change in the osmolality of extracellular and intracellular fluid per se that is the main signal that is used to regulate water balance (Ramsay, 1991). Potassium, which is the main osmotically active cation in the intracellular space, does not appear to play as pivotal a role as sodium in the maintenance of water balance.

4.1.1.3 FUNDAMENTALS OF FLUID AND SOLUTE ABSORPTION

Absorption of water and solutes occurs almost exclusively in the small intestine. Ingested fluids must cross the intestinal mucosal barrier before the water and constituent solutes can be integrated into the body pool (Sladen, 1972). In the stomach, there is little net absorption of water or solutes (Scholer and Code, 1954; Schütz and Kenedi, 1963); therefore the rate at which ingested fluid is delivered from the stomach to the absorptive surface of the small intestine will influence how quickly absorption will occur. Although some digestion of food occurs in the stomach, the main site of hydrolysis of carbohydrates, proteins, and fats is the small intestine. Prior to absorption, the complex components of the diet must be broken down into their simpler, smaller, constituent molecules. It is these smaller molecules that are absorbed across the intestinal mucosa and transported into the blood. Absorption of solute from the intestinal lumen occurs by diffusion along electro-chemical gradients and by specific transport mechanisms that are inserted in the brush border membrane of the epithelial cells of the intestinal villi. These transport mechanisms translocate the specific molecules from the intestinal lumen across the cell membrane and into the cytosol of the epithelial cell. A second carrier system, sited in the basolateral membrane of the cell, then transports the molecule into the interstitium and into the adjacent blood capillaries. Water uptake from the intestinal lumen is thought to be caused by the absorption of solutes, creating an osmotic gradient suitable for net water absorption.

In situations where rapid supply of exogenous nutrients or water is required, or where the presence of unabsorbed dietary material may cause gastrointestinal distress, it is essential that any ingested beverage is emptied quickly from the stomach and is rapidly and completely absorbed in the small intestine. The gastric emptying rate of liquids is faster than that of solids, and solutions with a low energy content empty more quickly than do those that are more energy dense. Therefore, nutrients and water supplied as drinks are more rapidly absorbed and assimilated than if solid foods are ingested. Properly formulated sports drinks are dilute carbohydrate solutions containing relatively simple carbohydrates and a small amount of sodium chloride. Their energy content ensures the minimum of delay in emptying from the stomach while being capable of providing both sufficient water to delay dehydration and enough carbohydrate to maintain blood sugar levels during prolonged exercise (Coyle and Montain, 1992). The carbohydrate composition of sports drinks is typically a mixture of glucose, sucrose, maltose, and maltodextrins. In the small intestine, glucose is directly absorbed by a specific transport carrier, while a range of enterocyte-bound hydrolytic enzymes rapidly digest the disaccharides and polysaccharides to their monomeric forms, which are then effectively transported across the mucosa by carrier systems.

The carbohydrate content of sports drinks is formulated to produce a solution that is essentially isotonic with normal human serum, while ensuring that sufficient active solute absorption occurs to establish suitable osmotic gradients that cause net water absorption in the small intestine. Although the inclusion of sodium chloride in sports drinks may not be necessary to promote water absorption (see Section 4.3.4.4 for discussion regarding this point), it appears to improve palatability and may be beneficial in maintaining the thirst response.

4.1.1.4 CONSERVATION OF WATER, NUTRIENTS, AND ELECTROLYTES BY THE INTESTINAL TRACT

At a conservative estimate, the small intestine receives about 7 to 10 liters of fluid daily. Water derived from food and drink, as well as salivary, gastric, pancreatic, biliary, and intestinal secretions, all contribute to this volume. The secretions are required in the digestion and absorption of food and to maintain normal intestinal function. If not reabsorbed, the secretions would constitute a massive loss of water and electrolytes. Most of the water that enters the small intestine is absorbed in the jejunum and ileum, and only about 600 ml of the total daily water load reaches the colon. Of this volume, only between 100 to 200 ml of water is normally lost from the body in the feces. Although the colon is thought to have a daily absorptive capacity of about 2 to 3 liters, the volume of water loss in the feces is influenced by the amount of non-digestible components of the diet and by other osmotically active solutes that constitute the fecal mass.

The digestion of foodstuffs mainly takes place in the proximal region of the small intestine. Although digestive enzymes are present in the lumen of the small intestine, the digestive enzymes bound to the brush border membrane of the enterocytes carry out most of the digestive process (Silk and Dawson, 1979). Before being absorbed, dietary carbohydrates must be hydrolyzed to monosaccharides, and proteins hydrolyzed to amino acids, dipeptides, and tripeptides. Absorption of the majority of nutrients is normally complete during the passage of the chyme through the jejunum. The products of digested nutrients are absorbed by specific transport carriers that are thought to lie in proximity to the sites of the membrane-bound digestive enzymes (Silk and Dawson, 1979). The enterocytes of the ileum also have the membrane-bound digestive enzymes and transport carriers of the jejunal cells, but this region of the intestine seems to act as a reserve in the event that not all the digestion and absorption has taken place in the jejunum. In this way, very little digestible carbohydrate or protein reaches the colon (Fordtran and Locklear, 1966; Phillips and Summerskill, 1967). In the ileum and colon, the luminal concentrations of glucose and amino acids are normally lower than those in the systemic circulation, but because of the relative impermeability of the distal intestinal mucosa, there is little movement of nutrients down their concentration gradients into the intestinal lumen.

The pre- and postprandial luminal contents of the healthy proximal small intestine rapidly reach isotonicity with respect to plasma, and isotonicity is maintained during passage along the entire small intestine, although the ionic constituents of the luminal contents do change (Fordtran and Locklear, 1966; Phillips and Summerskill, 1967). After a nutrient-dense food or beverage passes through the pylorus into the proximal small intestine, isotonicity is established by net movement of water and electrolytes along osmotic and electrochemical gradients (Turnberg, 1973). This process is facilitated by the relative permeability of the proximal small intestine to water and electrolytes. In the duodenum, the main ions are sodium and chloride, found in concentrations similar to that in serum (Table 4.1). During passage through the jejunum and ileum, sodium and chloride are reabsorbed along with water. Water and electrolyte reabsorption continues in the colon, resulting in almost complete conservation of the body's sodium and chloride pool. During this process, hydrogen and potassium ions are exchanged for sodium, and metabolically derived bicarbonate is exchanged for chloride (Turnberg, 1973).

TABLE 4.1
Approximate Daily Volume of Water and Electrolyte Concentration in the Regions of the Intestine

	Water (ml)	Sodium (mmol/l)	Potassium (mmol/l)	Chloride (mmol/l)	Bicarbonate (mmol/l)
Jejunum	8500	145	5	100	0–25
Ileum	600	125	9	60	74
Colon	100	40	90	15	30

4.2 GASTRIC EMPTYING OF FLUIDS

The stomach is the widest and most dilatable part of the alimentary canal; it receives ingested material from the esophagus and empties it in a highly controlled manner via the pylorus into the duodenum (Figure 4.3). Although varying in shape and position in response to changes in posture, the stomach generally forms a J-shaped sack, with the wide upper end near the diaphragm and the narrow lower end under the liver. The esophagus enters the upper end of the stomach on the lesser curvature by the cardiac orifice. Temporary relaxation of muscle tone in the area of the cardiac orifice allows ingested material to enter the stomach, but normally the orifice is closed to prevent air filling the stomach or acidic gastric reflux from damaging the esophageal mucosa. Above the level of the cardiac orifice lies the dome-shaped fundus, and below lies the body of the stomach. An angular notch about two-thirds down the lesser curvature marks the approximate division between the body and the pyloric region of the stomach. The pyloric region is further divided into the antrum and the pyloric canal. Three layers of smooth muscle cover the stomach: an outer longitudinal layer, a middle circular layer, and an inner oblique layer. The circular layer covers most of the stomach, while the oblique layer is present in only two bands lying on the anterior and posterior surfaces. Both the circular and longitudinal layers increase in thickness toward the pyloric region of the stomach.

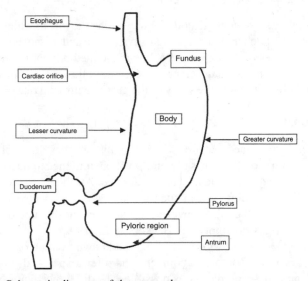

FIGURE 4.3 Schematic diagram of the stomach.

The stomach can alter in capacity from about 50 ml when empty to more than 1000 ml when fully distended with only minimal changes in gastric pressure. This occurs because the smooth muscle of the fundus and the proximal region of the body of the stomach relax to accommodate the ingested volume. The distal portion of the body of the stomach and pyloric region is less distensible, and this region is where the most active gastric peristaltic waves occur. The distal region of the stomach is where the ingestate is mixed, solid food particles are mechanically reduced in size, and the propulsive force is generated to empty the gastric contents into the duodenum.

Ingested food and fluids are not immediately available for assimilation into the body. The stomach stores the ingestate, initiates the degradation of complex food-stuffs, and controls the rate at which the ingestate is delivered into the small intestine. The rate at which food and beverage exits the stomach is regulated by central and enteric autonomic neural activity, and by local and systemic hormones (Minami and McCallum, 1984). These neural and hormonal influences govern the coordinated contractile activity of the musculature within the walls of the stomach and proximal small intestine (Burkes et al., 1985; Low, 1990), creating differences in pressure between the gastric antrum and the duodenum. Absorption of ingested water and the great majority of solutes occurs only in the small intestine; therefore, the rate of absorption of a drink will be greatly affected by the rate at which it is emptied from the stomach. Any delay in gastric emptying is detrimental to the effectiveness of a drink in situations where the constituents of the drink need to be rapidly utilized by the body. As discussed in detail later in this chapter, the volume of drink ingested and the composition of the drink are important factors regulating the rate of gastric emptying.

4.2.1   MEASUREMENT OF GASTRIC EMPTYING

There are several experimental methods for measuring the rate at which fluid empties from the stomach. Each method has its advantages and disadvantages, and the specific circumstances of the experiment dictate the method that is used to measure gastric emptying (Maughan and Leiper, 1996). The following sections describe the application of these methods to the study of the gastric emptying rate of sports drinks.

4.2.1.1   Intubation

There are several techniques that are included in this category. In all of the methods, a tube is passed either orally or nasally and positioned in the stomach or duodenum so that gastric or duodenal contents can be sampled. All the intubation methods are invasive, and the population used in such studies is a self-selected group who can tolerate the presence of the tube; however, the presence of the tube does not appear to affect the rate of gastric emptying (Beckers et al., 1992).

In the *single time point aspiration method*, a known volume of test beverage is either ingested or infused into the stomach, and after a specified time, the gastric contents are aspirated as completely as possible. The difference between the volume placed in the stomach and the volume aspirated from the stomach is taken as the volume emptied during that period. The accuracy of this method depends on the ability to recover all the volume in the stomach, and the ability to account for the addition of saliva and gastric secretions. It is possible to measure the volume of saliva and gastric secretions by adding a small amount of a non-absorbable marker such as phenol red to the test beverage. Even then, when the complete aspiration of gastric contents is used as a measure of gastric emptying rate, the assumption is that fluid empties from the stomach in a linear fashion. In fact, most solutions empty in exponential fashion (i.e., rapid emptying for the first few minutes followed by slower emptying as gastric volume diminishes) unless they have a high solute content (Maughan and Leiper, 1996).

The *serial time point method* is an adaptation of the single time point method, where the same volume of the same solution is repeatedly ingested and is completely aspirated from the stomach after different sampling times. This method is used in an attempt to identify the emptying curve of a given solution. This technique is limited by the fact that the rate of gastric emptying is influenced to an unknown extent by the fluid emptied into the intestine from the previous sample (via feedback from receptors in the small intestine and hepatic-portal vein). If the testing is carried out on different days, the day-to-day variability of the individual's response makes it difficult to place confidence in the results. Interestingly, all of the classical gastric emptying studies carried out by Hunt and his colleagues used these two aspiration techniques (Hunt and Knox, 1968).

The *double sampling aspiration technique* improves the ability to produce quantitative, reproducible data and has proved to be the most versatile method used in studying the gastric emptying of liquids (Maughan and Leiper, 1996). Following placement of a nasogastric tube, the stomach is washed with distilled water and the gastric residue removed. A known volume of test solution, labeled with phenol red, is then infused or ingested. Thereafter, following mixing of the stomach contents, a small sample is aspirated from the stomach and analyzed for phenol red concentration. Withdrawing small samples of the gastric contents at regular intervals (e.g., every 10 min), along with subsequent infusions of small volumes of phenol red of known concentration, allows for measurement of total gastric volume, gastric secretions, and the volume of fluid emptied from the stomach (Beckers et al., 1988). The double-sampling method has been successfully used in exercising subjects (Rehrer et al., 1989; Ryan et al., 1998), an approach that is critical in assessing the efficacy of sports drinks.

4.2.1.2 Scintigraphy

This is a non-invasive, indirect method of assessing gastric emptying that allows the use of relatively small volumes of test solution (200–250 ml). However, scintigraphy is limited by the requirement to minimize subject exposure to gamma radiation, but this technique has the advantage of being able to assess the emptying rates of solids and liquids simultaneously. In this technique, the test solution is labeled with a non-absorbable, gamma-emitting radionuclide, and it is the emptying of this label from the stomach into the small intestine that is monitored using a gamma camera. The method allows the emptying pattern to be followed almost continuously. By using either a dual head scanner or alternate anterior and posterior abdominal scans, corrections can be made for the effects of tissue attenuation and scatter, improving the precision of the method (Tothill, et al., 1978). The pattern of gastric emptying of test solutions is similar whether assessed by the double sampling aspiration method or by scintigraphy, although the actual rates tend to be slower when assessed by scintigraphy (Beckers,et al., 1992).

4.2.1.3 Epigastric Impedance

As with scintigraphy, this is a non-invasive, indirect method of estimating gastric emptying. A small electrical current is passed between skin surface electrodes sited in the epigastric region of the subject's torso. Changes in the impedance to this current depend on the conductivity of the ingested drink and the rate at which it empties from the stomach. Results using this method appear to correlate reasonably well with those obtained using scintigraphy and aspiration techniques (Maughan and Leiper, 1996). There are no known hazards involved with this technique, but the method is sensitive to body movements, reducing its application with physically active subjects.

4.2.1.4 Ultrasonography

This non-invasive, indirect method of determining gastric emptying uses real-time ultrasound to visualize the stomach or specific regions of the stomach. Changes in the calculated volume of the stomach are used to assess gastric emptying. Gastric emptying rate determined by ultrasound has been equated with those obtained by scintigraphy (Holt et al., 1986). A skilled operator is required to make the ultrasound scans, and the presence of gas in the stomach may make it difficult to obtain adequate images of the stomach. Measurements are usually made with the subject supine. There are no known hazards with this technique, but its use is limited to resting subjects.

4.2.1.5 Tracer Technique

The tracer technique is an indirect method of estimating gastric emptying that relies upon measures of the time taken for a specific marker substance to appear in the blood or breath (Maughan and Leiper, 1996). The marker is ingested with the test solution and it is assumed that the marker empties from the stomach at the same rate as that of the test solution, that it is not absorbed to any significant extent in the stomach, and that it is rapidly absorbed in the proximal small intestine. With tracer substances such as paracetamol or deuterium oxide, both of which can be detected in the blood, it is assumed that rate of disappearance of the tracer from the circulation is constant, and that there is little or no recirculation of the tracer from other pools within the body. Tracers such as carbon-labeled bicarbonate, acetate, or octanoic acid, which are detected in the breath using mass spectrometry, must first be metabolized, enter the body's bicarbonate pool, and then be excreted as carbon dioxide in the breath. With such tracers, the additional delay between being absorbed from the small intestine and appearing in the breath must be taken into account. The tracer method is relatively non-invasive (requiring only venipuncture) and lends itself to large-scale studies. However, the tracer method has not been compared with the more established methods of assessing gastric emptying.

4.2.1.6 Magnetic Resonance Imaging

Magnetic resonance imaging (MRI) is a non-invasive, non-radioactive method of producing a three-dimensional image of the total stomach and the ingested meal volume. The number of transaxial slices of the abdomen and the acquisition times greatly influence the sensitivity of the measurement. The time taken for a full scan of the abdomen precludes this method for measuring rapidly emptying solutions. The results of gastric emptying rates determined using MRI and both gastric aspiration and scintigraphy have been shown to be comparable (Maughan and Leiper, 1996). The costs of MRI, the relatively long acquisition times and the positioning of the magnetic coil will probably restrict the use of this technique to clinical use.

4.2.1.7   Radiography

This method of qualitatively estimating gastric emptying uses X-ray imaging and thereby increases the risk of subjects receiving high levels of radiation. A radio-opaque, heavy-metal contrast agent such as barium sulfate is ingested along with the test meal. Serial images of the abdominal area are made and the emptying of the radio-opaque compound from the stomach is recorded. The amount of contrast agent in the stomach cannot be accurately determined from the radiograph and the results are only qualitative (Minami and McCallum, 1984). In addition, it is by no means certain that the emptying rate of the contrast agent is the same as that of the test solution.

4.2.2   FACTORS AFFECTING GASTRIC EMPTYING

It is considered that the rate of gastric emptying is the main limiting factor in the assimilation of ingested fluids. This is a prudent design feature of the human gastrointestinal tract because if the rate of fluid delivery from the stomach were to exceed the absorptive capacity of the intestine, diarrhea would occur. Although gastrointestinal disturbances are not uncommon during exercise, diarrhea does not normally occur in most individuals during exercise.

Because of the complexity of the mechanisms that control the gastric emptying process, it is not surprising that there is considerable inter-individual variation in emptying rates (Beckers et al., 1991; Maughan and Leiper, 1996). However, most individuals do appear to be relatively consistent in the rate at which they empty the same solution on different occasions (Beckers et al., 1991). Many factors have been shown to influence the rate of gastric emptying of solutions.

Apart from the receptors responding to the volume of the stomach, the majority of receptors regulating gastric emptying are found in the duodenum (Hunt and Knox, 1968; Minami and McCallum, 1984) and ileum (Miller et al., 1981). These receptors appear to function primarily by initiating neural and hormonal responses that modify gastric and duodenal muscular tone and the frequency of contraction. The position of the receptors in the small intestine suggests that their main function is to inhibit gastric emptying and thus prevent the absorptive capacity of the intestine from being overwhelmed. Most of the information is derived from studies on resting individuals and many of these studies have used either single time point or serial time point aspiration techniques. Where possible, emphasis will be given to studies that used methods that more accurately follow the time course of emptying.

4.2.2.1   Gastric Volume

The exponential nature of the gastric emptying curve indicates the importance of the volume of the stomach in controlling the rate of emptying (Figure 4.4). Because the stomach acts as a reservoir, it must be able to distend to accommodate the ingestate while maintaining a relatively low intragastric pressure. This is accomplished by relaxation of the muscle tone in the fundus and upper body of the stomach. It is the slow, sustained contractions that sweep from the proximal to the distal regions of the stomach that mainly influence the pressure in the antral area of the stomach, and these remain unaffected by the muscle tone of the upper portion of the stomach (Wilbur and Kelly, 1973). Increasing the pressure in the antral region increases the rate of gastric emptying of fluids (Struntz and Grossman, 1978). Increasing the volume of the gastric contents stimulates the activity of the stretch receptors in the gastric mucosa, which in turn increases the intragastric pressure and promotes faster emptying (Hunt and Spurrell, 1951; Minami and McCallum, 1984; Noakes et al., 1991). It is the total volume in the stomach that is important; this includes the volume of drink ingested, plus the volume of gastric secretions and swallowed saliva.

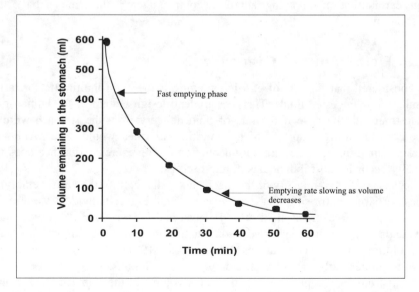

FIGURE 4.4   Typical gastric emptying pattern following ingestion of a single 600 ml bolus of a dilute energy-containing drink.

Using the single-time-point technique, Costill and Saltin (1974) measured the gastric volume 15 min after ingesting 200, 400, 600, 800, and 1000 ml of a 139 mmol/l glucose solution. A greater volume was emptied after ingestion of 600 ml compared with 400 ml, which was greater compared with 200ml; there was no difference in the volume emptied between 600 and 800 ml, but there was a tendency for less volume to be emptied after ingesting 1000 ml. This suggests that there may be an upper limit of gastric volume above which emptying rates may plateau or even slow (Noakes et al., 1991). It is also evident that the volume required to promote the maximum gastric emptying rate for a given test solution will be highly variable among individuals.

Research has demonstrated that repeated ingestion of test solutions will maintain a high gastric volume and result in faster rates of gastric emptying than would have been expected from the carbohydrate content of the drinks (Noakes et al., 1991). Following ingestion of a single bolus of a liquid, there is an initial fast phase of gastric emptying when the volume in the stomach is at its greatest and then the emptying rate becomes progressively slower as the volume in the stomach decreases. The rate of emptying is exponential, with a constant fraction of the volume in the stomach emptied per unit time (Hunt and Spurrell, 1951; Rehrer et al., 1989). By refilling the stomach at intervals, the volume in the stomach can be kept high and rates of gastric emptying equivalent to that of the initial phase of emptying can be maintained (Figure 4.5) (Rehrer et al., 1989; Mitchell and Voss, 1991). However, care must be taken that the stomach is not overfilled, as this may result in gastrointestinal distress and a reduction in the rate of gastric emptying.

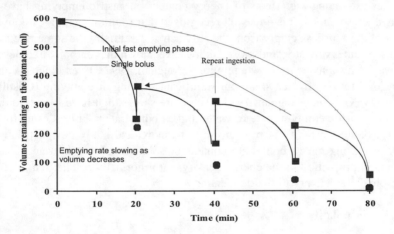

FIGURE 4.5 The effect on gastric emptying of maintaining a high gastric volume by repeated ingestion. Reher, et al., Gastric emptying with repeated drinking during running and bicycling, *Int. J. Sports Med.*, 29, 1725, 1988. Redrawn with permission.

4.2.2.2 Energy Density

Plain water empties rapidly from the stomach, while increasing the energy content of ingested solutions slows the rate of gastric emptying. Somewhat surprisingly, the rate of gastric emptying is regulated such that isoenergetic amounts of carbohydrates, proteins, fats, or alcohol (Hunt and Stubbs, 1975; Calbet and MacLean, 1997; Leiper et al., 1999) are delivered into the duodenum. The mechanisms whereby the regulatory system can detect as yet unmetabolized energy from a variety of sources is at present unknown, but it is not the osmolality of the duodenal chyme or of hydrolyzed meal nutrients that is the main factor (Brouns et al., 1995; Vist and

Maughan, 1995). It is widely accepted that the receptors responding to energy density lie outside the stomach; however, it is not known whether they are positioned on the luminal or serosal side of the small intestine, or whether they respond to the same stimulus for each nutrient (Thomas and Baldwin, 1968). While hyperglycemia can slow gastric emptying and hypoglycemia can accelerate the emptying of nutrients solutions, no hormone or gastrointestinal peptide has as yet been identified as the equivocal regulator of gastric emptying of energy sources (Schvarcz et al., 1997).

It has been proposed that the control of gastric emptying of nutrient-containing solutions ensures a constant rate of energy delivery of up to 9kJ/min (2.15 kcal/min) to the duodenum (Brener, et al., 1983; Hunt et al., 1985). This is clearly not the case for most beverages. The gastric emptying curve, other than when the energy density is extremely high, tends to be exponential. This implies that while feedback control from the duodenal receptors may operate to regulate a fixed rate of energy delivery to the small intestine, the effect of the decrease in gastric volume slows the rate of emptying to a greater extent than that mediated by the supply of nutrients.

The main nutrient source in most sports drinks is carbohydrate and the majority of studies examining the effects of energy content on gastric emptying have used carbohydrate solutions. It is now well recognized that solutions with a carbohydrate content of 2.5% or less empty from the stomach at essentially the same rate as that of equal volumes of water, and most studies have shown that carbohydrate levels at or above 6% unequivocally slow emptying (Maughan, 1997). Even glucose concentrations of 4 to 5% produce small but significant slowing of emptying (Costill and Saltin,1974; Vist and Maughan, 1994). There are studies that have found no difference in the gastric emptying rate of water and carbohydrate solutions of up to 10%, but most of this disparity is probably due to individual study design (Maughan, 1997). Increasing the carbohydrate content of solutions slows the rate of gastric emptying in proportion to the energy density, but it normally results in a faster rate of carbohydrate delivery to the duodenum.

4.2.2.3 Osmolality

J.B. Hunt recognized that energy density was crucial in the regulation of gastric emptying and that isoenergetic amounts of all the macronutrients were emptied at the same rate. He considered that it was the osmolality of the solution that was detected by the gut and proposed that osmoreceptors in the small intestine were instrumental in regulating emptying (Hunt and Knox, 1968). While it is clear that osmolality is a major controlling factor for solutions with no nutrient content, this is unlikely to be the case for fluids containing energy.

It can be argued that complex carbohydrate, proteins, and fats will have the same slowing effect on gastric emptying as isoenergetic solutions of their respective hydrolysis products if complete hydrolysis occurs before reaching the osmoreceptors. However, it is unlikely that isoenergetic amounts of the hydrolysis products of carbohydrates, proteins, and fats would each elicit the same osmotic response and, additionally, that this osmotic response would be the same as that of isoenergetic amounts of ethanol. This is because of the difference in energy content and molecular weight among carbohydrates, amino acids, fats, and alcohol. For example, a solution containing 1gram/l of glucose has an osmolality of 5.6 mosmol/kg and an energy content of 17.5 kJ/l (4.2 kcal/l), whereas a solution containing 1gram/l of ethanol has an osmolality of 21.7 mosmol/kg and energy content of 29.7 kJ/l (7.1 kcal/l).

Substitution of maltodextrins (glucose polymers) for glucose monomer reduces the osmolality of the solution while maintaining the total carbohydrate content. Several studies have examined the effect on gastric emptying of replacing glucose monomer with maltodextrin, but the findings are not consistent. Most investigations have found little or no difference in the rates of gastric emptying of isoenergetic solutions of glucose monomers compared with maltodextrins, despite the often large differences in osmolality (Maughan 1997; Brouns et al., 1995). This lack of difference implies that hydrolysis of the maltodextrins occurs before reaching the small intestinal osmoreceptors; therefore, the osmolality of the isoenergetic solutions are in fact equal at the point where they come in contact with the regulating osmoreceptors (Hunt and Knox, 1968). In one study, a 15% maltodextrin solution emptied faster than a 15% glucose monomer solution, but there was no difference in the emptying rates of 5% and 10% solutions of glucose monomer and maltodextrin, respectively. Furthermore, the differences in gastric emptying could not be explained solely by the differences in the initial osmolality of the solutions (Sole and Noakes, 1989). The addition of sodium chloride and potassium chloride with a combined osmolality of up to 336 mosmol/kg to a 15% maltodextrin solution with an initial osmolality of 114 mosmol/kg did not significantly affect gastric emptying compared with the maltodextrin solution without electrolytes (Rehrer et al., 1993). Consensus opinion at present is that the energy density of the solution exerts a greater effect than osmolality in the regulation of gastric emptying, and that substitution of maltodextrins for glucose monomer, especially at high energy densities, may slightly increase the rate of gastric emptying (Vist and Maughan, 1995).

4.2.2.4   Beverage Temperature

Nerve conduction and muscle motility are both sensitive to changes in temperature, which suggests that gastric emptying may be affected by the temperature of the ingested drink. Costill and Saltin (1974) found that gastric emptying, measured 15 min after ingestion of carbohydrate drinks, was slightly faster for cold solutions (5°C) than for warm (35°C). Others have reported that cold (4°C) or hot (50°C) drinks empty more slowly during the first 10 min after ingestion than does the same drink ingested at body temperature (Sun et al., 1988). Lambert and Maughan (1992) reported that there was a slightly greater blood concentration of the tracer used to estimate gastric emptying five min after ingesting the hot (50°C) solution than after drinking the same solution cold (4°C); thereafter, there was no difference in the circulating concentration of the tracer between the two treatments. This suggests that the intragastric temperature rapidly returns to normal body temperature (Sun et al., 1988) and that the temperature of the ingested solution has little effect on the overall rate of gastric emptying. The rate of recovery of intragastric temperature will depend on the temperature of the drink, the volume consumed, and the thermal capacity of the solution. In situations where the gastric volume is maintained at a high level by repeated ingestion, the temperature within the stomach may not be able to recover sufficiently and emptying may be inhibited, although this supposition has not yet been tested. An additional important factor, as described in Chapter 3, is that the palatability of drinks is influenced by the temperature at which they are served, and this will influence the volume that is voluntarily consumed.

4.2.2.5 Beverage pH

The pH within the stomach is normally acidic, and as the chyme moves into and along the proximal small intestine, the acid is neutralized by the duodenal and pancreatic secretions. In a series of experiments, Hunt and his colleagues demonstrated that it was not the pH of the fluid that determined the rate of gastric emptying, but the concentration and type of acids present (Hunt and Knox, 1968). Weak acids were not necessarily less effective than strong acids, but low-molecular-weight acids were associated with greater inhibition of gastric emptying than high-molecular-weight acids (Hunt and Knox, 1968). The types and concentrations of the mainly organic acids (e.g., citric acid) found in most sports drinks are unlikely to affect the gastric emptying rate of these beverages.

4.2.2.6 Exercise

Several mechanisms have been proposed whereby exercise intensity may affect the rate of gastric emptying, but there is little evidence to suggest which of these factors plays the major role (Murray, 1987). When discussing the possible effects of exercise on gastric emptying, the mode, intensity, and duration of the exercise are of fundamental importance. A number of studies have confirmed the findings of Costill and Saltin (1974) that cycle exercise at an intensity below about 70% of an individual's $VO_{2\,max}$ has little effect on gastric emptying; increasing the intensity above this level produces progressive, significant slowing of the emptying rates of ingested fluids (Maughan 1991). The majority of studies that have examined the effect of prolonged moderate exercise of up to 3 hours on gastric emptying have shown that high gastric emptying rates can be sustained during this type of exercise (Maughan, 1991), even in the heat (Ryan et al., 1989). One study has reported that a previously induced hypohydration of about 2.7% of body mass did not significantly affect gastric emptying or intestinal absorption of ingested fluids during cycle exercise at 65 % of $VO_{2\,max}$ (Ryan et al., 1998). Other studies, however, have indicated that both hypohydration and hyperthermia can slow gastric emptying (Neufer, et al., 1989; Rehrer et al., 1994

Upright exercise, such as walking or running, at intensities between 28% to 70% $VO_{2\,max}$ has been shown to stimulate gastric emptying compared with rest, but emptying was slower than at rest when running at 75% $VO_{2\,max}$ (Neufer, et al., 1989). Others, however, have found either no difference or a slowing in gastric emptying rates with treadmill running at relatively moderate exercise levels compared with rest (Maughan, 1991). The differences in findings among these studies may be due to variations in the composition of the drinks used or of the differences in study protocols. There are few studies that have directly compared gastric emptying during running and cycling exercise. The results from those that have done so suggest that there is no significant effect on gastric emptying of the mode of exercise (Rehrer et al., 1990).

At high levels of exercise intensity known to inhibit gastric emptying, the exercise duration is usually too short for any benefit to be derived from fluid ingested during the exercise (Maughan, 1991; Shi and Gisolfi, 1998). During many sports and other forms of physical activity, however, the period spent exercising is prolonged, while the exercise is intermittent and the intensity is varied. Many of the factors that have been shown to induce fatigue during prolonged constant-intensity exercise have the same effect on intermittent exercise of sufficient duration (Shi and Gisolfi, 1998). It has been assumed that in most forms of intermittent exercise, the time spent at relatively low levels of activity is sufficient to allow appropriate amounts of any ingested drink to be emptied from the stomach and absorbed, and that the time spent sprinting will have little effect. However, in many instances involving intermittent exercise, the overall intensity of physical activity might be expected to delay gastric emptying. For example, the average intensity of effort in top-level soccer has been reported to be above 70% $VO_{2\,max}$ (Bangsbo, 1994).

In a recent unpublished study in our laboratory, gastric emptying rates of a sports drink were measured while subjects sat at rest, exercised on a cycle ergometer at a constant power output equivalent to 66% of their $VO_{2\,max}$, or undertook intermittent high-intensity cycle exercise with an overall average intensity of either 66% or 75% of their $VO_{2\,max}$. The lower-intensity, intermittent exercise consisted of cycling at a power output of 60% $VO_{2\,max}$, interspersed every 10 min with three 30-second sprints at 100% $VO_{2\,max}$. The higher-intensity intermittent exercise consisted of cycling at a power output of 70% of $VO_{2\,max}$ interspersed every 10 minutes with three 30-second sprints at 100% $VO_{2\,max}$. Over the initial 10-minute period following ingestion, no difference in the volume remaining in the stomach could be detected among trials (Table 4.2). Thereafter, the rate of gastric emptying was similar on the rest and constant-power-output trials, which were both faster than on the low-intensity, intermittent exercise trial, which was faster than on the high-intensity, intermittent exercise trial. This study suggests that intermittent sprint exercise at intensities that might occur during many competitive sports can slow the rate of gastric emptying relative to rest and continuous moderate physical activity. Therefore, individuals may have to develop new drinking strategies when undertaking physical activity that includes bouts of high-intensity sprinting. The use of very dilute drinks that are known to empty rapidly, or practicing drinking while carrying out sprint training are possible solutions to this potential problem.

4.2.3 ADAPTATIONS TO CHANGES IN FLUID INTAKE AND NUTRIENT CONTENT

Anecdotal evidence suggests that, by practicing drinking larger volumes both at rest and during exercise, individuals can increase their gastric capacity and can improve their tolerance to exercising with a relatively full stomach. It is known that the gastrointestinal tract is a highly adaptable organ. Several studies in animals have indicated that the composition of the previous meal may influence the gastric emptying. In one study in humans, supplementing the normal diet with 440 g/d of glucose for between

TABLE 4.2
The Median Test Drink Volume in the Stomach at Each 10-Min Sampling Point

	Test Drink Volume Remaining in the Stomach (ml)			
Time (min)	R	C66	I66	I75
0	600	600	600	600
10	457	474	556	538
20	303	283	393	497
30	213	211	269	351
40	144	119	198	297
50	95	50	149	272
60	27	14	98	153

Note: R: rest trial; C66: the continuous steady state exercise trial at 66% $VO_{2\,max}$; I66: the intermittent exercise trial at 60% of $VO_{2\,max}$ with sprints at 100% of $VO_{2\,max}$; I75: the intermittent exercise trial at 70% of $VO_{2\,max}$ with sprints at 100% of $VO_{2\,max}$.

4 to 7 days promoted improved rates of gastric emptying of both glucose and fructose (Horowitz et al., 1996). It may be that some of the interindividual variation seen in gastric emptying may be caused by the previous diet of the individuals. It appears that the gastrointestinal tract can undergo a degree of training that might allow individuals to alter their usual gastric emptying pattern or overcome gastrointestinal distress during exercise. Any alteration in the volumes or type of beverage consumed is best practiced during training rather than in competition.

4.3   INTESTINAL ABSORPTION

The structure and functional architecture of the small intestine is ideally designed for absorption while presenting a barrier to potential noxious chemicals and organisms. The major barrier for transport across the intestinal mucosa is the phospholipid bilayer of the epithelial cells of the villi and the intercellular junctions between those cells (Sladen, 1972). Lipid-soluble solutes can readily permeate cell membranes, are translocated through the cell, and pass across the basal membrane on the serosal side into the lymphatics or portal vein (Dawson, 1972; Guandalini, 1988). Water and water-soluble solutes require different mechanisms to cross the intestinal mucosa. Embedded in the brush-border membrane of the enterocytes (in the columnar epithelial cells lining the intestinal villi) is a variety of transport carriers with different degrees of specificity. These transport carriers unidirectionally translocate carbohydrate monomers, amino acids, dipeptides, and tripeptides from the luminal surface into the cytoplasm of the cell (Crane, 1965; Silk and Dawson, 1979; Guandalini, 1988; Wright et al., 1986). This transport is often linked with sodium transport; in fact, sodium plays a pivotal role in the absorption of many organic and inorganic solutes (Murer and Burckhardt, 1983; Sladen, 1972) and, as an osmotically active transportable solute, it has a major influence on water absorption (Sladen, 1972). The current concept of net water movement is that water flux is passive and dependent on osmotic, hydrostatic, and filtration pressures. Water absorption from the intestine is considered to be a passive consequence of solute absorption, resulting from local osmotic gradients that promote net uptake of water from the lumen across the intestinal mucosa (Sladen, 1972; Hallbäck et al., 1980; Jodal and Lungren, 1986).

4.3.1 Measurement of Intestinal Absorption

Many methods have been described to study intestinal absorption in animals and man (Sladen, 1975). In man, both *in vivo* and *in vitro* techniques have been employed in intestinal studies.

4.3.1.1 Tissue Culture Techniques

In man, tissue material for study has been collected from biopsy of the intestinal mucosa or from resected segments of intestine. The tissue used, although morphologically normal, is often removed from patients with a localized disease of the intestine. However, the use of healthy animal tissue has confirmed the validity of these techniques. Absorption and transport have been studied using everted segments, rings, and sacs of intestine. Pieces and sheets of intestine, isolated enterocytes, and isolated brush-border vesicles have also been used. Measurement of absorption rates has involved detecting the movement of test solute and fluid from the mucosal to the serosal surfaces. The methods of detection have involved gravimetric, chemical and radio-isotopic methods, and measurement of transmucosal electrical fluxes. The use of short-circuit clamping has allowed the measurement of solute transport rates independent of the electrical gradients to be made.

In vitro tissue preparations are open to the criticism of having no blood, lymph, or nerve supply. Often there is no adequate removal of transported solute from the serosal surface and concentration gradients build up in the tissues; it is, therefore, only during the initial stages of transport that the kinetics can be accurately studied. However, *in vitro* methods have the advantage of there being only a limited number of uncontrollable variables, and basic cellular and subcellular mechanisms can be more thoroughly investigated.

4.3.1.2 Tracer Techniques

In conscious man, tracer methods involve measuring the disappearance of a test substance from the intestine or the appearance of the test substance in the blood, tissues, urine, or feces. These methods usually involve ingestion of a single bolus of the test solution containing the tracer followed by repeated sampling of blood, urine, or breath. Examples of tracers that have been used in this way are deuterium oxide as a marker for water, ^{13}C or ^{14}C labeled carbohydrates, and isotopically labeled electrolytes.

4.3.1.3 Whole Gut Balance Method

This method measures the difference between the amount of test substance ingested and the amount excreted, assuming that only minimal secretion of test substance occurs from the tissues. The test substance may be given as a single bolus or as repeated doses until steady state conditions are established. Such balance methods are dependent on complete collection of urine and feces, and the rate of colonic emptying is an important factor. Transit time through the gastrointestinal tract may be in excess of 5 days (Sladen, 1975). The effect of colonic bacteria in the degradation or synthesis of the test substance must also be considered.

4.3.1.4 Whole Body Retention Method

This technique usually involves the ingestion of a single bolus of a test substance containing a radioactive label. Using whole body counters, the activity of the label is measured at intervals. The unabsorbed material is excreted in the feces and the whole body count decreases. A steady plateau of activity is reached when all the unabsorbed test substance is excreted (Sladen, 1975). This method gives a direct estimate of the fractional retention of a substance in the body and does not require collection of blood. However, the method does not give a measure of absorption or recycling rates, and it is assumed that the labeled and non-labeled forms of the test substance are handled in the same way by the body.

4.3.1.5 Intestinal Segment Methods

These methods require the subject to be intubated, allowing fluid and solute absorption to be measured at various levels along the gastrointestinal tract. Absorption is measured as the difference between the amount of test substance introduced into the intestinal segment and the amount that is subsequently recovered further down the lumen. The use of non-absorbable markers allows studies to be made without quantitative recovery of all luminal contents. In the *single-bolus method*, after the correct placement of the collection tube in the intestine, the test solution with a non-absorbable marker is ingested. Small samples of the intestinal contents are subsequently aspirated via the tube at different sites along the intestine. The assumption is made that both test substance and marker mix uniformly in the intestine and that the sample fluid collected is representative of all the fluid passing the sample sites.

The *isolated segment method* utilizes two balloons set at a fixed distance apart along a tube positioned in the intestine. When the two balloons are inflated they effectively isolate a fixed length of intestine and the test solution containing a non-absorbable marker is then passed into the segment of intestine. Absorption rates can be calculated from changes in the marker concentration in the fluid that is recovered after a known time interval. Any leakage of fluid into or out of the segment invalidates the results. The distention of the intestine by the balloons may cause distress to the subject and may affect intestinal blood flow, motility, and hormone regulatory control of the intestine.

4.3.1.6　Intestinal Segment Perfusion Methods

The steady state perfusion technique is considered by many to be the only satisfactory method of studying regional absorption of water and rapidly transported solutes in the intact human (Sladen, 1975). Net absorption is the balance between the bi-directional transport of a substance from the intestinal lumen into the mucosa and from the mucosa into the intestinal lumen. Net absorption occurs only if the rate of influx is greater than the rate of efflux of the test substance.

The basic perfusion technique involves having the subject swallow the weighed end of a double lumen perfusion tube that is then positioned, under fluoroscopic control, in the part of the intestine under investigation. The test solution, warmed to 37°C and containing a non-absorbable marker, is perfused at a constant rate through the proximal orifice of the tube into the intestine. The test solution passes unimpeded through the intestine and is sampled via the distal orifice from another lumen of the tube. Once steady state conditions are established, absorption or secretion rates can be calculated from the perfusion rate and from the change in solute and marker concentration between the two orifices. The results are expressed per unit time per unit length of intestine perfused. To obviate the necessity for quantitative recovery of the luminal contents, the use of a non-absorbable marker and steady state conditions are essential. The period required to establish a steady state is variable and must be assessed in each experimental situation (Sladen, 1975). In steady state, the amounts of non-absorbable marker entering and leaving the intestinal segment are equal; therefore, differences in the concentration of the marker sampled between these two points are due to the net movement of water across the mucosa of the intestinal segment. True steady state conditions are rarely attained in the intestine and, in practice, collections of 10 to 15 min each are made over a prolonged period to minimize the effect of short term variations within the perfused intestinal segment. For practical purposes, steady state conditions can be said to exist when the concentration of the non-absorbable marker of consecutive collections deviates by 10% or less of the mean marker concentration of the samples (Sladen and Dawson, 1970). The accuracy of the perfusion method is affected by the uniformity of mixing of the test and marker substances with the intestinal contents, by changes in the flow and composition of the succus entericus above the perfusion orifice, and by variations in the reflux of the luminal contents (Sladen and Dawson, 1970; Modigliani and Bernier, 1971). Two modifications to the basic perfusion set have been used to reduce these problems.

The first modification was the introduction of a third tube to the perfusion set, and this tube carries a second aspiration port. Once this triple-lumen perfusion set is correctly positioned in the intestine, the test solution is perfused into the intestinal lumen via the proximal perfusion port and is sampled at two distal points, thereby allowing for mixing of both refluxing fluid and the proximal endogenous intestinal secretions with the perfusate. Sampling from the proximal aspiration port allows the composition and flow rate of fluid entering the test segment to be accurately determined. Absorption in the test segment is calculated from the difference between concentrations of solute collected from the proximal and distal aspiration ports

(Leiper and Maughan, 1988a). In this method, modifications to the original test solution occur to a variable extent so that rigid control of the composition and flow rate entering the test segment is impossible. However, these changes in the test solution are known, and absorption of water and solutes from the altered solution is easily calculated.

The second modification was the introduction of a balloon fixed proximal to the perfusion port. Once the perfusion set is correctly positioned, the balloon is inflated sufficiently to occlude the intestinal lumen above the test segment that is to be perfused. An aspiration port proximal to the balloon is used to collect the proximal intestinal secretions and is also used to inject a colored marker to test that the balloon is occlusive. Perfusion of the test solution and collection of the luminal contents that have passed through the perfused segment are made via the perfusion port. The use of the occlusion balloon excludes proximal intestinal secretions and proximal refluxing of the perfusate. There are criticisms of this technique. The adequacy of luminal occlusion must be continually checked and inflation of the balloon can cause intestinal distress to subjects. The presence of the inflated balloon may alter blood flow, hormonal regulation, and peristalsis.

However, no significant differences in the assessment of absorption have been demonstrated between the two techniques (Sladen and Dawson, 1970; Modigliani and Bernier, 1971). Compared with the occlusive-balloon technique, the triple-lumen perfusion method is considered simpler to manage and may cause less stress to the intestine, and for those reasons, this method has been extensively used. The steady state perfusion method has been used to study mechanisms of water absorption and solute exchange throughout the intestine both at rest (Sladen, 1975) and during exercise (Gisolfi et al., 1991). Although there are large interindividual variations in water and solute absorption, the reproducibility of the method appears good (Leiper and Maughan, 1991). The method is limited by the requirement to minimize the radiation dose given during fluoroscopic positioning of the perfusion set in the intestine and by the ability of individuals to successfully pass the perfusion set into their intestine and to tolerate its presence in their gastrointestinal tracts, particularly during exercise.

4.3.2 Regional Differences in Intestinal Function

The stomach contents that are delivered to the duodenum are rapidly brought into osmotic equilibrium with the circulating plasma. This appears to be brought about by movement of water and electrolytes into or out of the intestinal lumen along osmotic and electrochemical gradients (Sladen, 1972). The proximal small intestine, comprising the duodenum and upper jejunum, is relatively permeable to water and electrolytes, and movement in either direction across the mucosa is dependent on the prevailing gradient for the specific molecule. In comparison, the ileum is less permeable to water and electrolytes, and the colon is less permeable than the ileum. In the human jejunum, for example, net sodium absorption occurs only when the sodium chloride concentration of an isotonic solution is 127 mmol/l or greater, there being a net efflux of sodium into the jejunal lumen at lower concentrations. In the ileum, however, sodium is absorbed from luminal solutions of 115 mmol/l of sodium chloride (Phillips and Summerskill, 1967). The addition of relatively small amounts of actively transported sugars that need not be capable of being metabolized greatly enhances sodium uptake by the jejunal mucosa, but not by the ileal mucosa (Phillips and Summerskill, 1967). In the jejunum, absorption of chloride appears to be determined by water and sodium transport rather than by a specific transport mechanism. In the ileum, however, chloride is actively absorbed even against strong chemical gradients by a directly linked anion exchange mechanism, with chloride being exchanged for bicarbonate (Turnberg, 1973). This exchange mechanism does not operate in the jejunum, the predominant site of both chloride and bicarbonate absorption (Sladen, 1972).

4.3.3 ABSORPTIVE MECHANISMS

Two transcellular and one intercellular route have been proposed to explain the absorption of water and hydrophilic solutes across the intestinal mucosa of the proximal small intestine (Phillips and Summerskill, 1967; Sladen, 1972). Taking advantage of these routes of absorption is of critical importance in formulating sports drinks to optimize the rate of fluid and solute absorption.

One transcellular route is the *polar route via* water-filled pores that penetrate the enterocyte membrane. Studies using molecular probes of different dimensions have given estimates of an effective pore size of between 6.7 to 8.8 daltons in the jejunum and 3 to 3.8 daltons in the ileum (Fordtran et al., 1965). Because the surface of these pores carries an electrical charge, both the three-dimensional size and the charge of the molecule will influence the effective permeability. These pores are thought to be important routes that allow water and electrolytes to cross the mucosal barrier by osmotic and hydrostatic gradients and by diffusion along electrochemical gradients. The comparatively large physical size of monosaccharides and amino acids prevents their access via the polar route.

The second transcellular route involves the *carrier mediated transporter systems* that are embedded in the brush-border membrane of the enterocytes. These carriers are thought to bind to solutes on the luminal surface, translocate them across the brush border membrane, and release the solute within the cell cytosol. The carrier molecule, freed from its substrate, then relocates itself to the luminal side of the membrane (Turnberg, 1973). Carrier transport is specific to individual molecules or to a group of similar molecules. For example, the carrier mechanism that transports glucose is equally effective in transporting galactose, but is not involved in the transport of fructose or lactose. There are families of carrier mechanisms that have different specificities for neutral, acidic, and branched chain amino acids, and for small peptides (Silk and Dawson, 1979). Movement of solute against an electrical or concentration gradient requires energy, and the term *active transporters* has been used to describe carrier mediated systems that are energy dependent and capable of moving solute against a concentration gradient. Active transporters use the electrochemical potential gradient of a co-transported cation, which is usually sodium, to supply the required energy; therefore, they are ultimately dependent on the activity of the sodium potassium ATPase pump located in the basolateral membrane of the enterocytes (Crane, 1965; Silk and Dawson, 1979; Guandalini, 1988; Wright et al.,

1986). Other carriers, termed *diffusion facilitated transporters*, are driven by concentration differences favoring absorption of a specific solute, but the carrier mechanism increases the rate of transport compared with simple diffusion (Gould and Holdman, 1993; Silk and Dawson, 1979). Facilitated diffusion transporters are energy- and sodium-independent, but they are less efficient, especially at relatively low solute concentrations, than are the active transporters. While glucose is mainly absorbed by being actively co-transported with sodium by the transporter SGLT1, the facilitated diffusion transporter GLUT5 absorbs fructose. In addition to the brush-border transporter systems, there are a number of electrically neutral ion exchange mechanisms and ion co-transport systems sited in the enterocyte membrane. In the jejunum, sodium and chloride are transported into the enterocyte via a dual-coupled antiport system involving hydrogen and bicarbonate ions (Murer and Burckhardt, 1983). In the ileum, chloride enters the enterocyte in exchange for bicarbonate (Murer and Burckhardt, 1983).

The *intercellular route* occurs through the tight junctions between the enterocytes at the luminal side of the lateral edge of the cells. The outer leaves of the adjacent plasma membranes appear fused and no intercellular space can be discerned. This area is often referred to as the *tight junction*. Below this junction, the lateral membranes diverge to form the intracellular lateral space that opens into the interstitial space of the villus core. The perijunctional actomyosin ring of the intestinal tight junctions can be activated to increase or decrease the permeability of the intercellular junction. Activation of any of the active transporters causes the tight junctions to become more permeable to water and solute (Madara and Pappenheimer, 1987).

Water absorption from isotonic luminal fluid is mainly a passive consequence of solute absorption that establishes a local osmotic gradient that promotes the net uptake of water from the intestine. A number of different models have been proposed that couple solute and water absorption in the absence of, or against, moderate osmotic gradients. In each paradigm, active uptake of nutrients and/or sodium initiates an osmotic gradient that causes an increase in the lumen-to-mucosa water flux (Curran and MacIntosh, 1962, Fordtran et al., 1968; Jodal and Lungren, 1986; Pappenheimer and Reiss, 1987). The main differences among the various models are the influence that sodium has on establishing the osmotic gradient (Fordtran et al., 1968; Jodal and Lungren, 1986) and the relative importance of the paracellular convective flow of water, produced by the osmotic gradient, in determining overall absorption rates (Fordtran et al., 1968; Jodal and Lungren, 1986; Pappenheimer and Reiss, 1987). It is, however, clearly established that the intestinal absorption of solutes, such as glucose, does promote net water uptake, which in turn increases the non-selective transport of additional solute from the intestinal lumen. This knowledge underscores the importance of glucose as a key functional ingredient in a sports drink.

4.3.4 FACTORS AFFECTING INTESTINAL ABSORPTION

The majority of studies that have investigated the factors that affect intestinal absorption in man have used steady state perfusion methods in a segment of intestine. While the presence of the perfusion tubes in the intestine is not thought to influence the results (Modigliani and Bernier, 1971), measurements are made in a relatively short segment of the intestine and it is unlikely that the steady state conditions required by the technique normally occur post-prandially in the intestine. Absorption of solute by active and passive means promotes water absorption, and the flow of water through the tight junction can act as a conduit conveying a heterogeneous sample of the intestinal contents across the intestinal mucosa by solvent drag. Therefore, absorption of both water and solute are closely related and each can assist the absorption of the other.

4.3.4.1   Intestinal Flow Rate

As previously mentioned, the normal pattern of gastric emptying is exponential following ingestion of a beverage. Therefore, the flow rate through the intestine is variable. In the steady state perfusion method, although the rates of perfusion (5 to 15 m/min) are similar to gastric emptying rates, the flow rate is held constant. It is also possible for subjects to ingest beverages at a frequency and volume that maintain relatively constant rates of gastric emptying that can be relied upon for calculating fluid and solute flux in the proximal small intestine (Lambert et al., 1996).

Perfusion studies have shown that increasing the perfusion rate in the intestinal segment produces greater absorption of water and solute; however, this phenomenon appears to be due to the increase in the absolute solute load in the intestine rather than the greater fluid volume (Modigliani and Bernier, 1971).

4.3.4.2   Nutrient Type and Concentration

The major nutrient source in sports drinks and oral rehydration solutions is carbohydrate in the form of glucose monomer or polymer (i.e., maltodextrins). Several studies have shown that the rate of increase of glucose absorption in the human jejunum appears to plateau as the glucose monomer content in the lumen approaches about 200 mmol/l (Sladen and Dawson, 1969; Modigliani and Bernier, 1971). Although greater glucose monomer concentrations are associated with luminal hypertonicity and reductions in water absorption, rates of glucose absorption still tend to increase, at least up to a glucose concentration of around 555 mmol/l (Pappenheimer and Reiss, 1987). It is thought that the majority of glucose absorption up to the 200 mmol/l concentration is due to the active Na^+-glucose transporters (SGLT1), which become fully saturated above this concentration; thereafter, the gradual increase in glucose absorption is caused either by diffusion down the concentration gradient or by solvent drag. Whether the additional glucose uptake is the result of diffusion or solvent drag, it is likely that the route of absorption is through the tight junctions. Although glucose absorption tends to increase with increasing luminal concentration, the main effect on glucose and water absorption occurs with perfusion solutions with a glucose content of about 200 mmol/l (i.e., 3.6% glucose wt/vol).

The substitution of disaccharides or maltodextrins for equimolar amounts of glucose monomers has been reported to increase glucose absorption (Jones et al., 1987; Silk and Dawson, 1979). While most hypotheses have stressed an improved rate of binding between the Na$^+$-glucose transporter and the hydrolysis products of maltodextrins, others have suggested that membrane-bound digestion results in a high local concentration of glucose monomer from which non-specific paracellular (intercellular) absorption occurs. However, it is not a universal finding that glucose absorption is faster from maltodextrins than from equivalent concentrations of glucose monomers (Shi et al., 1995; Sladen and Dawson, 1969). The majority of evidence would suggest that glucose absorption is similar from glucose monomer solutions and mixtures of maltodextrin solutions that are equimolar and isotonic. Because solutions containing maltodextrins have a lower osmolality than those of equivalent amounts of glucose monomer, water uptake is faster from the low-osmolality maltodextrin solution and more carbohydrate may be non-specifically absorbed by solvent drag (Leiper et al., 1994).

Sucrose has been suggested as a disaccharide that may potentiate carbohydrate absorption because fructose, one of its two hydrolysis products, is absorbed by a facilitated transport mechanism (GLUT5), which is not utilized for glucose uptake (Shi et al., 1995; Gray and Ingelfinger, 1966). Therefore, it is less likely that the Na$^+$-glucose transporters will become saturated and each of the two different monosaccharides will not interfere with the absorption of the other. The results from perfusion studies using sucrose or mixtures of glucose and fructose have been equivocal on this issue. Total carbohydrate uptake from sucrose or the monosaccharide mixtures tends to be similar to that from equimolar amounts of glucose monomer (Gray and Ingelfinger, 1966; Jones et al., 1987; Leiper et al., 1996). One study, however, reported faster carbohydrate uptake from a mixture of glucose and fructose than from an equivalent amount of either glucose or sucrose (Shi et al., 1995). Some studies have shown that water absorption from sucrose solutions is slower than from equimolar glucose solutions (Leiper et al., 1996; Wheeler and Banwell, 1986). This may result from an increase in luminal osmolality produced by an accumulation of fructose (fructose is absorbed at about two-thirds the rate of an equivalent concentration of glucose) or because the transporter GLUT5 does not co-transport sodium, resulting in less total solute absorption and a reduced osmotic gradient. This is not a universal finding, however, as others have shown that water uptake can be faster from sucrose solutions than from solutions with an equivalent amount of glucose (Shi et al., 1995). The ingestion of large amounts of fructose should be avoided, as the human intestine has a relatively limited capacity to absorb this monosaccharide and gastrointestinal distress and diarrhea may result.

The incorporation of amino acids into carbohydrate solutions has been suggested to potentiate nutrient and water absorption. Amino acids that are actively co-transported with sodium by carrier systems other than that of the Na$^+$-glucose transporter would appear to be ideally suited to promote solute uptake and thereby stimulate greater water absorption. While faster rates of water absorption have been detected in some animal models with the addition of amino acids, the results in human studies have been disappointing. In many studies, the presence of amino acids in carbohydrate solutions has inhibited water absorption or has failed to promote increases. This is often caused by the increase in osmolality resulting from the addition of the amino acids (Cunha Ferreira et al., 1992). Others have postulated that the reduced rate of absorption is due to competitive inhibition between glucose and the amino acids for sodium, and that luminal sodium concentrations in excess of 90 mmol/l are needed to meet the requirements of the two substrates (Semenza, 1972).

4.3.4.3 Intestinal Osmolality

In a fasted individual, the normal osmolality of the luminal contents of the small intestine is usually between 270 and 290 mosmol/kg, which is isotonic with respect to human serum. Following ingestion of a food or beverage, the osmolality of the duodenum and jejunum changes in accordance with the osmolality of the gastric contents and the rate at which those contents are emptied into the small intestine. Thereafter, luminal osmolality is eventually returned to isotonicity, due to the movement of water and electrolytes into and out of the proximal intestine. After the luminal contents have been made isotonic, they remain that way during the process of absorption. The time required to achieve isotonicity varies with the osmolality and nutrient load of the gastric efflux. For example, water is rapidly made isotonic within the duodenum and proximal jejunum by the influx of sodium and other electrolytes, whereas beverages such as fruit juices and soft drinks that contain 10% to 16% carbohydrate require a greater period of time and thereby traverse a greater length of small intestine.

Solutions with an osmolality of greater than 290 mosmol/kg initially cause a net efflux of water into the intestinal lumen. The time required to achieve isotonicity reduces the rate of net water absorption. As noted above, the rate of water efflux increases in proportion to the level of hyperosmolality of the luminal contents (i.e. the greater the osmotic gradient between the lumen and the intestinal cells, the greater the net efflux of water). Hypertonic solutions are eventually absorbed, but this occurs farther down the small intestine after the solution has been made isotonic. This delay, coupled with the initial net movement of water from the circulation to dilute the luminal contents, renders hypertonic solutions ineffective in promoting rapid rehydration.

Absorption of solute from isotonic solutions can produce local osmotic gradients that are sufficient to promote net water absorption from the intestinal lumen. If the luminal contents have an osmolality of less than 270 mosmol/kg, water will follow the osmotic gradient and move from the lumen across the mucosa. Therefore, hypotonicity of the luminal content can be an additive factor to that of solute absorption for promoting net water absorption (Sladen, 1972; Shi et al., 1995). Many studies have demonstrated that faster rates of intestinal water absorption in the jejunum occur from hypotonic than from isotonic carbohydrate-electrolyte solutions (Wapnir and Lifshitz, 1985; Cunha Ferreira et al., 1992; Shi et al., 1995). It would follow that drinking water or mineral waters that are markedly hypotonic (with osmolalities generally between 5 and 15 mosmol/kg) would be expected to promote high rates of water absorption. However, water absorption is actually faster from isotonic carbohydrate-electrolyte solutions than from water in the jejunum (Sladen, 1972; Gisolfi et al., 1991).

The main reason for the relatively poor rate of water absorption from the infusion of plain water is thought to be due to the resulting efflux of electrolytes, mainly sodium, down concentration gradients, causing some body water to cross the mucosa into the jejunal lumen. Most studies have shown that both glucose-containing and nutrient-free solutions with an osmolality of less than 200 mosmol/kg produce slower rates of water absorption in the jejunum than do similar solutions with an osmolality between 200 and 260 mosmol/kg (Soergel et al., 1968; Hunt et al., 1992). This is true even when carbohydrate and sodium are present. Therefore, the most effective osmolality range for rehydration solutions appears to be relatively narrow because even small differences in osmolality have marked effects on water absorption. For example, in one study where the total carbohydrate and sodium content of the perfusion solutions were similar but osmolality differed, net water absorption was about twice as fast from a moderately hypotonic (229 mosmol/kg) solution than from an isotonic (277 mosmol/kg) solution (Figure 4.5; Leiper et al., 1994). Water absorption from a moderately hypertonic (352 mosmol/kg) solution was significantly less than from the isotonic solution. There was an increased rate of glucose absorption associated with the faster rates of water absorption from the hypotonic solution, while there was no difference in solute absorption between the isotonic and hypertonic solutions (Figure 4.5).

4.3.4.4 Electrolyte Content

In the jejunum of fasted humans, sodium is absorbed only against low electrochemical gradients. However, sodium is actively co-transported with a variety of sugars, amino acids, peptides and pyrimidines, organic acids, and bile salts (Sladen, 1972). Bicarbonate ions promote sodium absorption in the jejunum by a pH-independent, dual-coupled antiport system that involves chloride and hydrogen ions (Murer and Burckhardt, 1983). Sodium absorption appears pivotal to the establishment of the osmotic gradients that are essential for net water uptake. No other electrolyte appears to affect water absorption to such a significant extent. Because of the essential role of sodium in active nutrient transport, it has been thought necessary to have it included in oral rehydration solutions. However, because sodium from the blood rapidly effluxes into the proximal small intestine, it has been argued that exogenous sodium is not required to activate nutrient transporters. Perfusion studies have shown that the exclusion of sodium from glucose solutions does not have a detrimental effect on water absorption. However, substitution of mannitol or magnesium for sodium results in 23% and 45% reductions, respectively, in glucose uptake (Saltzman et al., 1972). In addition, enhanced carbohydrate absorption from solutions containing maltose and maltodextrins has been associated with luminal sodium concentrations greater than 100 mmol/l (Jones et al., 1987). It is known that net sodium uptake from isotonic carbohydrate-electrolyte solutions is marginal when the luminal sodium concentration is below 60 mmol/l. In a study utilizing deuterium as a tracer for water, the addition of 50 mmol/l of sodium chloride had little effect on the gastric emptying of 200 mmol/l of either glucose or fructose as assessed by the double-sample aspiration technique. However, the rate of accumulation of the deuterium tracer in the circulation was faster from the glucose solution with sodium than without sodium, although there was no difference in uptake between the sodium-containing and sodium-free fructose solutions. In addition, the inclusion of sodium in the glucose solution, but not the fructose solution, increased the glycaemic response (Leiper et al., 1995). This suggests that the presence of exogenous sodium in glucose solutions, but not in fructose solutions, can enhance the carbohydrate and water absorption.

The other major electrolytes of the body (e.g., potassium, magnesium, calcium), are absorbed down electrochemical gradients or by carrier-mediated processes. The inclusion of electrolytes in rehydration solutions, with the exception of sodium, increases the osmolality of the solution and their presence does not have a discernable impact on water absorption. The majority of studies that have investigated the effect of sodium on water absorption have used chloride as the accompanying anion. In the jejunum, the transport of chloride follows more closely that of sodium and water than its own concentration gradient (Fordtran et al., 1968). In the ileum, however, chloride is actively absorbed via an antiport system where chloride is being exchanged for bicarbonate (Murer & Burckhardt, 1983). Some studies have shown that other anions such as acetate or citrate can enhance water absorption from glucose-sodium solutions containing bicarbonate (Leiper and Maughan, 1988c). In all of these studies, however, the major anion in the intestinal lumen has always been chloride. For reasons of palatability, chloride is probably the anion of choice to be included in drinks that contain sodium.

4.3.4.5 Beverage Temperature

The stomach rapidly equilibrates the temperature of ingested beverages to approximate internal body temperature and so it is unlikely that significant amounts of either markedly hot or cold fluid are emptied into the duodenum. There is one study in which a non-nutrient electrolyte solution was perfused at different temperatures into the small intestines of human volunteers. In this investigation, perfusion temperatures above 37°C induced approximately a 25% increase in water and sodium absorption compared with solutions at 37°C, while lowering the perfusion temperature to between 17 and 25°C caused about a 32% reduction in water and sodium absorption compared with that at 37°C (Love, 1966). The differences in absorption rates are presumably due to differences in blood flow through the intestinal segment caused by the temperature effects.

4.3.4.6 Beverage pH

Several studies in animals have examined the effect of alterations in acid–base balance on water and solute absorption in the small intestine (Charney et al., 1989). These investigations have demonstrated that a reduction in the arterial pH increased water, sodium, and chloride absorption in the rat ileum, but did not alter glucose absorption. Less work has been carried out in humans, but in one study, perfusing the jejunum with a carbohydrate-electrolyte solution containing 23 mmol/l bicarbonate produced a pH of 6.6(0.8) in the luminal contents. This was higher than the pH produced in the same solution than when tartrate was substituted for the bicarbonate. Water absorption was faster from the bicarbonate solution (14.1(6.2) ml/cm/hour) than from the tartrate solution (9.7(6.7) ml/cm/hour), and glucose uptake was also faster from the bicarbonate solution (1.2 (0.5) mmol/cm/hour) than from the tartrate solution (0.8 (0.4) mmol/cm/h) (Leiper and Maughan, 1988b). However, it is unclear from this study whether the improved absorption rates were due directly to bicarbonate uptake's enhancing intestinal transport or to a buffering effect's increasing active absorption of glucose. Sports drinks, fruit juices, soft drinks, tea, coffee, and most alcohol-containing beverages are acidic with little buffering capacity. Therefore, the pH of the intestinal luminal contents is little affected by the levels of acidity present in drinks.

4.3.4.7 Exercise

There have been relatively few studies that have investigated the effect of exercise on intestinal absorption. This is largely due to the practical difficulties associated with perfusing the small intestine in individuals who are exercising. In one study, treadmill exercise at 70% of $VO_{2\,max}$ had no discernible effect on intestinal absorption of water, glucose, or electrolytes (Fordtran and Saltin, 1967). Another study reported no difference in absorption rates between rest and cycle exercise at 30%, 50%, and 70% $VO_{2\,max}$ from either water or a carbohydrate-electrolyte solution (Gisolfi et al., 1991). However, cycle exercise designed to increase heart rate about 50% above resting values produced a small but significant reduction in water and electrolyte absorption from an electrolyte solution that contained no carbohydrate (Barclay and Turnberg, 1988). The reduction in absorption in this study was of a similar order to that elicited by psychological stress or mild pain.

Using a water tracer technique, the rate of accumulation in the circulation of the tracer decreased in proportion to the exercise intensity, and the time to peak tracer concentration in the blood was greater with increasing exercise intensities in the range 40% to 80% $VO_{2\,max}$ (Figure 4.6). This study was carried out with the subjects ingesting the same carbohydrate-electrolyte labeled solution with the tracer on each of the trials. The results suggest a decreased availability of ingested fluids during exercise, but whether the main cause was due to changes in the rate of gastric emptying or intestinal absorption could not be ascertained (Maughan et al., 1990).

The mechanisms by which exercise might affect intestinal absorption are thought to be related to increased circulating catecholamine levels and reduced perfusion of the splanchnic vascular bed. It is highly probable that intermittent high-intensity sprinting will reduce absorption at least to the same extent as it affects gastric emptying. However, the validity of this supposition awaits testing.

4.3.5 ADAPTATIONS TO CHANGES IN NUTRIENT INTAKE

The gastrointestinal tract is a highly adaptable organ that alters its functional ability depending on dietary intake. The digestive enzymes and the nutrient, vitamin, and mineral transporters are regulated in part by composition of the diet (Ferraris and Diamond, 1989). This means that any substantial change in an individual's diet will cause alterations in the levels of brush border digestive enzymes and transporters that will allow the gut to increase its ability to absorb the components of subsequent meals of similar composition.

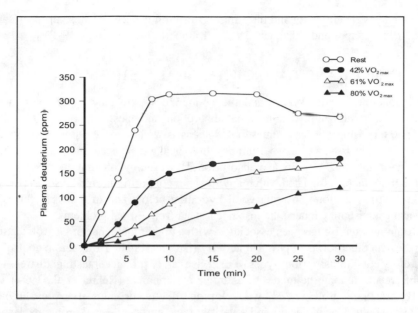

FIGURE 4.6 Plasma deuterium accumulation at rest and during exercise at 42, 61, or 80% VO_{2max} after ingestion of drinks containing deuterium oxide. (Maughan et al., Effects of exercise intensity on absorption of ingested fluids, *Experimental Physiology,* 1990; redrawn with permission.)

By practicing drinking and experimenting with different drink formulations during training, it should be possible to establish the best drinking strategies for the specific sporting events and environmental conditions that are likely to occur. To allow the body to adapt and benefit from changes in dietary intake, alterations in the diet should be made well in advance of any competition.

4.4 INTEGRATION OF MEASURES OF GASTRIC EMPTYING AND INTESTINAL ABSORPTION

The use of isotopic tracers was introduced in the early 1960s to differentiate the effects of the bidirectional fluxes of water and sodium on the specific rates of the net absorption of each. Other studies measured both gastric emptying rates and intestinal absorption rates separately and gave estimates of the relative importance of each in determining the incorporation of beverage constituents in the body pools (Fordtran and Saltin, 1967; Davis et al., 1987; Lambert et al., 1996). Although the isotopic technique does not determine net rates of gastric emptying or intestinal fluid absorption, comparison of the unidirectional flux of the tracer appears to give a measure of the relative rates of absorption from different drinks. Several studies comparing the unidirectional accumulation rate in the circulation of a tracer for water from various drinks have shown differences among beverages that reflect the combined gastric emptying and intestinal absorption patterns of those drinks (Davis et al., 1987; Leiper and Maughan, 1988a; Lambert and Maughan, 1992).

4.5   EXERCISE AND GASTROINTESTINAL DISTRESS

The autonomic nervous system and the endocrine system play major roles in the regulation of gastric emptying, intestinal absorption, and intestinal motility. It is therefore not surprising that gastrointestinal distress is a commonly reported complaint among individuals who exercise. Both psychological and physical stress are known to affect gastrointestinal motility and absorption. However, hypohydration appears to be an important factor associated with many instances of gastrointestinal distress (Rehrer et al., 1990). Therefore, ensuring good hydration before and in the early stages of physical exercise may reduce the instances of gastrointestinal problems.

Running exercise has been associated with a higher incidence of gastrointestinal distress than other forms of physical activity (Brouns, 1991). However, in controlled laboratory conditions, various types of exercise rarely produce intestinal distress and no differences among the modes of exercise are apparent (Rehrer et al., 1994).

By practicing drinking and by developing effective drinking strategies, an individual can reduce the incidence and severity of any gastrointestinal problems. Experimentation with different formulations of beverages may also help. Increasing the volume of fluid in the stomach stimulates gastric emptying. Therefore, the rate at which any drink is emptied into the small intestine is maximized by the intake of a large volume of the drink and by maintaining this volume in the stomach by frequent ingestion of the drink. Maintaining a large volume of fluid in the stomach throughout exercise may cause difficulty in some individuals; however, empirical evidence suggests that by repeatedly exercising with a full stomach, adaptations will occur that reduce problems with gastrointestinal discomfort.

4.6   SUMMARY

There is no doubt that the gastric emptying and intestinal absorption characteristics of sports drinks are critical elements in their effectiveness. Rapid gastric emptying is promoted by ingesting large volumes of a beverage of low energy content. The beverage energy content appears to be the main inhibitory regulator of gastric emptying, and increasing the amount of energy proportionally decreases the rate of gastric emptying. Carbohydrates are the main energy source in sports drinks, but other nutrients such as proteins, fats, and alcohol slow emptying by the same extent. Increased beverage osmolality also slows gastric emptying to some extent, but this effect is secondary to the energy density of the beverage.

The effects of drink temperature, electrolyte content, and pH are relatively unimportant in the regulation of gastric emptying, but all play important roles in the palatability of a drink and the volume of it that is voluntarily consumed. While low intensity walking may increase the rate of gastric emptying compared with that at rest, similar rates of gastric emptying have been reported in running and cycling at the same levels of intensity. Exercise at a steady power output, however, has little effect on gastric emptying at intensities of less than about 70% $VO_{2\,max}$. Relatively few bouts of high intensity sprinting appear to be required to cause significant slowing of gastric emptying. However, the gastrointestinal tract appears to be capable of undergoing some degree of adaptation to fluid ingestion that can allow for greater fluid intake to be tolerated during exercise and an increase in the potential benefit of the beverages consumed.

Many of the factors that alter the rate of gastric emptying have a similar effect on intestinal absorption. The most obvious difference is osmolality, which has a greater effect on the rate of intestinal water and solute absorption than it does on the gastric emptying rate. The presence of carbohydrate in a beverage will promote water absorption in addition to supplying an energy source to the working muscles. Increasing the carbohydrate content of a drink will slow gastric emptying.

Markedly hypertonic drinks will initially cause water to move from the body tissues into the intestinal lumen and will result in poor rates of water absorption. Carbohydrate beverages with an osmolality between about 200 and 260 mosmol/kg will promote rapid rates of water uptake, and these beverages can be formulated with adequate amounts of carbohydrate to maintain blood glucose levels during prolonged exercise. No other nutrients in addition to carbohydrates and sodium appear to be required to stimulate water absorption. Temperature, pH, and the presence of other electrolytes have little effect on intestinal absorption, but their effect on palatability may mean that they are factors that need to be considered in the formulation of sports drinks.

REFERENCES

Barclay, G.R. and Turnberg, L.A., Influence of physical and psychological stress on fluid and electrolyte absorption in the human jejunum *in vitro, Gut,* 26, 554, 1985.

Bangsbo, J., Fitness Training in Football — A Scientific Approach. Bagsvaerd, Denmark: HO+Storm, 1994. pp. 57, 1994.

Beckers, E.J., Leiper, J.B., and Davidson, J., Comparison of aspiration and scintigraphic techniques for the measurement of gastric emptying rates of liquids in man. *Gut* 33: 115, 1992.

Beckers, E.J., Rehrer, N.J., Brouns, F., ten Hoor, F., and Saris. W.H.M., Determination of total gastric volume, gastric secretion and residual meal volume using the double sampling technique of George. *Gut* 29: 1725,1988.

Beckers, E.J., Rehrer, N.J., Saris, W.H.M., Brouns, F., ten Hoor, F., and Kester, A.D.M., Daily variation in gastric emptying when using the double sampling technique. *Med. Sci. Sports Exerc.* 23: 1210, 1991.

Blundell, J.E., and MacDiarmid, J.L., Fat as a risk factor for overconsumption: satiation, satiety, and patterns of eating. *J. Am. Diet. Assoc.* 97 (supplement 7): S63, 1997.

Burkes, T.F., Galligan, J.J., Porrela, F., and Barber, W.D., Regulation of gastric emptying. *Fed. Proc.* 44: 2897, 1985.

Brener, T., Hendrix, T.R., and McHugh, P.R., Regulation of gastric emptying of glucose. *Gastroenterology* 85:76, 1983.

Brouns, F., Etiology of gastrointestinal disturbances during endurance events. *Scand. J. Med. and Sci.* 1: 66, 1991.

Brouns, F., Seden, J., Beckers, E.J., and Saris, W.H.M., Osmolality does not affect the gastric emptying rate of oral rehydration solutions. *J. Enter. and Parental Nutr.* 19: 403, 1995.

Burkes, T.F., Galligan, J.J., Porrela, F., and Barber, W.D., Regulation of gastric emptying, *Fed. Proc.* 44, 2897, 1985.

Calbet, J.A.L. and MacLean, D.A., Role of caloric content on gastric emptying in humans. *J. Physiol.* 498: 553, 1997.

Charney, A.N., Ingrassia, P.M., Thaler, S.M., and Keane, M.G., Effect of systemic pH on models of altered ileal transport in the rat. *Gastroenterology*, 96: 331, 1989.

Costill, D.L. and Saltin, B., Factors limiting gastric emptying during rest and exercise. *J. Appl. Physiol.* 37: 679, 1974.

Coyle, E.F. and Montain, S.J., Carbohydrate and fluid ingestion during exercise: are there trade-offs? *Med. Sci. Sports Exerc.*, 24, 671, 1992.

Crane, R.K., Na^+-dependent transport in the intestine and in other animal tissues. *Fed. Proc.*; 24: 1000, 1965.

Cunha Ferreira, R.M.C., Elliott, E.J., Watson, A.J.M., Brennan, E., Walker-Smith, J.A., and Farthing, M.J.G., Dominant role for osmolality in the efficacy of glucose and glycine-containing oral rehydration solutions: studies in a rate model of secretory diarrhoea. *Acta Paediatrica* 81: 46, 1992.

Curran, P.F. and MacIntosh, J.R., A model system for biological water transport. *Nature, London*, 193: 347, 1962.

Davis, J.M., Lamb, D.R., Burgess, W.A., and Bartoli, W.P., Accumulation of deuterium oxide (D_2O) in body fluids following ingestion of D_2O-labeled beverages. *J. Appl. Physiol.* 63: 2060, 1987.

Dawson, A.M., A review of fat transport, in *Transport Across the Intestine*, Burland, W.L. and Samul, P.K., (Eds.), Churchill Livingston, London. 1972, 210.

Ferraris, R.P. and Diamond, J.M., Specific regulation of intestinal nutrient transporters by their dietary substrates. *Ann. Rev. Physiol.* 51: 125, 1989.

Fordtran, J.S. and Locklear, T.W., Ionic constituents and osmolality of gastric and small intestinal fluids after eating. *Am. J. Digest. Diseases* 11: 503, 1966.

Fordtran, J.S., Rector, F.C., and Carter, N.W., The mechanisms of sodium absorption in the human small intestine. *J. Clinic. Invest.* 47: 884, 1968.

Fordtran, J.S., Rector, F.C., Ewton, M.F., Soter ,N., and Kinney, J., Permeability characteristics of the human small intestine. *J. Clinic. Invest.* 44: 1935, 1965.

Fordtran, J.S. and Saltin, B., Gastric emptying and intestinal absorption during prolonged severe exercise. *J. Appl. Physiol.* 23: 331, 1967.

Gisolfi, C.V., Summers, R.W., Schedl, H.P., Bleiler, T.L., and Oppliger, R.A., Human intestinal water absorption: direct vs. indirect measurements. *Am. J. Physiol.* 258: G216, 1990.

Gisolfi, C.V., Spranger, K.J., Summers, R.W., Schedl, H.P., and Bleiler, T.L., The effects of exercise on intestinal absorption in humans. *J. Appl. Physiol.* 7: 2518, 1991.

Gould, G.W. and Holdman, G.D., The glucose transporter family: structure, function and tissue specific expression. *J. Biochem.* 295: 329, 1993.

Gray, G.M. and Ingelfinger, F.J., Intestinal absorption of sucrose in man: interrelation of hydrolysis and monosaccharide product absorption. *J. Clinic. Invest.* 45: 388, 1966.

Guandalini, S., Intestinal ion and nutrient transport in health and infectious diarrheal diseases. In: *Drugs* 36 (supplement 4), Bank, S., Farthing, M.J.G. (Eds.), 26, 1988.

Hallbäck, D.-A., Jodal, M., Sjöqvist, C., and Lundgren, O., Villous tissue osmolality and intestinal transport of water and electrolytes. *Acta Physiologica Scandinavica*: 110: 95, 1980.

Holt, S., Cervantes, J., Wilkinson, A.A., and Wallace, J.H.K., Measurement of gastric emptying rate in humans by real-time ultrasound. *Gastroenterology* 90: 918, 1986.

Horowitz, M., Cunningham, K.M., Wishart, J.M., Jones, K.L., and Read, N.W., The effect of short-term dietary supplementation with glucose on gastric emptying of glucose and fructose and oral glucose tolerance in normal subjects. *Diabetologia* 39: 481-486, 1996.

Hunt, J.B., Elliott, E., Fairclough, P.D., Clark, M.L., and Farthing, M.J.G., Water and solute absorption from hypotonic glucose-electrolyte solutions in human jejunum. *Gut* 33: 479, 1992.

Hunt, J.N. and Knox, M.T., Regulation of gastric emptying. *Handbook of Physiology.* Section 6: alimentary canal. Volume IV. *Motility.* American Physiological Society, Washington, D.C. pp. 1917, 1968.

Hunt, J.N. and Spurrell, W.R., The pattern of emptying of the human stomach. *J. Physiol.* 133: 157, 1951.

Hunt, J.N. and Stubbs, D.F. The volume and energy content of meals as determinants of gastric emptying. *J. Physiol.* 245: 209, 1975.

Hunt, J.N., Smith, J.L., and Jiang, C.L. Effect of meal volume and energy density on the gastric emptying rate of carbohydrates. *Gastroenterology* 89: 1326, 1985.

Jodal, M. and Lungren, O., Countercurrent mechanisms in the mammalian gastrointestinal tract. *Gastroenterology;* 91: 225, 1986.

Jones, B.J.M., Higgins, B.E., and Silk, D.B.A., Glucose absorption from maltotriose and glucose oligomers in the human jejunum. *Clinic. Sci.* 72: 409, 1987.

Lambert, C.P., Ball, D., Leiper, J.B., and Maughan, R.J., The use of a deuterium tracer to follow the fate of ingested fluids: effects of drink volume and tracer concentration and content, *Experimental Physiol.*, 84, 391, 1999.

Lambert, G.P., Chang, R.T., Joensen, D., Shi, X., Summers, R.W., Schedl, H.P., and Gisolfi, C.V., Simultaneous determination of gastric emptying and intestinal absorption during cycle exercise. *Int. J. Sports Med.* 17: 48, 1996.

Lambert, C.P. and Maughan, R.J., Accumulation in the blood of a deuterium tracer added to hot and cold beverages. *Scandin. J. Med. Sci. in Sports* 2: 76, 1992.

Leiper, J.B., The use of beverages as ergogenic aids. In: *The Clinical Pharmacology of Sport and Exercise,* Reilly,T. and Orme, M. (Eds.) Elsevier Science B.V., Amsterdam, 1997, pp. 233, 1998.

Leiper, J.B., Thirst Physiology. In: *Encyclopaedia of Human Nutrition*, Sadler, M., Caballero, B., and Strain, S. (Eds.), Academic Press, London, 1998, pp. 1870.

Leiper, J.B. and Maughan, R.J., Experimental models for the investigation of water and solute transport in man: Implications for oral rehydration solutions. In: *Drugs* 36 (supplement 4), Bank, S. and Farthing, M.J.G. (Eds.), 65, 1988.

Leiper, J.B. and Maughan, R.J, Jejunal water transport in man: effects of bicarbonate or tartrate. *Proc. Nutr. Soc.* 47: 9A, 1988a.

Leiper, J.B. and Maughan, R.J., Effect of bicarbonate or base precursor on water and solute absorption from a glucose-electrolyte solution in the human jejunum. *Digestion* 41: 39, 1988b.

Leiper, J.B., Brouns, F., and Maughan, R.J., The effect of osmolality on absorption from carbohydrate-electrolyte solutions (CES) in the human jejunal perfusion model. *J. Physiol.* 479: 59P, 1994.

Leiper, J.B., Brouns, F., and Maughan, R.J., Effects of variation in the type of carbohydrate on absorption from hypotonic carbohydrate-electrolyte solutions (CES) in the human jejunal perfusion model. *J. Physiol.* 495, 128P, 1996.

Leiper, J.B., Brouns, F., and Maughan, R.J., A comparison of the gastric emptying rate of carbohydrate and ethanol solutions in man: regulation by osmolality or energy density. *J. Physiol.* 515P, 87, 1999.

Leiper, J.B., Vist, G.E., and Maughan, R.J., The effect of carbohydrate type, sodium and osmolality on unidirectional water uptake from ingested solutions in man. *J. Physiol.* 481, 52P, 1995.

Love, A.H.G., The influence of the temperature of intraluminal contents on fluid transit and absorption in the human intestine. *J. Physiol.* 185: 80P, 1966.

Low, A.G., Nutritional regulation of gastric secretion, digestion and emptying. *Nutr. Res. Rev.* 3: 229, 1990.

Mack, G.W., Recovery after exercise in the heat factors influencing fluid intake, *Int. J. Sports Med.*, 19, supplement 2, S139, 1998.

Madara, J.L. and Pappenheimer, J.R., Structural basis for physiological regulation of paracellular pathways. *J. Membr. Biol.* 100: 149, 1987.

Maughan, R.J., Carbohydrate-electrolyte solutions during prolonged exercise. In: *Perspectives in Exercise Sciences and Sports Medicine, Vol 4, Ergogenics-Enhancement of Performance in Exercise and Sport*, Lamb, D.R., Williams, M.H. (Eds.), Benchmark Press, Carmel, IN,1991, 35.

Maughan, R.J., Optimizing hydration for competitive sport. In: *Perspectives in Exercise Science and Sports Medicine, Vol 10, Optimizing Sport Performance,* Lamb, D.R., Murray, R., (Ed.), Cooper: Carmel, IN, pp. 139, 1997.

Maughan, R.J and Leiper, J.B., Methods for the assessment of gastric emptying in humans: an overview. *Diabetic Med.* 13: S6, 1996.

Maughan, R.J., Leiper, J.B., and McGaw, B.A., Effects of exercise intensity on absorption of ingested fluids, *Exper. Physiol.*, 75, 419, 1990.

Miller, L.J., Malagelada, J.R., Taylot, W.F., and Go, V.L., Intestinal control of human postprandial gastric function: the role of components of jejunoileal chyme in regulating gastric secretion and gastric emptying, *Gastroenterology*, 80, 763, 1981.

Minami, H. and McCallum, R.W. (1984). The physiology and pathophysiology of gastric emptying in humans. *Gastroenterology* 86: 1592-1610.

Mitchell, J.B. and Voss, K.W., The influence of volume on gastric emptying and fluid balance. *Med. Sci. Sports Exerc.* 23; 314, 1991.

Modigliani, R. and Bernier, J.J., Absorption of glucose, sodium, and water by the human jejunum studied by intestinal perfusion with a proximal occluding balloon and at variable flow rates. *Gut* 12: 184, 1971.

Murer, H. and Burckhardt, G., Membrane transport of anions across the epithelia of mammalian small intestine and kidney proximal tubule. *Reviews of Physiology, Biochemistry and Pharmacology*; 96: 1, 1983.

Murray, R., The effects of consuming carbohydrate-electrolyte beverages on gastric emptying and fluid absorption during and following exercise. *Sports Med.* 4; 322, 1987.

Neufer, P.D., Young, A.J., and Sawka, M.N., Gastric emptying during exercise: effects of heat stress and hypohydration. *Europ. J. Appl. Physiol.* 58: 433, 1989.

Noakes, T.D., Rehrer, N.J., and Maughan, R.J., The importance of volume in regulating gastric emptying. *Med. and Sci. in Sports and Exerc.* 23: 307, 1991.

Pappenheimer, J.R. and Reiss, K.Z., Contribution of solvent drag through intercellular junctions to absorption of nutrients by the small intestine. *J. Membr. Biol.* 100: 123, 1987.

Phillips, S..F and Summerskill, W.H.J., Water and electrolyte transport during maintenance of isotonicity in human jejunum and ileum. *J. Laboratory Clinical Med.* 70: 686, 1967.

Ramsay, D.J., The importance of thirst in the maintenance of fluid balance. In: *Water and Salt Homeostasis in Health and Disease*, Bayliss, P.H. (Ed.) Bailliere Tindall, London, 1989, (*Clinical Endocrinology and Metabolism,* vol 3, No. 2), 371.

Rehrer, N.J., Beckers, E.J., Brouns, F., Saris, W.H.M., and ten Hoor, F., Effects of electrolytes in carbohydrate beverages on gastric emptying and secretion. *Med. Sci. Sports Exerc.* 25: 42, 1993.

Rehrer, N.J., Beckers, E.J., Brouns, F., and ten Hoor, F., Effects of dehydration on gastric emptying and gastrointestinal distress while running. *Med. Sci. Sports Exerc.* 22: 790, 1990.

Rehrer, N.J., Brouns, F., Beckers, E.J., and Saris, W.H.M., The influence of beverage composition and gastrointestinal function on fluid and nutrient availability during exercise. *Scandin. J. Med. and Sci. in Sport* 4; 159, 1994.

Rehrer, N.J., Brouns, F., Beckers, E.J., ten Hoor, F., and Saris, W.H.M., Gastric emptying with repeated drinking during running and bicycling. *Int. J. Sports Med.* 11: 238, 1990.

Ryan, A.J., Bleiler, T.L., Carter. J.E., and Gisolfi, C.V., Gastric emptying during prolonged cycling exercise in the heat. *Med. Sci. Sports Exerc.* 21: 51, 1989.

Ryan, A.J., Lambert, G.P., Shi, X., Chang, R.J., Summers, R.W. and Gisolfi, CV., Effects of hypohydration on gastric emptying and intestinal absorption during exercise. *J. Appl. Physiol.* 84: 1581, 1998.

Saltzman, D.A, Rector, F.C., and Fordtran, J.S., The role of intraluminal sodium in glucose absorption in vitro. *J. Clinic. Invest.* 51: 876, 1972.

Shi, X. and Gisolfi, C.V., Fluid and carbohydrate replacement during intermittent exercise. *Sports Med.* 3: 157,1998.

Schvarcz, E., Palmer, M., Aman, J., and Berne, C., Accelerated gastric emptying during hypoglycaemia is not associated with changes in plasma motilin levels. *Acta Diabetologica* 34: 194, 1997.

Scholer, J.F. and Code, C.F., Rate of absorption of water from the stomach and small bowel of human beings. *Gastroenterology* 27: 565, 1954.

Schütz, H.B. and Kenedi, T., Water exchange through the stomach wall. *Scandin. J. Clinic. Invest.*; 15: 445, 1963.

Semenza, G. Some aspects of intestinal sugar transport. In: *Transport Across the Intestine*, Burland, W.L. and Samuel, P.K. (Eds.), Churchill Livingstone, London, 1972, 78-92.

Shi, X., Summers, R.W., Schedl, H.P., Flanagan, S.W., Chang, R., and Gisolfi, C.V., Effects of carbohydrate type and concentration and solution osmolality on water absorption. *Med. Sci. Sports and Exerc.* 27: 1607, 1995.

Silk, D.B.A. and Dawson, A.M., Intestinal absorption of carbohydrate and protein in man. In: *International Review of Physiology. Gastrointestinal Physiology II.* Vol 19, Crane, R.K. (Ed.), University Park Press, Baltimore, 1979, pp. 151.

Sladen, G.E.G., A review of water and electrolyte transport. In: *Transport Across the Intestine*, Burland, W.L. and Samuel, P.K. (Eds.), Churchill Livingstone, London, 1972, pp. 14.

Sladen, G.E.G. Methods of studying intestinal absorption in man. In: *Intestinal Absorption in Man*, McColl, I. and Sladen, G.E.G. (Eds.), Academic Press, London. pp. 1, 1975.

Sladen, G.E.G. and Dawson, A.M., Further studies on the perfusion method for measuring intestinal absorption in man: the effects of the proximal occlusive balloon and a mixing segment. *Gut* 11: 947,1970.

Soergel, K.H., Whalen, G.E. and Harris, J.A., Passive movement of water and sodium across the small intestinal mucosa. *J. Appl. Physiol.* 24: 40, 1968.

Sole, C.C. and Noakes, T.D., Faster gastric emptying for glucose-polymer and fructose solutions than for glucose. *Europe. J. Appl. Physiol.* 58: 605, 1989.

Struntz, U.T. and Grossman,M.I., Effect of intragastric pressure on gastric emptying and secretion. *Am. J. Physiol.* 234: E552, 1978.

Sun, W.M., Houghton, L.A., Read, N.W., Grundy, D.G., and Johnson, A.G., Effect of meal temperature on gastric emptying of liquids in man. *Gut* 29: 302, 1988.

Thomas, J.E. and Baldwin, M.V., Pathways and mechanisms for the regulation of gastric motility. *Handbook of Physiology*. Section 6: alimentary canal. Volume IV. *Motility*. American Physiological Society; Washington, D.C. pp. 1937,1968.

Tothill, P., McLoughlin, G.P. and Heading, R.C., Techniques and errors in scintigraphic measurement of gastric emptying. *J. Nucl. Med.* 19: 256, 1978.

Turnberg, L.A., Absorption and secretion of salt and water by the small intestine. *Digestion* 9: 357, 1973.

Verbalis, J.G., Inhibitory controls of drinking: satiation of thirst. In: *Thirst: Physiological and Psychological Aspects*, Ramsay, D.J. and Booth, D.A., (Eds.), *ILSI Human Nutrition Reviews*, Springer-Verlag, London, 1990, pp. 313.

Vist, G.E. and Maughan, R.J., Gastric emptying of ingested solutions in man: effect of beverage glucose concentration. *Med. and Sci. in Sports and Exerc.* 26: 1269, 1994.

Vist, G.E. and Maughan, R.J. The effect of osmolality and carbohydrate content on the rate of gastric emptying. *J. Physiol.* 486: 523, 1995.

Wapnir, R.A. and Lifshitz, F., Osmolality and solute concentration—their relationship with oral rehydration solution effectiveness: An experimental model. *Pediatric Res.* 19: 894 1985.

Wheeler, K. and Banwell, J.G., Intestinal water and electrolyte flux of glucose-polymer electrolyte solutions. *Med. Sci. Sports Exerc.* 18: 436, 1986.

Wilbur, B.G. and Kelly, K.A., Effect of proximal gastric, complete gastric and truncal vagotomy on canine gastric electrical activity, motility and emptying. *Ann. Surg.*, 178: 295-303, 1973.

Wright, J.K., Seckler, R., and Overath, P., Molecular aspects of sugar:ion co-transport. *Ann. Rev. of Biochem.*; 55: 225, 1986.

5 Physiological Responses to Fluid Intake During Exercise

Ronald J. Maughan

CONTENTS

5.1 INTRODUCTION

It is well recognized that fluid ingestion can benefit performance in many exercise situations, and an extensive literature is devoted to the various performance-enhancing effects of different beverage formulations. The interest of the athletic community in sports drinks is largely confined to their potential for improved performance. To the scientist, however, the administration of drinks of varying composition during exercise offers a tool for the study of the normal physiological response to exercise. Indeed, exercise itself is often used as a model for the investigation of normal physiological function, a scientific approach that also benefits the athlete. If the normal responses to exercise are understood, and if the sequelae of fluid ingestion are also known, then predictions can be made that will allow optimizsation of the formulation of drinks intended to improve performance.

Many studies of the effects of fluid replacement on exercise performance have lacked the physiological and biochemical measurements that would allow insights into the underlying mechanisms by which performance is improved. However, there has not been any standardization of the control against which responses to different carbohydrate-electrolyte solutions should be compared, whether a no-drink trial, a trial where plain water is given, or a flavored water placebo in those studies where flavored drinks have been used. Many of these studies, especially those funded by the sports drinks industry, have involved comparisons of different candidate formulations in which various combinations of carbohydrate and electrolytes have been administered. These studies are clearly focused on the potential performance benefits of different formulations, and the measurement of performance itself gives valuable information on the subjective response to exercise and on the impact of different rehydration strategies. In that regard, it is important to understand the factors that may limit exercise performance in different conditions; only if this is done can effective strategies to delay fatigue and enhance performance be identified.

This chapter will review the normal cardiovascular and thermoregulatory responses to exercise and then consider the effects of fluid ingestion on exercise performance and on those responses.

5.2 CARDIOVASCULAR AND THERMOREGULATORY RESPONSES TO EXERCISE

5.2.1 BLOOD AND PLASMA VOLUME

The normal response to exercise is a reduction in blood volume, but the pattern of response and the underlying mechanisms are far from clear in all situations. The exercise intensity and duration, and the posture — upright in running, sitting with legs dependent in cycling, and sitting with legs raised in rowing, for example — are key factors that will influence the blood volume response to exercise. In high-intensity exercise, which is inevitably of short duration, plasma volume falls because of an internal redistribution of water that draws water out of the vasculature into surrounding muscle tissue. Within the active muscle cells, glycogen is broken down and the concentration of the products of glycogenolysis is increased. The primary

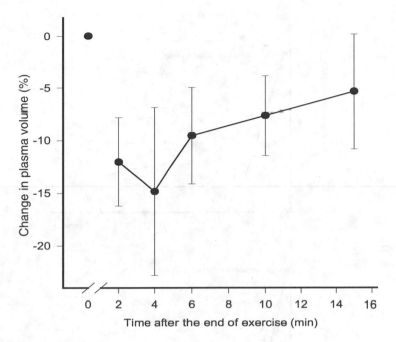

FIGURE 5.1   Reduction in blood and plasma volumes in response to high intensity exercise.

end point of the glycolytic pathway is lactate, but there are also increases in the concentration of pyruvate and of the phosphorylated intermediates of glycolysis. This large increase in the osmolality of the cells draws water from the extracellular space, and the plasma volume declines (Figure 5.1). A reduction in plasma volume occurs even in the absence of any change in the total body water content. When the exercise intensity is very high (about 100% of VO_{2max}), leading to exhaustion within a few minutes, the peak decrease in plasma volume is typically observed to occur at about 2 to 4 min after the end of exercise and to amount to about 10 to 12% of the pre-exercise volume. Given that the plasma volume amounts to about 41 to 44 ml/kg body mass,[1] this amounts to a loss of about 300 to 400 ml from the vascular space in a typical 70-kg individual. These average values, of course, conceal the variability that occurs among subjects; a decrease in plasma volume of up to 20% or even more can occur in subjects exercising to the point of fatigue in very high intensity exercise (Maughan, unpublished data).

     In prolonged exercise, there is generally an initial fall in plasma volume (and hence in blood volume) because of a movement of water into the active muscles, but this picture is reversed to some extent over time and plasma volume may return to close to the pre-exercise value in the later stages of moderate intensity exercise (Figure 5.2). There is a tendency for a greater restoration of plasma volume in running exercise than in cycling, but the interpretation of many of these studies is complicated by a failure of the investigators to ensure that the pre-exercise baseline measurement was made with subjects in an appropriate posture. If the pre-exercise blood sample is drawn with the subject in a sitting or supine position, a fall in plasma

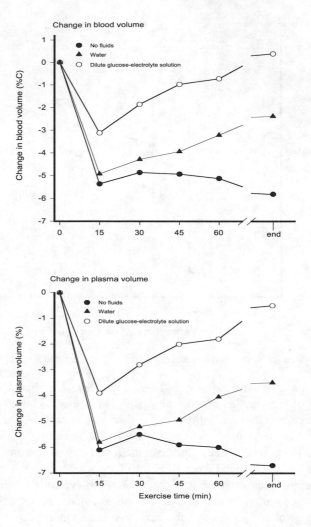

FIGURE 5.2   Blood and plasma volume changes during prolonged cycling exercise at about 70% of VO_{2max} when subjects received no fluids, water, or a dilute carbohydrate electrolyte drink at intervals throughout exercise. Data from Maughan et al. (1996).

volume of 5 to 15% is likely to occur within 15 to 20 min of assuming a standing position, even in the absence of any exercise. This reduction in plasma volume is due to an increase in hydrostatic pressure that forces water out of vessels in the legs as a person moves from a sitting to standing position. When exercise begins, the response that is observed will depend primarily on the exercise intensity and on the environmental temperature and humidity, as these factors will largely determine the sweat loss that is incurred. A high exercise intensity and a high rate of sweat loss combine to produce the greatest reduction in plasma volume.

If sweat loss is not matched by fluid intake, there will be a decrease in the total body water content and some of this water will be derived from the vascular space.

Costill[2] calculated that about 10 to 11% of sweat loss is derived from plasma water at all levels of dehydration, and that when sweat loss exceeds about 2% of body mass, the intracellular space accounts for about half of the total sweat loss. Nose et al.[3] found that the sweat sodium concentration was an important factor in determining the distribution of body water losses; changes in body fluid compartments were assessed 1 h after mild (2.3% of body mass) dehydration induced by exercise in the heat. In both of these studies, however, the time at which the measurements were made would have been a significant factor in the results obtained, as some redistribution of fluid between body compartments will take place over time.

In summary, a decline in blood volume accompanies both short-term high-intensity exercise and more prolonged exercise at lower intensities. This can be reduced by ingesting fluid during exercise to maintain important cardiovascular and thermoregulatory responses.

5.2.2 HEART RATE, STROKE VOLUME, AND CARDIAC OUTPUT

The heart rate response to exercise is determined primarily by the relative exercise intensity expressed as a fraction of the individual's maximum aerobic capacity, although the relationship is not quite linear at the highest power outputs. However, this relationship is good enough to allow prediction of maximum oxygen uptake from measurements of heart rate at submaximal exercise intensities. Endurance-trained individuals have a lower heart rate than their sedentary counterparts at any given absolute power output, reflecting the increased stroke volume of the endurance athlete.[4] Maximum heart rate is little affected by training status, but declines by about 1 beat per year of age from a peak of about 200 beats/min at the age of 20 years.

After the initial few (3 to 4) min of exercise, during which heart rate increases rapidly, something approaching a steady state is reached. If the exercise is prolonged and moderately intense, however, a steady upward drift of heart rate is normally observed to occur, even when the external power output remains constant.[5] This "cardiovascular drift" is generally ascribed to a falling stroke volume due to fluid loss from the vascular space, resulting in the need to increase heart rate to maintain cardiac output. Part of the progressive rise in heart rate may also be attributed to an exercise-induced rise in core temperature. There may be a need for an increase in cardiac output over time to meet an increasing need for skin blood flow to promote heat loss, while maintaining the blood flow to the exercising muscles. When dehydration occurs, however, an increase in heart rate may be necessary to compensate for a falling stroke volume resulting from the decreased return of blood to the heart.

There is no doubt that increasing the levels of dehydration and hyperthermia that are associated with strenuous exercise in the heat causes a reduction in stroke volume and an increased heart rate. Even then, cardiac output is not normally maintained in the latter stages of exercise, with the result that thermoregulatory capacity is impaired.[6] The fact that the increase in heart rate and the fall in cardiac output are attenuated by fluid ingestion is strong supportive evidence for the suggestion that the reduction in blood volume is responsible for these effects. When the extent of the dehydration incurred during prolonged exercise in a warm environment is manipulated by ingestion of graded volumes of fluid, the elevation of heart rate is proportional to the amount of dehydration.[7] By inducing dehydration prior to exercise and then allowing different degrees of rehydration during a 2-h recovery period prior to a second exercise test, Heaps et al.[8] were able to show that the magnitude of the cardiovascular drift was proportional to the whole body fluid deficit, but not to the blood volume, which was the same when euhydrated and at the two levels of induced hypohydration.

Recent evidence suggests that skin blood flow does not increase substantially after the first 15 min of a 60-min moderate-intensity (57% of peak VO_2) cycling exercise test in a warm (27°C) environment, and that preventing the rise in heart rate by administration of a beta-adrenoreceptor blocking agent also prevented the decline in stroke volume that occurred on the control trial.[9]

In summary, heart rate, stroke volume, and cardiac output all increase during exercise to levels required to meet the needs of active muscles for an increased supply of oxygen and nutrients and to fill the vessels of the skin with enough blood to assure adequate heat loss to the environment. Dehydration ultimately reduces cardiac output and compromises the ability of the cardiovascular system to meet the demands of both muscle and skin for an increased blood flow. Preventing dehydration by adequate fluid intake during exercise helps maintain these important cardiovascular responses.

5.2.3 BLOOD VOLUME, TISSUE BLOOD FLOW, AND MAINTENANCE OF BLOOD PRESSURE

Heat produced in the working muscles is lost from the body surface by various mechanisms as discussed below. This requires a high rate of blood flow to the skin to convect heat from the warm body core and from the exercising muscles to the skin. Muscle blood flow must also be maintained throughout exercise to ensure an adequate supply of oxygen and substrate. There is clearly the possibility, when cardiac output is limited, of a large part of the total blood volume being relocated to the periphery, leading to a decreased venous return and a potentially catastrophic fall in central venous pressure. This can be avoided by peripheral vasoconstriction in the capillary beds of the muscle or of the skin, or of both these tissues, but each of these options also has negative consequence for exercise performances and thermoregulation.

The negative effects of dehydration, hyperthermia, and exercise in the heat on endurance performance are well established, but the role of changes in cardiovascular function in this impairment of exercise performance is less clear. There may be some reduction in cardiac output during exercise in the heat, especially in the latter stages of prolonged moderately intense exercise in a warm environment, but there has been some debate as to whether this translates to a reduction in blood flow to the active muscles (which might affect substrate delivery) or to the skin (which would affect heat loss from the body).

Data from Gonzalez-Alonso et al.[10] clearly indicate a reduction in muscle blood flow during hyperthermia and hypohydration. Their subjects cycled to exhaustion at 62% of VO_{2max} in the heat (35°C) while drinking a small volume (200 ml) of concentrated carbohydrate, and repeated this later with sufficient dilute carbohydrate-electrolyte solution to match sweat losses and to provide the same amount of carbohydrate. Maintaining euhydration resulted in a markedly lower core temperature at fatigue (38.2°C) than on the dehydrated trial (39.7°C). Cardiac output, mean arterial pressure, and leg blood flow declined after the first 20 min of exercise when subjects became dehydrated and hyperthermic, but these reductions were prevented when euhydration was maintained. Cardiac output was about 3 l/min lower at the end of exercise in the dehydrated state; about 2 l/min of this was accounted for by a reduction in flow to the exercising legs. Skin blood flow, measured on the forearm, also fell progressively after the first 20 min of exercise on the dehydrated trial, but tended to increase over time when fluid intake was high.

Mora-Rodriguez et al.,[11] beginning after 30 min of exercise, infused saline, adrenaline (epinephrine), or glucose into subjects performing prolonged (120 to 150 min) moderate-intensity (65% of VO_{2max}) cycle exercise in the heat (33°C). Adrenaline infusion markedly increased the plasma adrenaline concentration, but glucose infusion suppressed both adrenaline and noradrenaline concentrations. After 30 min of exercise, core (esophageal) temperature was the same on all three trials, but thereafter, temperature was higher when adrenaline was infused than on the other trials and was lower with glucose infusion. Mean skin temperature fell during the first 30 min of exercise and thereafter was better maintained on the glucose infusion trial than with saline or adrenaline infusion. Skin temperature fell sharply within 10 min of adrenaline infusion but returned to the pre-infusion value within 10 min. Heart rate was higher with adrenaline infusion than with saline and increased less on the glucose infusion trial, but stroke volume and cardiac output were not different between trials. Forearm skin blood flow declined sharply at the onset of adrenaline infusion and remained at a reduced level for the remainder of the exercise period. Taking these data together with those of Febbraio et al.,[12] which show a smaller rise in circulating catecholamine levels when water is ingested during exercise, it is possible to suggest a mechanism by which fluid intake might limit the rise in core temperature during exercise and thus promote an increased endurance capacity.

5.2.4 THERMOREGULATION

All the body's metabolic processes involve heat production, and the rate of heat production is directly related to the rate of energy metabolism. A relatively constant fraction of about 20 to 22% of energy is available to perform external work, but the remainder appears in the body as heat. At rest, energy metabolism is low, and the energy requirement is met by aerobic metabolism at a rate that requires about 4 ml of oxygen per kg body mass per min. The rate of heat production is correspondingly low, amounting to about 60W for a 70-kg individual. Body temperature is maintained at a relatively constant level, although this varies somewhat among individuals, fluctuates with circadian rhythm, and also varies across the female menstrual cycle. A combination of physiological responses (regulation of skin blood flow, shivering) and behavioral responses (adjusting the amount of clothing, seeking shade or shelter, adjusting environmental conditions) ensure that the deep body temperature is maintained within narrow limits, although the skin temperature is allowed to fluctuate more widely.

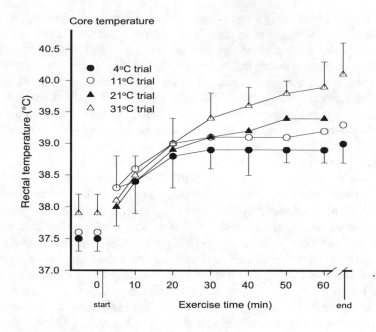

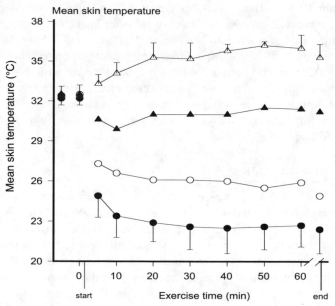

FIGURE 5.3 Effect of exercise at a fixed power output on the core (rectal) and mean skin temperature responses to exercise in eight men exercising to fatigue at different ambient temperatures. Reproduced with permission from Galloway and Maughan (1997).

During exercise, the energy demand increases in proportion to the exercise intensity and the rate of heat production increases correspondingly. In the simple locomotor activities (walking, running, swimming, cycling) the rate of energy expenditure is approximately linearly related to speed, although the relationship becomes exponential at higher speeds as the impact of air or water resistance becomes more important. In sprinting and short-duration activities, the metabolic rate is very high, but the large body mass and the high specific heat of body tissues mean that there is little change in body temperature before fatigue ensues. In longer-duration exercise, however, a progressive rise in body temperature is seen. This generally follows an exponential pattern, indicating that heat production exceeds heat loss in the early stages and that a balance is achieved in the latter stages such that the rate of heat loss rather precisely matches the rate of heat production. As the energy cost is more or less constant throughout exercise, there must be an increase in the rate of heat loss until this matches the rate of heat production. The avenues of heat loss (conduction, convection, radiation, and evaporation of sweat) and their magnitudes are described in all standard physiology textbooks.

The time course of the change in core temperature during exercise and its magnitude depend on several factors, the most important of which are the exercise intensity, the ambient temperature and humidity, and the insulating qualities of the clothing worn. The importance of ambient temperature is shown in Figure 5.3. In warm (21°C) or hot (30°C) environments, time to fatigue in cycling exercise at about 70% of VO_{2max} is less than that achieved in a cool (11°C) environment,[13] and it seems unlikely that depletion of muscle glycogen is the cause of fatigue during prolonged exercise in a warm environment. Much more likely is some change related to the hyperthermia per se; Nielsen et al.[14] have postulated a reduced motor drive in the hyperthermic state, but have not clearly identified a mechanism by which this might operate.

Several lines of evidence support a thermoregulatory, rather than metabolic or cardiovascular, limitation to prolonged exercise. Among these is the observation that exercise can be prolonged if subjects are exposed to a cold stimulus prior to exercise[15,16] and that performance is reduced if body temperature is elevated by warm water immersion prior to exercise.[17] Supporting evidence comes from the observation that the improvements in endurance performance that accompany heat acclimation are associated with a reduced resting core temperature.[14]

5.3 EFFECTS OF FLUID INTAKE DURING EXERCISE

The cardiovascular, thermoregulatory, and metabolic responses to exercise are profoundly affected by the hydration status of the individual. For the scientist, fluid administration during exercise is a tool that allows hydration status to be manipulated to investigate the regulatory processes involved. Measurement of exercise performance offers more pieces of useful information. For the athlete, fluid ingestion is seen as a way to improve performance in training and, more importantly, in competition. An understanding of the effects of fluid ingestion on responses to exercise is fundamental to the efforts of both the athlete and the scientist.

5.3.1 Effects of Fluid Ingestion on The Cardiovascular and Thermoregulatory Responses to Exercise

Given the negative effects of dehydration on exercise performance and on cardio-vascular and thermoregulatory function, restoration of euhydration offers the prospect of improved performance and better homeostatic control. Oral ingestion of fluids during exercise can be effective in replacing losses in sweat and in supplying fuel substrates. Carbohydrate-electrolyte solutions are usually the fluid of choice during prolonged exercise, and much interest has focused on the metabolic fate of the ingested carbohydrate, but this section will focus on the replacement of water and electrolyte losses. The effects of carbohydrate ingestion are covered in detail in Chapter 6.

Pitts et al.[18] conducted one of the first studies into the effects of prolonged exercise (4 h) with or without fluid replacement. They observed that the increases in heart rate and in core temperature that occurred were both attenuated by drinking fluid, and that plain water, dilute saline (0.2% NaCl), and dilute (3.5%) glucose solutions were all equally effective. When the subjects drank fluid in excess of the amount voluntarily consumed, but sufficient to match the rate of sweat loss, there were more-pronounced positive effects than when fluid intake was allowed on a voluntary basis. Many studies have since confirmed these observations and have demonstrated that fluid intake is also effective in reducing the negative impact of heat and dehydration on exercise performance.[19]

Many of the early studies were confounded by inadequate methodology for the assessment of cardiovascular function. In an elegant series of studies, Coyle and his colleagues have looked at the changes that occur during prolonged exercise and at the effects of varying levels of dehydration on cardiovascular and thermoregulatory mechanisms. Many of these results were summarized by Coyle and Montain,[6] but much new information has been added since then. For example, Hamilton et al.[20] showed that fluid replacement, in a volume sufficient to replace water loss, during 2 h of exercise at about 10 to 75% of VO_{2max} was effective in preventing the fall in stroke volume and reversing the fall in cardiac output that developed over time when no fluid was given. When fluid intake was prescribed, cardiac output and heart rate increased progressively over the exercise period. On both the water and no-fluid trials, oxygen consumption also increased over time. Nielsen et al.[21] had previously shown, using measurements of oxygen uptake across the exercising legs, that this upward drift of oxygen consumption was not occurring in the working muscles.

The idea that fluid replacement improved thermoregulatory function and exercise performance by minimizing any decrease in blood volume was challenged by Montain and Coyle.[22] In this study, their subjects exercised for 2 h in a hot (33°C) environment and were given either no fluid, a volume of a carbohydrate-electrolyte drink sufficient to replace about 80% of sweat loss (about 2.4 l in total), or an intravenous infusion of about 400 ml of an artificial plasma volume expander. Blood and plasma volumes on the oral replacement trial were generally intermediate between those on the other two trials: at the end of exercise, plasma volume had fallen by about 2% with the intravenous infusion, about 6% with oral fluids, and by about 9% on the trial where no fluid was given. Oral fluid replacement was effective in attenuating the rise in core temperature that was observed on the other two trials, suggesting that this effect is mediated by a mechanism other than one involving blood volume.

In another important study using the same conditions as those described above, Montain and Coyle[23] exposed subjects to graded levels of dehydration by prescribing different volumes (0, 20, 50, and 80% of sweat loss) of the same carbohydrate-electrolyte drink. The decline in stroke volume and cardiac output, and the increase in heart rate and core temperature, were all related to the magnitude of the fluid deficit incurred. In a third study in this series by Montain and Coyle[24], a close relationship was observed between the exercise-induced increase in core temperature and the decrease in forearm skin blood flow. The same group of authors later confirmed that preventing dehydration by ingestion of sufficient fluid to meet 95% of the sweat loss was effective in preventing the progressive decline in cardiac output and the small but significant decrease in mean arterial pressure that was seen when subjects were allowed to become dehydrated.[25] Fluid intake was also effective in limiting the rise in core temperature. Systemic vascular resistance and cutaneous vascular resistance increased over time in the dehydrated trial, but did not change after the first 20 min of exercise when euhydration was maintained. The reduced skin blood flow in the dehydrated condition is surprising, given the higher core temperature on this trial, but presumably reflects the higher circulating catecholamine concentrations.

McConnell et al.[26] used a similar experimental model, but conducted their study in a cooler (21°C) environment; during 2 h of cycle exercise at 69% of VO_{2max}, their subjects received no fluid, sufficient water to prevent a decrease in body mass, or 50% of this amount of water. They also added a performance ride to exhaustion at 90% of VO_{2max} after the initial 2 h of exercise. Fluid replacement attenuated the increases in heart rate, rectal temperature and plasma sodium concentration and the decrease in plasma volume, with the larger fluid intake having a greater effect. Endurance time in the performance ride was longer with the large fluid volume (328 sec) than the no-fluid trial (171 sec), and was intermediate on the 50% replacement trial (248 sec). Taken together, these studies suggest that the ability to maintain a high skin blood flow is a key factor in limiting the rise in core temperature that occurs during exercise in the heat, and that hydration status plays a vital role in this process.

In contrast to the findings of Montain and Coyle, there are several reports that suggest that plasma volume expansion may alter the thermoregulatory response to exercise. Coyle and Montain[6] suggested that the differences in observed responses may be attributed to differences in training and acclimation status of subjects and to differences in environmental conditions. In particular, skin temperature may be an important variable, and this is strongly influenced by ambient temperature and humidity and by air movement, which will affect the rate of evaporation from the skin surface. High tissue osmolality and sodium concentrations can impair heat dissipation by reducing skin blood flow and sweating responsiveness,[27] and a close relationship is seen between the plasma sodium concentration and the steady state core temperature during exercise.[28] Although there are obvious links between blood volume and thermoregulatory function in exercise, this suggests another mechanism by which fluid replacement might promote heat loss.

Maintaining a high skin temperature is important in promoting the evaporation of sweat from the skin surface. The higher the skin temperature, the greater the vapor pressure gradient between the skin surface and the environment, and it is this vapor pressure gradient that drives the evaporation of water from the skin surface. If skin temperature falls because of a reduction in skin blood flow, skin temperature will fall and evaporative capacity will be reduced.

5.3.2   EFFECTS OF FLUID INGESTION ON THE METABOLIC RESPONSE TO EXERCISE

Muscle glycogen depletion is commonly accepted as the most likely limiting factor to performance in prolonged (1 to 3 h duration) exercise performed in temperate environmental conditions, even though there is compelling evidence that this is not the case at higher ambient temperatures. The primary purpose of the ingestion of carbohydrate-containing drinks in this situation is to slow the rate of muscle glycogen utilization and thus delay the point at which a critically low value is reached.

Hargreaves et al.[29] investigated the effects of water ingestion on muscle glycogen utilization during 2 h of cycling exercise at 67% of peak VO_2 at an ambient temperature of 20 to 22°C. On one trial, no fluid was allowed and on the other, sufficient water was ingested to maintain body mass. Water ingestion resulted in a lower heart rate throughout exercise and in lower rectal and muscle temperatures at the end of exercise. The total amount of glycogen used was 16% less on the trial where water was ingested than on the no-fluid trial. Water ingestion was accompanied by a smaller rise in circulating catecholamine levels during the second hour of exercise, which might, at least in part, be responsible for the lower rate of glycogenolysis.[30] The lower muscle temperature when fluids were ingested may also be partly responsible for the lower rate of glycogen breakdown.[12]

The finding of an increased rate of carbohydrate use during prolonged cycling in the heat when subjects are deprived of fluid has been confirmed by Gonzalez-Alonso et al.[17] When a small volume of fluid (0.2 l orally of a concentrated carbohydrate solution and 0.6 l of saline by infusion) was provided, blood flow to the exercising legs declined in the latter stages of exercise, but it tended to increase during this time when subjects drank a volume (3.7 l) of a dilute carbohydrate-electrolyte solution sufficient to prevent a decline in body mass. Carbohydrate intake was matched on the two trials. In spite of the lower leg blood flow on the dehydrated trial, glucose delivery was the same on both trials. Muscle glycogen utilization was, however, higher by 45% on the dehydrated trial. In the conditions of this study, however, muscle glycogen did not reach critically low levels at the end of exercise, and was excluded as a cause of fatigue.

Several other studies have confirmed that exercise in the heat is not likely to be limited by the availability of muscle glycogen. The significance of the increased rate of carbohydrate utilization in conditions of hyperthermia and dehydration therefore remains to be established.

5.3.3 EFFECTS OF ADDITION OF ELECTROLYTES TO DRINKS CONSUMED DURING EXERCISE

There has been much debate as to the value of the addition of electrolytes to fluids ingested during exercise, and the argument remains unresolved. Dill et al.[31] recalculated the original data reported by Adolph et al.[32] and reported that saline ingestion during prolonged walking in a hot environment resulted in a higher fluid intake and less urine output than on trials where plain water was consumed; positive fluid balance (by 110 ml) was maintained on saline trials as opposed to a negative balance of 600 ml with plain water. However, experimental data reported by Dill et al.[31] tended to suggest that plasma volume was better maintained when saline was ingested than on trials where water was consumed.

Because the sodium concentration of sweat is invariably less than that of plasma, the normal response to large sweat losses incurred during exercise is a rise in the plasma sodium concentration and in plasma osmolality. These responses are largely responsible for driving the thirst mechanism that stimulates fluid intake. Physicians dealing with individuals in distress at the end of long-distance races have become accustomed to dealing with hyperthermia associated with dehydration and hypernatremia, but it is now well documented that a small number of individuals at the end of very prolonged events may be suffering from hyponatremia in conjunction with either hyperhydration or hypohydration. The experimental evidence for this was reviewed by Maughan.[33]

All the reported cases of hyponatremia have been associated with ultramarathon or prolonged triathlon events; most have occurred in events lasting in excess of 8 h, although there are few reports of cases where the exercise duration is less than 4 h. These cases are characterized by low plasma sodium, usually in the range of about 115 to 125 mmol/l, and a high intake of fluids with low electrolyte content during exercise. That a dilutional hyponatremia should occur during exercise when sweat losses are significant should not perhaps be too surprising. Hyponatremia as a consequence of ingestion of large volumes of fluids with a low sodium content has also been recognized in resting individuals. Flear et al.[34] reported the case of a man who drank 9 l of beer, with a sodium content of 1.5 mmol/l, in the space of 20 mins; plasma sodium fell from 143 mmol/l before to 127 mmol/l after drinking, but the man appeared unaffected. In these cases, there is clearly a replacement of water in excess of losses with inadequate electrolyte replacement. In competitors in the Hawaii Ironman Triathlon who have been found to be hyponatremic, however, dehydration has also been reported to be present,[35] and this observation is more difficult to explain.

These reports are interesting and indicate that some supplementation with sodium chloride may be required in prolonged events where large sweat losses can be expected and where there are opportunities to consume large volumes of fluid. Athletes training hard in hot environments, especially those training more than once per day, will also incur large water and electrolyte losses. This should not, however, divert attention away from the fact that electrolyte replacement during exercise is not a priority for most participants in most sporting events, although it is certainly helpful after the event to restore body water and electrolyte content (see Chapter 7).

5.3.4 Effects of Temperature of Ingested Beverages

It is well recognized that the temperature of ingested fluids can affect a variety of sensory and physiological functions. The most important effect of temperature may be on beverage palatability, which, in turn, will affect voluntary fluid intake. Cool drinks are generally preferred, and the volume of water ingested on a voluntary basis decreases as the water temperature increases, although this effect may be overcome when the physiological stimuli (plasma osmolality, sodium concentration) are strong.[36] The preferred temperature for fluid intake seems to be about 15°C; the studies on which this observation is based have been reviewed by Hubbard et al.[37] The effect of temperature on fluid intake is discussed further in Chapter 3.

Although the effects of drink temperature in influencing the volume of fluid ingested may be more important, there are also potential effects on physiological function. The temperature of ingested drinks may influence the rate of gastric emptying and subsequent intestinal absorption, but this effect is generally rather small (see Chapter 4).

There have been a limited number of investigations of the effect of ingesting beverages at different temperatures on the thermoregulatory response to exercise. Wimer et al.[38] studied the response to ingestion of water at a temperature of 0.5°C, 19°C, or 38°C on the responses to 2 h of low-intensity exercise (51% VO_{2max}) at an ambient temperature of 26°C. The cold drink (0.5°C) was effective in attenuating the rise in core temperature, forearm blood flow, and sweat rate relative to the trial where the warm (38°C) water was ingested. The cool (19°C) drink also reduced the rate of rise in core temperature relative to the trial where the warm water was ingested. Irrespective of the temperature of the drinks, however, ingestion of water on all trials reduced the rate of rise of core temperature relative to the trial where no fluid was ingested. These data suggest two important roles of fluid intake. First, fluid ingestion itself can help to maintain thermoregulatory function by attenuating or reversing the normal exercise-induced contraction of blood volume. Second, a bolus of cold fluid represents a heat deficit, and heat energy must be added to the ingested fluid to raise it to body temperature. This latter effect is often ignored, but it will help to increase exercise capacity by delaying the point at which a critical core temperature is reached. Dill et al.[31] showed that ingestion of 2.4 l of water at a temperature of 15°C reduced body temperature during exercise by an amount very close to the calculated 1°C.

5.4 EFFECTS OF FLUID INGESTION ON EXERCISE PERFORMANCE

The effects of feeding different types and amounts of beverages on exercise performance have been investigated using a wide variety of experimental models. Not all of the published studies have shown a positive effect of fluid ingestion on performance, but, with the exception of a few investigations where the composition or volume of the drinks administered was such as to result in gastrointestinal disturbances or subjective discomfort, there are no studies showing that fluid ingestion will have an adverse effect on performance. It must, of course, be recognized that scientific journals are less likely to publish studies that are perceived as failing to produce a positive effect.

5.4.1 Assessment of Exercise Performance

Until very recently, laboratory investigations into the ergogenic effects of the administration of carbohydrate-electrolyte drinks generally relied on changes in exercise time to exhaustion at a fixed work rate as a measure of performance. This approach has several advantages. The constant power output allows measures of physiological function to be compared between trials in the early stages of exercise. Performance is also relatively reproducible; repeatability of performance is generally better in well-trained individuals, but is also repeatable in subjects who are not highly trained athletes, provided that suitable familiarization trials are allowed before the subjects take part in experimental trials. In a study by Maughan et al.,[39] subjects completed two trials to exhaustion under the same experimental conditions, with these trials separated by 5 weeks during which various other fluid replacement strategies were evaluated; the mean of the differences in exercise time between the two trials was 5.9%, but the mean exercise time for the two trials was 72.2 min for the first trial and 71.5 min for the second. These results contrast markedly with those of Jeukendrup et al.,[40] who reported a coefficient of variation of 27% when 10 well-trained subjects performed five tests to exhaustion at a constant power output of 75% of maximal workload. These results seem remarkable; with a mean exercise time for all subjects over all trials of 61.8 min, the inter-individual range was 27.5 to 83.8 min, even though all subjects were supposedly exercising at the same fraction of their maximum. Likewise, most subjects showed a twofold range between trials. This is not the common experience, provided that precautions are taken to standardize the pre-exercise conditions and to ensure that subjects are completely familiar with the exercise task.

Even allowing for fluctuations in performance, there are difficulties in extrapolating results obtained in trials at constant speed or effort to a race situation where the workload is likely to fluctuate as the pace, the weather conditions, and the topography vary, and where tactical considerations and motivational factors are involved. It is possible to demonstrate large differences in the time for which a fixed power output can be sustained in laboratory tests when carbohydrate solutions are given during exercise. For example, Coyle et al.[41] reported a 30% increase in endurance capacity (from 3 to 4 h) in response to carbohydrate administration, and Maughan et al.[39] observed an increase in endurance time from 70.2 min when no fluid was given to 91 min when a dilute carbohydrate-electrolyte solution was administered at intervals throughout exercise. In a simulated race situation, where a fixed distance had to be covered as fast as possible, the advantage would translate to no more than a few percent, and in a real competition it would probably be even less. Even a few percent, however, is often the difference between a world class performance and a mediocre one; in running, 5% represents about 10 sec over 1500 meters and 7 min over the marathon distance at world-class level.

In an attempt to make their results more relevant to competitive athletes, some recent investigations have used exercise tests involving intermittent exercise, simulated races, or prolonged exercise with intermediate sprints and with a sprint finish. The repeatability of time trial performances in the laboratory over distances of 20 km and 40 km was measured and was compared with performance in a road time trial by Palmer et al.[42] Time taken for the rides was found to be highly reproducible, with a coefficient of variation of about 1%. Jeukendrup et al.,[40] as part of the same study referred to above, found a rather larger coefficient of variance of 3.4% for a 1-h cycling time trial. Schabort et al.[43] used a 100-km cycling time trial with intermediate sprints. They found, as was already well known, that performance improved from trial 1 to trial 2, but that there was little or no change between trials 2 and 3. The test was found to be highly reliable (coefficient of variation of 1.7%), and performance in the inter-mediate sprints showed a similarly small variability. The same authors[44] also examined the variability in performance of a 60-min time trial run on a treadmill. They concluded that, though the variability was again small (about 2.7%), the test was not sufficiently reproducible to detect meaningful changes in performance without using unrealistically large numbers of subjects. Jeukendrup et al.[40] also looked at the variability of an exercise model where subjects exercised for 45 min at 70% of maximum power output followed by a 15-min time trial where they completed as much work as possible. Their CV was about the same (3.5%) as for the 60-min time trial. It must be noted that these trials all involved well trained competitive runners or cyclists, and it is highly unlikely that the typical laboratory subject would perform well in time trial tests, which demand a good sense of pace and effort.

5.4.2 LABORATORY STUDIES — CYCLING TO FATIGUE AT CONSTANT POWER OUTPUT

Ingestion of water alone or of carbohydrate-electrolyte solutions can improve per-formance in a variety of exercise situations, but even when the exercise model used is apparently similar, different results have been obtained. In some cases, the studies are unreliable; poor choice of experimental model, lack of appropriate controls, and failure to familiarize subjects with the experimental procedures prior to testing invalidate some of the published studies. Even where appropriate control is evident, the presence of different mixtures of carbohydrates in varying concentrations along with various electrolytes, often in unspecified concentrations, and different flavoring agents makes interpretation of the results of many of the published studies difficult. Added to this are differences between studies in the choice of the exercise test used, the training and acclimation status of the subjects, and the environmental conditions, making comparisons between studies even more difficult. Variations in the volume and temperature of fluid prescribed, the frequency of intake, and the extent of dehydration incurred further complicate the picture. These studies have been the subject of a number of extensive reviews that have concentrated on the effects of administration of carbohydrate, electrolytes, and water on exercise performance. Maughan and Shirreffs[45] have reviewed the recent literature and have referred to a number of excellent reviews of the earlier literature.

For the same commercial reasons that have driven so many of these studies, there have been surprisingly few studies of cycling exercise where the effect of water administration has been compared with trials where no fluid was allowed. Some studies, however, have included both plain water and no-drink trials in their comparisons. In the study of Maughan et al.,[46] 12 male subjects exercised to fatigue at about 70% of VO_{2max} on four occasions after appropriate familiarization tests. When subjects ingested plain water (100 ml every 10 min) median exercise time was longer (93 min) than when no drink was given (81 min). Subjects also completed trials where dilute carbohydrate-electrolyte drinks were given and these also extended exercise time compared to the no-drink trial.

In more prolonged exercise at low intensity, water may be as effective as dilute saline solutions[47] or nutrient-electrolyte solutions[48] in maintaining cardiovascular and thermoregulatory function. It is clear, however, that the addition of carbohydrate has a number of potential benefits, including a reduction in the rate of decline of muscle glycogen concentration, which may be important for performance. Studies where carbohydrate has been added to ingested fluids will be discussed in detail in the following chapter.

5.4.3 OTHER LABORATORY STUDIES — CYCLING

Several studies have employed an experimental model consisting of prolonged intermittent exercise followed by a brief high-intensity sprint, and again the results are not altogether consistent. Most of these studies have tested various combinations of carbohydrate and electrolytes, and have failed to compare trials with no fluid and with the ingestion of plain water. Below et al.[49] used an experimental model where subjects performed 50 min of exercise at about 80% of VO_{2max} followed by a time trial where a set amount of work had to be completed as fast as possible. During the initial 50 min of exercise, subjects were given either a small volume (200 ml) of water, a small volume of water with added carbohydrate (40% solution, 79 g of maltodextrin), a large volume (1330 ml) of flavored water, or a large volume of water with the same amount of carbohydrate as in the other carbohydrate trial (a 6% solution). They found water ingestion to be effective in improving performance; exercise time was 11.34 min on the placebo trial and 10.51 min on the water trial. Exercise time on the carbohydrate trial was 10.55 min, indicating that carbohydrate provision during exercise acted independently to improve performance, and the effects were found to be additive, with the shortest time (9.93 min) when the 6% carbohydrate drink was given.

5.4.4 OTHER LABORATORY STUDIES — RUNNING

As with studies during cycling exercise, many different exercise models have been used to investigate the effects of the administration of carbohydrate-electrolyte solutions during walking and running. Macaraeg[50] compared endurance time during running at 85% of maximum heart rate when subjects were given no fluid, water, or a 7% carbohydrate-electrolyte solution which provided 84 g of carbohydrate in a volume of 1.2 l. Mean running times were 56 min with no drink, 78 min with water, and 102 min with the carbohydrate-electrolyte drink. The environmental conditions were not specified in this study, but it does indicate that plain water can improve endurance capacity, and that addition of carbohydrate and electrolytes confers a further benefit, a pattern similar to that observed by Below et al.[49] in cycling.

Williams[51] and Williams et al.[52] have used an experimental model in which the subject is able to adjust the treadmill speed while running; the subject can then be encouraged either to cover the maximum distance possible in a fixed time or to complete a fixed distance in the fastest time possible. They showed that ingestion of 1 l of a glucose polymer-sucrose (50 g/l) solution did not increase the total distance covered in a 2-h run, but running speed was greater over the last 30 min of exercise when carbohydrate was given compared with a placebo trial.[51] They also observed a similar effect when a carbohydrate solution (50 grams of glucose-glucose polymer, or 50 grams of fructose-glucose polymer) or water was given in a 30-km treadmill time trial.[52] In this study, running speed decreased over the last 10 km of the water trial, but was maintained throughout the whole distance on the other two runs; there was no significant difference among the three trials in the time taken to cover the total distance. As with cycling exercise, the conclusion must be that ingestion of carbohydrate-containing drinks is generally effective in improving performance relative to trials where plain water or water-placebo is given. This does not tell us whether water alone is effective in this experimental model.

Not all studies have shown beneficial effects of ingestion of carbohydrate-electrolyte drinks on exercise performance. In a further variation of the running model, the subjects of Nassis et al.[53] performed two prolonged, intermittent, high-intensity shuttle runs at an unspecified ambient temperature; on one trial, subjects ingested a flavored water placebo and on the other trial they ingested a 6.9% carbohydrate-electrolyte drink. Exercise performance was not different between trials: subjects ran for an average of 113 min on the placebo trial and 110 min when drinking the sports drink.

5.4.5 FIELD STUDIES

There are many practical difficulties associated with the conduct of field trials to assess the efficacy of ergogenic aids, which accounts for the fact that few well controlled studies of the effects of administration of carbohydrate-electrolyte solutions have been carried out in this way. The main problem is with the design of an adequately controlled trial. In competitive events where a benefit of fluid ingestion might be anticipated, it is unrealistic to expect competitors to repeat the same effort, and where a crossover design is used, this is likely to be confounded by changes in the environmental conditions between trials. The use of parallel control and test groups (i.e., matched groups) raises the difficulties of recruiting an adequate number of experimental subjects and of appropriately matching the groups. Many of the early studies purporting to show beneficial effects of ingestion of carbohydrate-containing solutions on performance in events such as cycling, canoeing, and soccer were so poorly designed that the results are of no value.

Cade et al.[54] gave subjects no fluids or approximately 1 l of hypotonic saline or a glucose-electrolyte solution during a 7-mile course consisting of walking and running at an ambient temperature of 32 to 34°C. None of the subjects completed the course when no fluid was given, and the mean distance covered was 4.7 miles; when saline was given, they covered a mean distance of 5.5 miles, and all subjects completed the 7-mile course when given the glucose-electrolyte solution. These results imply a benefit from ingestion of saline and a further benefit from the addition of carbohydrate. Apart from the early studies of prolonged walking in the heat by Adolph et al.[32] and Pitts et al.,[18] there are few studies in which these comparisons are made.

Studies where matched groups of competitors consumed 1.4 l of either water or a glucose-electrolyte solution during a marathon race[55] or 1.4 l of different carbo-hydrate-containing drinks during marathon and ultramarathon races[56] have shown no differences between the groups in finishing time. In the study of Maughan and Whiting,[55] subjects were matched on the basis of their anticipated finishing times. Many of these individuals had not previously completed a marathon, so these times must be considered unreliable. Nonetheless, mean finishing time for the runners (n = 43) drinking the carbohydrate-electrolyte solution was 220 ± 40 min compared with a predicted finishing time of 220 ± 35 min; for the group drinking water (n = 47) actual finishing time was 217 ± 32 min and predicted time was 212 ± 32 min. Twenty four runners (60%) in the carbohydrate-electrolyte group ran faster than expected, compared with 19 (40%) in the water group.

More recently, Tsintzas et al.[57] gave runners in a simulated road race held over a distance of 30 km either a commercially formulated 5% carbohydrate solution or plain water and found an improved (by a mean of 2.9 min) performance on the trial where the carbohydrate solution was given. The mean time to complete 30 km (about 130 min) indicates that the subjects in this study were not well trained. This study does not tell us whether administration of plain water would improve performance in this experimental model relative to a trial where no fluid was given. The absence of information on environmental temperature and humidity also makes it difficult to place this study in the context of laboratory studies, which are normally carried out under well-defined conditions.

5.4.6 OTHER EXERCISE MODELS

Performance is more difficult to assess in complex tasks such as those involved in most sports, but the common assumption is that an improved exercise tolerance will lead to an improved playing performance — especially in the latter stages when fatigue is more pronounced. In many sports, however, the ability to continue to perform skilled movements is more important than simple endurance capacity, and several studies have been conducted to look at performance of specific components of various sports activities. In most of the studies that have been conducted, carbo-hydrate-containing solutions have been compared with placebo drinks or with no-drink trials; there are few studies where all the options (no drink, water, water plus carbohydrate) have been compared. Shephard and Leatt[58] gave 1 l of a 7% glucose polymer solution or a flavored placebo to football (soccer) players during a practice game. During the match, the group who had been given carbohydrate utilized 31% less glycogen than the placebo group. No measure of performance of the two groups was made, but it was proposed that the players taking the glucose polymer would experience a beneficial effect in the latter stages of the game. Nicholas et al.[59] simulated the running pattern of ball games using an intermittent high-intensity shuttle running test. Ingestion of a carbohydrate-electrolyte drink was effective in improving performance compared with a trial where a non-carbohydrate placebo was given. In contrast to these findings, Zeederberg et al.[60] reported that ingestion of a glucose polymer drink before and at half time in a soccer game played in a cool (13 to 15°C) environment had no effect on most measures of playing performance, and players achieved fewer successful tackles when drinking the glucose polymer than on the control trial.

5.5 SUMMARY

Prolonged exercise is accompanied by a loss of fluid and electrolytes from the body due to the sweating response. Plasma volume falls, in part because of sweat loss and in part because of a redistribution of fluid between the body water compartments. Increasing levels of dehydration result in a decrease in cardiac stroke volume and, in spite of an increased heart rate, cardiac output may fall. Muscle and skin blood flow fall as the level of dehydration increases. Fluid intake can serve to maintain the plasma volume and also allows better maintenance of thermal homeostasis by promoting evaporative cooling. Fluid provision also has metabolic effects: there is a decreased rate of glycogenolysis when water is ingested, perhaps due to the lower circulating catecholamine levels. Addition of electrolytes to ingested fluids helps maintain plasma volume and may be important when sweat losses are large. Water ingestion has been shown to improve exercise performance in many studies using different experimental models, but relatively few studies have looked at the effects of water itself without the addition of carbohydrate and other compounds.

REFERENCES

1. Lentner, C., *Geigy Scientific Tables*. Volume 3. *Physical Chemistry, Composition of Blood, Hematology, Somatometric Data.* 8th ed. Ciba-Geigy, Basle. p 65, 1984.
2. Costill, D.L., Sweating: its composition and effects on body fluids. *Ann. NY Acad. Sci.* 301, 160-174, 1977.
3. Nose, H., Mack, G.W., Shi, X.R., and Nadel, E.R., Shift in body fluid compartments after dehydration in humans. *J. App. Physiol.* 65, 318-324, 1988.
4. Maughan, R.J., Aerobic function. *Sport Sci. Rev.* 1, 28-42, 1992.
5. Rowell, L.B., *Human Circulation*. Oxford University Press, 1986, NY.
6. Coyle, E.F., Montain, S.J., Thermal and cardiovascular responses to fluid replacement during exercise, in *Exercise, Heat and Thermoregulation*, Gisolfi, C.V., Lamb, D.R., and Nadel, E.R., Eds., Brown and Benchmark, Carmel, IN, 1993, Chap. 5.
7. Coyle, E.F., Montain, S.F., Benefits of fluid replacement with carbohydrate during exercise. *Med. Sci. Sports Exerc.* 24, S324-S330, 1992.
8. Heaps, C.L., Gonzalez-Alonso, J., and Coyle, E.F., Hypohydration causes cardiovascular drift without reducing blood volume. *Int. J. Sports Med.* 15, 74-79, 1994.
9. Fritzsche, R.G., Switzer, T.W., Hodgkinson, B.J., Coyle, E.F., Stroke volume decline during prolonged exercise is influenced by the increase in heart rate. *J. App. Physiol.* 86, 799-805, 1999.
10. Gonzalez-Alonso, J., Calbet, J.A.L., Nielsen, B., Muscle blood flow is reduced with dehydration during prolonged exercise in humans. *J. Physiol.* 513, 895-905, 1998.

11. Mora-Rodriguez, R., Gonzalez-Alonso, J., Below, P.R., and Coyle, E.F., Plasma catecholamines and hyperglycaemia influence thermoregulation in man during prolonged exercise in the heat. *J. Physiol.* 491, 529-540, 1996.

12. Febbraio, M.A., Carey, M.F., Snow, R.J., Stathis, C.G., and Hargreaves, M., Influence of elevated muscle temperature on metabolism during intense, dynamic exercise. *Am. J. Physiol.* 271, R1252-R1255, 1996.

13. Galloway, S.D.R., Maughan, R.J., Effects of ambient temperature on the capacity to perform prolonged cycle exercise in man. *Med. Sci. Sports Exerc.* 29, 1240-1249, 1997.

14. Nielsen, B., Hales, J.R.S., Strange, S., Christensen, N.J., Warberg, J., and Saltin, B., Human circulatory and thermoregulatory adaptations with heat acclimation and exercise in a hot, dry environment. *J. Physiol.* 460, 467-486, 1993.

15. Booth, J., Marino, F., and Ward, J.J., Improved running performance in hot humid conditions following whole body precooling. *Med. Sci. Sports Exerc.* 29, 943-949, 1997.

16. Schmidt, V. and Bruck, K., Effect of a precooling maneuver on body temperature and exercise performance. *J. App. Physiol.* 50, 772-778, 1981.

17. Gonzalez-Alonso, J., Teller, C., Andersen, C. L., Jensen, F.B., Hyldig, T., and Nielsen, B., Influence of body temperature on the development of fatigue during prolonged exercise in the heat. *J. App. Physiol.* 86, 1032-1039, 1999.

18. Pitts, R.F., Johnson, R.E., and Consolazio, F.C., Work in the heat as affected by intake of water, salt and glucose. *Am. J. Physiol.* 142, 253-259, 1944.

19. Nadel, E.R., Mack, G.W., and Nose, H., Influence of fluid replacement beverages on body fluid homeostasis during exercise and recovery. Fluid homeostasis during exercise, Gisolfi, C.V. and Lamb, D.R., Benchmark, Carmel, IN, 1990, chap. 5.

20. Hamilton, M.T., Alonso, J.G., Montain, S.J., and Coyle, E.F. Fluid replacement and glucose infusion during exercise prevents cardiovascular drift. *J. App. Physiol.* 71, 871-877, 1991.

21. Nielsen, B., Savard, G., Richter, E.A., Hargreaves, M., and Saltin, B., Muscle blood flow and muscle metabolism during exercise and heat stress. *J. App. Physiol.* 69, 1040-1046, 1990.

22. Montain, S.J. and Coyle, E.F., Fluid ingestion during exercise increases skin blood flow independent of increases in blood volume. *J. App. Physiol.* 73, 903-910, 1992.

23. Montain, S.J.and Coyle, E.F., Influence of graded dehydration on hyperthermia and cardiovascular drift during exercise. *J. App. Physiol.* 73, 1340-1350, 1992.

24. Montain, S.J. and Coyle, E.F., Influence of the timing of fluid ingestion on temperature regulation during exercise. *J. App. Physiol.* 75, 688-695, 1993.

25. Gonzalez-Alonso, J., Mora-Rodriguez, R., Below, P.R., and Coyle, E.F., Dehydration reduces cardiac output and increases systemic and cutaneous vascular resistance during exercise. *J. App. Physiol.* 79, 1487-1496, 1995.

26. McConnell, G.K., Burge, C.,M., Skinner, S.L., and Hargreaves, M., Influence of ingested fluid volume on physiological responses during prolonged exercise. *Acta Physiologica Scandinavica* 160, 149-156, 1997.

27. Fortney, S.M., Wenger, C.B., Bove, J.R., and Nadel, E.R., Effect of hyperosmolality on control of blood flow and sweating. *J. App. Physiol.* 57, 1688-1695, 1984.

28. Greenleaf, J.E., Convertino, V.A., Stremel, R.W., Bernauer, E.M., Adams, W.C., Vignau, S.R., and Brock, P.J., Plasma $[Na^+]$ and $[Ca^{2+}]$, and volume shifts and thermoregulation during exercise in man. *J. App. Physiol.* 43, 1026-1032, 1977.

29. Hargreaves, M., Dillo, P., Angus, D., and Febbraio, M., Effect of fluid ingestion on muscle metabolism during prolonged exercise. *J. App. Physiol.* 80, 363-366, 1996.

30. Febbraio, M.A., Lambert, D.L., Starkie, R.L., Proietto, J., and Hargreaves, M., Effect of epinephrine on muscle glycogenolysis during exercise in trained men. *J. App. Physiol.* 84, 465-470, 1998.

31. Dill, D.B., Yousef, M.K., and Nelson, J.D., Responses of men and women to 2-h walks in desert heat. *J. App. Physiol.* 35, 231-235, 1973.

32. Adolph, E.F. and Associates. *Physiology of Man in the Desert*. Interscience, NY, 1947.

33. Maughan, R.J. Carbohydrate-electrolyte solutions during prolonged exercise, in *Ergogenics Enhancement of Performance in Exercise and Sport*, Lamb, D.R. and Williams, M.H., Eds., Brown and Benchmark, Carmel, IN, Chap. 2. 1993.

34. Flear, C.T.G., Gill, C.V., and Burn, J,. Beer drinking and hyponatraemia. *Lancet* 2, 477, 1981.

35. Hiller, W.D.B., Dehydration and hyponatraemia during triathlons. *Med. Sci. Sports Exerc.* 21, S219-S221, 1989.

36. Armstrong, L.E., Costill, D.L., and Fink, W.J., Changes in body water and electrolytes during heat acclimation: effects of dietary sodium. *Aviation Space and Environ. Med.* 58, 143-148, 1987.

37. Hubbard, R.W., Szlyk, P.C., and Armstrong, L.E., Influence of thirst and fluid palatability on fluid ingestion during exercise. *Fluid homeostasis during exercise in Perspectives in Exercise Science and Sports Medicine Volume 3: Fluid Homeostasis During Exercise*. Gisolfi, C.V. and Lamb, D.R., Eds., Brown & Benchmark, Carmel, IN, 1990.

38. Wimer, G.S., Lamb, D.R., Sherman, W.M., and Swanson, S.C., Temperature of ingested water and thermoregulation during moderate-intensity exercise. *Can. J. App. Physiol.* 22, 479-493, 1997.

39. Maughan, R.J., Fenn, C.E., and Leiper, J.B., Effects of fluid, electrolyte and substrate ingestion on endurance capacity. *Europ. J. App. Physiol.* 58, 481-486, 1989.

40. Jeukendrup, A., Saris, W.H.M., Brouns, F., and Kester, A.D.M., A new validated endurance performance test. *Med. Sci. Sports Exerc.* 28, 266-270, 1996.

41. Coyle, E.F., Coggan, A.R., Hemmert, M.K., and Ivy, J.L., Muscle glycogen utilization during prolonged strenuous exercise when fed carbohydrate. *J. App. Physiol.* 61, 165-172, 1986.

42. Palmer, G.S., Dennis, S.C., Noakes, T.D., and Hawley, J.A., Assessment of the reproducibility of performance testing on an air-braked cycle ergometer. *Int. J. Sports Med.* 17, 293-298, 1996.

43. Schabort, E.J., Hawley, J.A., Hopkins, W.G., Mujika, I., and Noakes T.D. A new reliable laboratory test of endurance performance for road cyclists. *Med. Sci. Sports Exerc.* 30, 1744-1750, 1998a.

44. Schabort, E.J., Hopkins, W.G., and Hawley, J.A. Reproducibility of self-paced treadmill performance of trained endurance runners. *Int. J. Sports Med.* 19, 48-51, 1998b.

45. Maughan, R.J.and Shirreffs, S.M. Fluid and electrolyte loss and replacement in exercise. In: Harries, M., Williams, C., Stanish, W.D., and Micheli, L.L., Eds. *Oxford Textbook of Sports Medicine*. 2nd. ed., Oxford University Press, NY, 1998. pp 97-113.

46. Maughan, R.J., Bethell, L.R., and Leiper, J.B., Effects of ingested fluids on exercise capacity and on cardiovascular and metabolic responses to prolonged exercise in man. *Experimental Physiol.* 81, 847-859, 1996.

47. Barr, S.I., Costill, D.L., and Fink, W.J., Fluid replacement during prolonged exercise: effects of water, saline or no fluid. *Med. Sci. Sports Exerc.* 23, 811-817, 1991.

48. Levine. L., Rose, M.S., Francesconi, R.P., Neufer, P.D., and Sawka, M.N., Fluid replacement during sustained activity: nutrient solution vs. water. *Aviation Space Environ. Med.* 62, 559-564, 1991.

49. Below, P.R., Mora-Rodriguez, R., Gonzalez-Alonso, J., and Coyle, E.F., Fluid and carbohydrate ingestion independently improve performance during 1 h of intense exercise. *Med. Sci. Sports Exerc.* 27, 200-210, 1995

50. Macaraeg, P.V.J., Influence of carbohydrate electrolyte ingestion on running endurance, in: *Nutrient Utilization During Exercise*, Fox, E.L., Ed., Ross Laboratories, Columbus, pp 91-96, 1983.

51. Williams, C., Diet and endurance fitness. *Am. J. Clinic. Nutr.* 49, 1077-1083, 1989.

52. Williams, C., Nute, M.G., Broadbank, L., and Vinall, S., Influence of fluid intake on endurance running performance. A comparison between water, glucose and fructose solutions. *Europ. J. App. Physiol.* 60, 112-119, 1990.

53. Nassis, G.P., Williams, C., and Chisnall, P., Effect of a carbohydrate-electrolyte drink on endurance capacity during prolonged intermittent high intensity running. *Brit. J. Sports Med.* 32, 248-252, 1998.

54. Cade, R., Spooner, G., Schlein, E., Pickering, M., Dean, R., Effect of fluid, electrolyte, and glucose replacement on performance, body temperature, rate of sweat loss and compositional changes of extracellular fluid. *J. Sports Med. and Physical Fitness* 12, 150-156, 1972.

55. Maughan, R.J. and Whiting, P.H., Factors influencing plasma glucose concentration during marathon running, in: *Exercise Physiology. Volume 1*, Dotson, C.O. and Humphrey, J.H., Eds., AMS Press, NY, 87-98, 1985.

56. Noakes, T.D., Lambert, E.V., Lambert, M.I., McArthur, P.S., Myburgh, K.H., and Benade, A.J.S,. Carbohydrate ingestion and muscle glycogen depletion during marathon and ultramarathon racing. *Europ. J. App. Physiol.* 57, 482-489, 1988.

57. Tsintzas, K., Liu, R., Williams, C., Campbell, I., and Gaitanos, G., The effect of carbohydrate ingestion on performance during a 30-km race. *Int. J. Sport Nutr.* 3, 127-139, 1993.

58. Shephard, R.J., Leatt, P.B., Carbohydrate and fluid needs of the soccer player. *Sports Med.* 4, 164-176, 1987.

59. Nicholas, C.W., Williams, C., Lakomy, H.K., Phillips, G., and Nowitz, A., Influence of ingesting a carbohydrate-electrolyte solution on endurance capacity during intermittent, high intensity shuttle running. *J. Sports Sci.* 13, 283-290, 1995.

60. Zeederberg, C., Leach, L., Lambert, E.V., Noakes, T.D., Dennis, S.C., and Hawley, J.A., The effect of carbohydrate ingestion on the motor skill proficiency of soccer players. *Int. J. Sport Nutr.* 6, 348-355, 1996.

6 Metabolic and Performance Responses to Carbohydrate Intake During Exercise

Luis F. Aragón-Vargas

CONTENTS

6.1 INTRODUCTION

During exercise, an adequate supply of substrates is required for the continuing resynthesis of ATP in working muscles. Muscle fibers have limited stores of creatine phosphate, glycogen, and triglycerides and so must also be able to extract glucose and free fatty acids from the blood to meet the overall energy needs of the contracting fiber. Oxidization of protein usually makes only a small contribution to energy production, although protein can be an important source of energy under extreme circumstances. To maintain the homeostasis and to assure that adequate fuel is available to sustain contraction of muscle fibers, utilization of carbohydrate, fatty acids, and protein is carefully balanced by an orchestra of hormones and enzymes.

An adequate supply of carbohydrate (in the form of blood glucose and muscle glycogen) is clearly related to exercise performance. Human performance involves a variety of biomechanical, physiological, and psychological factors. From a physiological point of view, performance is strongly related to the ability to produce or sustain a large power output to overcome resistance or drag while protecting the homeostasis of cells and organ systems.[1] Maintaining a given power output requires an appropriate supply of energy to the working muscle fibers and, as explained below, this requires the availability of carbohydrate as fuel. Because carbohydrate stores in the human body are not very large (about 300 to 500 grams), and because carbohydrate is a predominant fuel during many types of exercise, ingestion of various forms of carbohydrate before, during, and after exercise has been systematically studied as a means of extending that fuel supply for a longer period of time. This research has repeatedly shown an improvement in exercise performance. For excellent reviews on this topic, particularly related to prolonged endurance exercise, see Coggan and Coyle (1991),[2] Coyle (1997),[3] Hargreaves (1999),[4] and Maughan (1991).[5]

Understanding the metabolic and performance responses to carbohydrate intake during exercise is critical in understanding one important aspect of sports drink efficacy: the ability of the beverage to improve exercise performance. For this reason, this chapter will focus on the metabolic and performance effects of carbohydrate consumption during exercise with special attention devoted to recent research on the effects of consuming sports drinks during intermittent high intensity exercise.

6.2 CARBOHYDRATE, FAT, AND PROTEIN AS FUELS DURING EXERCISE

The relative contribution of protein, fat, and carbohydrate fuels during exercise depends on the exercise intensity and duration, as well as level of fitness and the nutritional status of the individual. As an example, fasting will promote lipolysis from adipose tissue and higher circulating levels of free fatty acids, promoting a greater reliance on fats and protein for energy. Another example is that endurance training increases the ability of muscles to oxidize fats for energy. Nevertheless, almost regardless of the nuances of exercise, fitness, and nutritional status, carbohydrate is the most important energy source during vigorous exercise.

Although protein contributes only a small portion of the total energy needs of active muscles, amino acids may provide between 5% and 10% of substrate supply during prolonged exhausting exercise (see Brooks, et al.,1996, Chapter 8).[6] Amino acids released from muscle and other tissues can supply substrates to the liver for gluconeogenesis, the production of glucose from amino acids and other substrates. This glucose can be released from the liver, taken up by active muscle, and oxidized for energy. Oxidization of branched chain amino acids (leucine, isoleucine, and valine), and alanine, glutamate, and aspartate also occurs in muscle and can serve as a direct provider of a small amount of the ATP required for muscle contraction. The contribution of protein oxidation to energy metabolism increases when muscle glycogen stores are depleted,[7] but the major problem with using amino acids for energy production is that they must be retrieved from protein in skeletal muscle or from the tissues of the gut, as there are no amino acid stores in the body. Under most circumstances, it is obviously preferable to spare muscle protein.

Fat, in the form of triglycerides, is stored in small amounts within muscle fibers and in large amounts in adipose tissue. During exercise, these triglycerides can be hydrolyzed to glycerol and free fatty acids. Free fatty acids play an important role as a fuel, mainly during prolonged endurance exercise, but because adipose tissue provides an almost unlimited source of free fatty acids, fatigue is not related to depletion of fats. In addition, the rate at which fatty acids can be oxidized is so limited that if skeletal muscle were to rely solely on fat as fuel, maximal energy expenditure would be limited to about 60% VO_{2max}. It is not entirely clear why the muscle has a limited ability to oxidize fat.[3]

Carbohydrate is available to the muscle fibers from muscle glycogen and from glucose circulating in the blood. Muscle glycogen stores are rather limited, although they can be improved by diet and training. Plasma glucose is even more limited, but euglycemia during exercise is carefully maintained under most circumstances by liver glycogenolysis and gluconeogenesis. During prolonged exercise (e. g., > 2 h), muscle glycogen can be depleted and liver glycogen stores may not be able to maintain blood glucose levels. Under those circumstances, fatigue will quickly ensue. It should also be noted that muscle glycogen stores can be quickly depleted during intense intermittent exercise; prolonged exercise is not the only circumstance in which carbohydrate stores can be problematic. Fortunately, blood glucose levels can be maintained by absorption of ingested glucose from the intestine, a critical consideration in supplementing the body's limited carbohydrate reserves.

Not all the metabolic effects of carbohydrate intake during exercise are directly related to substrate utilization for energy delivery to working muscles. Some scientists have suggested that carbohydrate feeding may have a positive effect on the concentrations of brain neurotransmitters related to the perception of pain and central fatigue.[5,8,9] Central fatigue, or fatigue of the central nervous system, is "… a failure to maintain the required or expected force or power output, associated with specific alterations in central nervous system function that cannot reasonably be explained by dysfunction within the muscle itself" (Davis and Bailey, 1997, page 46).[8] These alterations include increased concentrations of serotonin, resulting from an increase in plasma free tryptophan or in the ratio of free tryptophan to branched-chain amino acids. While it is difficult to distinguish between the positive effects of carbohydrate feedings on central vs. peripheral mechanisms of fatigue, ingestion of carbohydrate during exercise has been shown to attenuate the rise in plasma free tryptophan while delaying fatigue considerably.[8] In other words, ingesting carbohydrate during prolonged exercise may influence neurotransmitter production in the brain in a way that delays the onset of "central fatigue" in addition to the positive metabolic effects on the working muscles.

6.2.1 EXERCISE INTENSITY

At low exercise intensities, most of the energy needed for exercise comes from plasma free fatty acids, but as exercise intensity increases, muscle glycogen and plasma glucose provide an increasing contribution (Figure 6.1). At 25% VO_{2max}, most of the energy comes from oxidation of free fatty acids; blood glucose makes only a small contribution.[3] When exercise intensity is at 40% VO_{2max}, the respiratory exchange ratio is about 0.85, suggesting a contribution of 50% carbohydrate and 50% fats.[6] Romijn et al.[10] have shown that when intensity increases to 65% VO_{2max}, the relative contribution of plasma free fatty acids decreases to about 54% of total energy needs. The decrease in fat oxidation is even more pronounced at 85% VO_{2max}. As fatty acid oxidation decreases, plasma glucose uptake and muscle glycogen oxidation increase in relation to exercise intensity.[10] Thus, carbohydrate is essential for exercise at moderate intensities or higher.

6.2.2 EXERCISE DURATION

In the early stages of prolonged exercise at moderate intensity (about 65% VO_{2max}), carbohydrate and fat each provide about 50% of the energy. Muscle glycogen makes the major carbohydrate contribution, while energy from fat is obtained in similar amounts from plasma free fatty acids and muscle triglycerides. As exercise continues and muscle glycogen stores decline, blood glucose becomes progressively more important as a carbohydrate source for muscle fibers. Plasma free fatty acids also become a more important source of fuel later in exercise (Figure 6.2).[3] During prolonged exercise at moderate intensity, time to fatigue is usually associated with the time when glycogen stores are depleted and blood glucose may approach hypoglycemic levels (see below).[11]

6.2.3 FITNESS LEVEL

A clear, consistent effect that results from endurance training is an increase in the mitochondrial content of skeletal muscle. This larger mitochondrial mass facilitates aerobic metabolism, including the muscle's ability to use free fatty acids as fuel. The greater ability to generate ATP and citrate from beta oxidation inhibits key enzymes in the glycolytic pathway and slows the catabolism of glucose and glycogen.[6] Martin proposes that this increased contribution of free fatty acids to energy production comes primarily from intramuscular triglycerides.[12] The end result is a gradual shift from less to more reliance on fat as fuel as aerobic fitness improves. Nevertheless, as pointed out by Coyle (1997)[3], fitness improvements also allow an

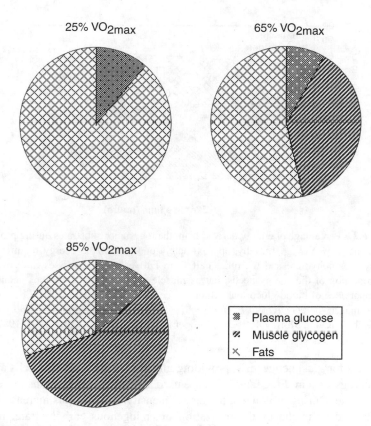

FIGURE 6.1   Percent contribution of fuels to total energy expenditure at different exercise intensities, after 30 min of exercise and an overnight fast. (Drawn from data in Romijn, J.A., Coyle, E.F., Sidossis, L.S., Gastaldelli, A., Horowitz, J.F., Endert, E., and Wolfe, R.R., *Am. J. Physiol.,* 265, E380, 1993).

individual to exercise more intensely, and therefore the reliance on carbohydrate as a fuel source during intense exercise remains.

6.2.4 NUTRITIONAL STATUS

Fasting has a significant effect on the utilization of carbohydrate as fuel during moderate intensity exercise.[13] During the postabsorptive phase, humans rely heavily on liver glycogenolysis for blood glucose homeostasis. Consequently, liver glycogen tends to be low after an overnight fast. When exercise is performed under these conditions, blood glucose homeostasis must be maintained despite liver glycogen depletion and the increased demand of working muscle for glucose.[14,15] Maintenance of blood glucose is partially achieved by gluconeogenesis and by a greater reliance by active muscles on free fatty acids for fuel.[13] During the early stage of fasting (24 hours to 3 days), there is an increased lipolysis from adipose tissue and protein breakdown from the body stores (skeletal muscle at rest, or the gut if the muscles are active). Circulating glycerol and amino acids are taken up by the liver and used

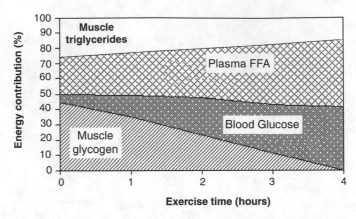

FIGURE 6.2 Percentage of energy derived from the four major substrates during prolonged exercise at 65–75% VO_{2max}. Initially, approximately one-half of the energy requirement is derived from carbohydrate and the other half from fat. As time progresses, fat provides a greater proportion of the energy needs, but as muscle glycogen concentrations decline, the relative importance of blood glucose as a fuel source increases. (From Coyle, E.F., Fuels for sport performance, *Perspectives in Exercise and Sports Medicine: Optimizing Sport Performance*, Lamb, D.R. and Murray, R. (Eds.), Cooper Publishing Group, Carmel, IN, 1997. With permission).

as precursors for gluconeogenesis, providing glucose for the red blood cells and the central nervous system. Free fatty acids are used as fuel for other organs, especially skeletal muscle. During prolonged, moderate intensity exercise, this increase in free fatty acid oxidation reduces the utilization of endogenous carbohydrate; that is, muscle glycogen is spared.[16]

At the other extreme, ingestion of a high-glycemic carbohydrate bolus results in an elevation of plasma insulin and suppression of adipose tissue lipolysis that is still observable 4 hours after the meal. Carbohydrate oxidation is elevated and fat oxidation is reduced for about the first hour of moderate intensity exercise, although the suppression of fat oxidation is slowly reversed as exercise duration increases.[17] Some authors have warned that this higher reliance on carbohydrate may have detrimental effects on performance, or simply blunt any potential ergogenic effect of carbohydrate ingestion, because glycogen stores may be depleted faster.[18] This should not be a problem, provided that the meal contains enough carbohydrate to supply all the excess carbohydrate that will be oxidized. In fact, most of the studies on the performance effects of carbohydrate ingestion prior to exercise show either a positive response or no effect.[3,4]

A key factor in the regulation of the balance between free fatty acid/carbohydrate oxidation is plasma insulin.[3] Because plasma insulin is sensitive to the ingestion of even small amounts of carbohydrate, the pre-exercise diet plays a very important role in the utilization of carbohydrate during exercise.

When the regular diet does not contain sufficient carbohydrate for the demands of physical activity, glycogen stores will be depleted and insufficiently restored during the hours following exercise. Low muscle glycogen levels result in a higher utilization of protein for fuel during exercise,[7] the necessary amino acids being obtained from breakdown of skeletal muscle protein. It is possible that ingestion of carbohydrate during exercise, even if glycogen stores are low, may result in higher oxidation of exogenous carbohydrate and sparing of muscle protein breakdown. For example, a recent study using carbohydrate supplementation after resistance exercise showed that the ingestion of carbohydrate was able to reduce myofibrillar protein breakdown and urinary urea excretion, resulting in a more positive body protein balance.[19]

6.2.5 CARBOHYDRATE SOURCES DURING EXERCISE

As mentioned previously, the body's primary carbohydrate stores are liver and muscle glycogen. The other source of carbohydrate is blood glucose, but the total amount of glucose that is in the blood at any given time is very low, the equivalent of only 20 kcal. To maintain euglycemia during physical activity, humans rely on liver glycogenolysis and gluconeogenesis and, if ingesting sports drinks or solid carbohydrate supplements, on glucose absorption from the gut.

Lactate can also play an important role as a source of carbohydrate during exercise. On one hand, lactate (and pyruvate) produced and released by skeletal muscle can be used by the liver to synthesize new glucose that, in turn, can be used by skeletal muscle to resynthesize ATP.[6] Lactate can also be used as fuel by some muscle fibers, in the so-called "lactate shuttle. " Some evidence for this mechanism has been provided in a study of simulated marathon running,[20] where the estimated total carbohydrate utilization could not be accounted for by glycogen stores and circulating blood glucose. The role of lactate as a glycogen precursor was recently evaluated by Bangsbo et al.[21] They concluded that while muscle glycogenesis from lactate can occur in humans, this substrate only contributes a minor portion of glycogen synthesis, even when muscle and blood lactate concentrations are high.

6.2.5.1 Glycogen Utilization, Glycogen Stores, and Performance

Glycogen stores in skeletal muscle are very important for performance, but they are relatively small. Overall muscle glycogen is about 300 to 500 grams, or about 1200 to 2000 kcal of energy. Both the carbohydrate content of the diet and training status influence the amount of glycogen stored; between 10 and 30 grams of glycogen can be stored in one kilogram of skeletal muscle.[3] Regardless, these values are an overestimate of the amount of muscle glycogen that is actually available during specific forms of exercise because only glycogen from active muscle fibers can be used.

In 1967, Bergstrom et al. showed a clear relationship between diet, pre-exercise muscle glycogen stores, and endurance performance.[22] In this paper, subjects were fed three different but isoenergetic diets for 3 days: low-carbohydrate, mixed diet, and high-carbohydrate. Resulting muscle glycogen stores before exercise were low, normal, and high, and corresponded with shorter, intermediate, and longer times to fatigue during cycling. At the point of fatigue, muscle glycogen levels were similar in all conditions. From this and many other similar studies, it is clear that the initial muscle glycogen content is strongly related to endurance performance (see Conlee, 1987, for a review on this topic).[23] Because muscle glycogen depletion can be associated with fatigue during prolonged strenuous exercise,[11,24] high initial glycogen stores and reduced glycogen utilization for fuel are viewed as very positive factors for an improved performance. Although the ingestion of carbohydrate via a sports drink during exercise has a debatable effect on muscle glycogen stores, the fact that muscle glycogen status is such a powerful determinant of performance is evidence of the importance of carbohydrate as a key source of energy during vigorous exercise.

6.2.5.2　Fate of Ingested Carbohydrate During Exercise

Studies of the utilization of exogenous carbohydrate during exercise rely mainly on the analysis of labeled carbon after ingesting different forms of carbohydrate. Different methodologies cause some difficulties in the estimations, but there is basic agreement that ingested carbohydrate may provide between 10% and 30% of total carbohydrate oxidation.[25] Adopo et al.[26] estimated that the oxidation of ingested carbohydrates can provide around 16% to 20% of total energy expenditure. They noted that when carbohydrate is given as 50 g glucose plus 50 g fructose rather than 100 g glucose, the combined hexoses allow for a greater contribution to total energy expenditure ($21.9 \pm 1.6\%$ vs. $15.7 \pm 2.9\%$) during 2 hours of cycling at 60% VO_{2max}. In the early stages of exercise, the amount of exogenous carbohydrate oxidized is very small: only about 32% of the carbohydrate emptied from the stomach is oxidized during the first 80 to 90 minutes of exercise. This is about 20 g of exogenous carbohydrate oxidized during the first hour of exercise.[25] Later in exercise, the situation is different, as blood glucose becomes the major carbohydrate fuel source.[2] The fate of the exogenous carbohydrate that is not oxidized during exercise is still an open question, although there are suggestions that some of it may be incorporated into the glycogen stores of inactive muscle fibers.

The metabolic effects of carbohydrate ingestion during exercise vary with exercise duration and intensity. When carbohydrate is ingested during low intensity exercise, blood glucose levels and plasma insulin levels reach higher values compared with control conditions. The resulting hyperglycemia and hyperinsulinemia cause a higher rate of muscle glucose uptake, compared with exercise in a fasted state. However, when carbohydrate is ingested during moderate intensity exercise (50% to 75% VO_{2max}), the alterations in substrate metabolism are not as obvious. Plasma insulin levels are only slightly higher or the same as during exercise in the fasted state, and the reduction in free fatty acid oxidation is not as marked as during low intensity exercise.[2]

During prolonged strenuous exercise, glucose output by the liver is reduced by ingestion of carbohydrate, while muscle glucose uptake is increased. The greater muscle uptake of glucose potentially favors a reduced net glycogen utilization, but this only appears to happen under specific conditions (see below).[4] Ingestion of carbohydrate during exercise also results in lower levels of plasma free fatty acids,[27,28] although this does not affect fat oxidation to the same extent as when carbohydrate is ingested before exercise.[4]

According to DeMarco et al. (1999),[29] there is a clear and strong relationship between blood glucose levels at various points in time, and ratings of perceived exertion (RPE) and respiratory exchange ratio (RER). This is further evidence that higher blood glucose concentrations promote an increased utilization of carbohydrate as a fuel. Provided there is a good supply of exogenous glucose, this would be an advantage for performance.

A key positive effect of carbohydrate ingestion during exercise is often manifested late during exercise of 2 hours or more. Utilization of plasma glucose increases with exercise duration in the fasted state, and this seems to be related to a steady decrease in the rate of muscle glycogenolysis. When muscle glycogen stores are high, blood glucose provides only about 25% of carbohydrate fuel, but late in exercise, when glycogen levels are low, blood glucose oxidation accounts for most of the carbohydrate oxidation. During the latter stages of prolonged exercise of low or moderate intensity, blood glucose concentration decreases due to a reduced liver glucose output and performance is impaired to the extent that carbohydrate plays an important role as fuel at that time. This decrease in blood glucose may be prevented by the ingestion of carbohydrate during exercise.[2,11,30]

Based on the above findings, Coyle and colleagues[11] have proposed a well-documented model of the absolute rate of carbohydrate oxidation from different sources during prolonged cycling at a constant intensity of 70% to 75% VO_{2max} (Figure 6.3). According to this model, the rate of muscle glycogen utilization during exercise is the same when fasted or when fed carbohydrate. During prolonged exercise, blood glucose becomes more and more important, while muscle glycogen contributes less and less to energy production as time progresses. After about 3 hours of exercise in the fasted state, fatigue occurs due to an insufficient rate of carbohydrate oxidation resulting from a decrease in blood glucose concentration. Ingestion of carbohydrate maintains blood glucose availability and prevents this decrease in carbohydrate oxidation, even when muscle glycogen is almost depleted, enabling exercise to be continued for an additional hour or so.

6.2.5.3 Blood Glucose Availability and Muscle Glycogen Utilization

A reduction in carbohydrate availability is associated with fatigue during prolonged strenuous exercise. Because muscle glycogen stores — one of the two major sources of carbohydrate for the exercising muscle — are limited, scientists have been interested in the effect of exogenous glucose on glycogen utilization. Glycogen utilization depends on glycogen phosphorylase activity, which is potentially reduced by an increase in the concentrations of glucose and glucose-6-phosphate inside the muscle. Intramuscular glucose accumulation can be increased, in turn, by carbohydrate ingestion.[31] On the other hand, as indicated above, carbohydrate ingestion causes high plasma glucose and insulin concentrations at exercise intensities below about 70% to 75% VO_{2max}, thus inhibiting lipolysis and reducing the availability of free fatty acids, resulting in a greater reliance on carbohydrate for exercise. If this need for additional carbohydrate is supplied by muscle glycogen because of insufficient glucose availability, an ergolytic rather than an ergogenic effect results. If sufficient

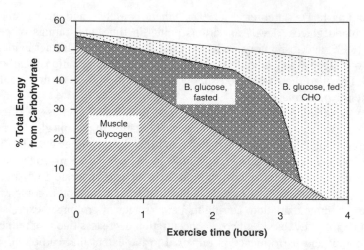

FIGURE 6.3 Model of carbohydrate oxidation and fatigue. Percentage of energy and absolute rate of carbohydrate oxidation from various sources during prolonged cycling at 70–75% VO_{2max} when fasted or when fed carbohydrate throughout exercise. (From Coyle, E. F., Coggan, A. R., Hemmert, M. K., and Ivy, J. L., Muscle glycogen utilization during prolonged strenuous exercise when fed carbohydrate, *J. Appl. Physiol.*, 61, 165, 1986. Figure 5, page 170. With permission).

amounts of sports drinks or other sources of carbohydrate are ingested at regular intervals throughout exercise, this should not be a concern.

A net reduction in muscle glycogen utilization with carbohydrate ingestion has been observed in prolonged treadmill running at 70% VO_{2max},[24,32] but not in prolonged cycling at 70% to 75% VO_{2max}.[11,31] Interestingly, variable intensity cycling protocols have been shown to allow for glycogen sparing.[33,34] Thus, blood glucose availability can influence the net rate of glycogen utilization, but this depends on the mode and intensity of exercise, amount and type of carbohydrate ingested, and pre-exercise nutrition and training status.[35] During prolonged strenuous cycling exercise, any ergogenic effect of carbohydrate ingestion must act through a mechanism other than sparing of muscle glycogen.

6.3 PERFORMANCE RESPONSE TO CARBOHYDRATE INGESTION DURING EXERCISE

According to Hargreaves,[4] "perhaps one of the most studied areas in sports nutrition has been the metabolic and performance responses to carbohydrate ingestion during exercise" (p. 100). As early as 1924,[36–38] scientists were beginning to publish evidence supporting the important role of an exogenous source of carbohydrate during prolonged exercise. The success of commercial sports drinks and other nutritional supplements gave momentum to research in this area in the 1980s and 1990s, resulting in a considerable amount of evidence in favor of the ergogenic effects of carbohydrate ingestion on different types of exercise.

6.3.1 GENERAL CONSIDERATIONS

Because the relative importance of carbohydrate as fuel depends on exercise intensity and duration, as well as fitness level and nutritional status, all those factors will also bear on performance responses to carbohydrate ingestion during exercise. A nice example of the role of nutrition status can be found in a study by Neufer et al.[39] on four different occasions. Ten well-trained male cyclists reported to the laboratory 24 hours after a glycogen depletion session and after a 12-hour fast. They cycled for only 45 minutes at 80% VO_{2max} and were then requested to generate as much work as possible on an isokinetic cycle ergometer for 15 minutes. These subjects, who started the tests with low muscle glycogen levels, performed significantly better when fed carbohydrate right before the tests than when using a placebo. Furthermore, if a light carbohydrate feeding was also given 4 hours before the test in addition to the pre-test carbohydrate, performance was improved even more, although the increase in pre-exercise glycogen concentration of 15% was not statistically significant. The authors concluded that when initial endogenous carbohydrate stores are less than optimal, the ingestion of 45 grams of carbohydrate immediately before high intensity exercise will improve performance during the final 15 minutes of a 1-hour exercise bout.

Performance responses to different ergogenic aids are typically measured in one of three ways:

1. time to fatigue at a constant exercise intensity
2. mean power output (or total work performed) generated in a fixed amount of time
3. a time trial (time required to cover a particular distance)

The latter two are very similar, since both depend on average power output, although attempting to complete as much work as possible in a fixed period of time is not as intuitive a task for most subjects as is trying to complete a task as fast as possible. The type of performance test must be selected according to the hypothesis to be tested. Sometimes, the question of interest relates to understanding a particular physiological mechanism; at other times, what matters is whether a specific sport performance can be improved, and the performance test is selected to mimic the demands of that sport. Interpretation of the research should take these issues into consideration.

6.3.2 PROLONGED EXERCISE

It is reasonable to expect that an exogenous fuel supply in the form of carbohydrate should have a greater effect on prolonged exercise, where fuel stores and fuel availability often limit performance. Shorter efforts (under 15 minutes) are usually assumed to be powered by endogenous fuel sources, with the limiting factor to performance being the ability of the metabolic pathways to use the available fuel without large disturbances to homeostasis. For this reason, most of the earlier research on carbohydrate intake and performance involved prolonged, steady-state exercise. Because of the different relative contributions of carbohydrate and fat as fuels during exercise, subjects performing low intensity (25% to 30% VO_{2max}) and moderate intensity (70% to 75% VO_{2max}) exercise respond very differently to carbohydrate supplementation.

6.3.2.1   Low intensity Exercise

Most of the energy necessary for steady-state exercise at 25% VO_{2max} comes from plasma free fatty acids. To be used as fuel, lipids (from adipose tissue or intramuscular triglycerides) must undergo mobilization, circulation via the bloodstream, and uptake by muscle, followed by activation, translocation, beta oxidation, and finally mitochondrial oxidation and production of ATP.[6] Because the processes of lipid utilization are slow to be activated, the contribution of fats is small at the onset of exercise, although little plasma glucose is used because of the low intensity of the exercise. After 30 minutes, plasma free fatty acids and muscle triglycerides provide about 85% of all fuel for low intensity exercise.[10] As time goes on, the relative contribution of free fatty acids becomes more and more important,[3] but body stores of fat are so large that it is more likely that carbohydrate remains as the limiting factor; there are no reports of complete depletion of intramuscular or adipose tissue lipid stores. Ingestion of carbohydrate in the early stages of this type of exercise is not warranted, though, because it is well documented that carbohydrate ingestion at this low intensity of exercise will suppress free fatty acid mobilization from adipose tissue and total fat oxidation by skeletal muscle,[40] resulting in a greater reliance on carbohydrate fuels. While this effect should not be detrimental to performance as long as carbohydrate ingestion is maintained, the major benefit of carbohydrate ingestion during low intensity activities would be apparent only after several hours of exercise, if the effort is long enough to deplete muscle glycogen stores. In addition, carbohydrate intake during low intensity exercise will prevent hypoglycemia and the neuroglucopenia that can negatively affect the function of the central nervous system.

6.3.2.2   Moderate Intensity Exercise.

There is compelling evidence that carbohydrate ingestion during exercise improves performance of prolonged moderate intensity exercise.[2,4,41] This typically represents more than 2 hours of exercise, but the effects have been observed in exercise of about 1-hour duration, especially if muscle glycogen stores are low.[42] Long-distance runners and cyclists have relied on this scientific finding for years, as evidenced by their frequent use of sports drinks as a source of carbohydrate and fluids during exercise.

The positive effect of carbohydrate ingestion occurs independent of the performance measure. For example, time to fatigue at a constant intensity of exercise has been improved by anywhere from about 20 minutes to an hour.[11,24,27,30,43–47] Average power output for a fixed distance or time has also been improved by carbohydrate ingestion during the exercise.[28,48–50] Although the physiological mechanism responsible for an improved performance with carbohydrate ingestion may vary with mode of exercise, the ergogenic effect has been found both in running[24,46,47,50] and cycling.[2,43,49]

What is the underlying mechanism for the improved performance seen with carbohydrate ingestion during exercise? According to Nicholas et al.,[51] "... the mechanisms responsible for improving endurance capacity have been linked with the prevention of hypoglycemia, maintaining a high rate of carbohydrate oxidation and, in some studies, glycogen sparing" (p. 288). In well-trained cyclists, moderate intensity cycling (about 70% VO_{2max}) typically can be continued for more than 2 hours. In an elegant series of experiments, Coggan and Coyle[2] have collected compelling evidence showing that carbohydrate ingestion improves performance of this type of exercise primarily by maintaining the availability and oxidation of blood glucose, especially late in exercise. Their model is valid only for prolonged strenuous cycling, where glycogen sparing has been shown not to occur.[11] During prolonged strenuous running, blood glucose levels do not fall as low as during cycling, but a reduced net muscle glycogen utilization, thanks to higher blood glucose availability, is observed.[24,32] It is not clear whether the difference between running and cycling is due to the relative importance of blood glucose vs. muscle glycogen as carbohydrate fuel sources or to differences in muscle fiber total recruitment or recruitment patterns.[4]

Carbohydrate ingestion during this type of exercise seems to be unable to improve performance under certain conditions. Performance is often improved in the absence of hypoglycemia but, in agreement with the model of Coyle et al.,[11] those subjects who are able to maintain blood glucose levels throughout exercise without carbohydrate supplementation do not benefit from carbohydrate ingestion. This is often the case when subjects have good liver and muscle glycogen stores and duration is relatively short,[42] but it may also occur in some subjects who have a better ability to regulate their blood glucose.[27] Aside from these few exceptions, ingestion of carbohydrate during long duration, moderate intensity exercise is normally expected to have a positive effect on performance. Sports drinks are seen as a convenient and effective way to ingest carbohydrate during this type of exercise, because they fulfill a double purpose by also helping to prevent dehydration.

6.3.3 Higher Intensity, Shorter Duration Exercise

Until the early 1990s, the main focus of research on carbohydrate feeding during exercise was on prolonged continuous exercise. As recently as 1996, an American College of Sports Medicine position stand on exercise and fluid replacement stated: "During exercise lasting less than 1 h, there is little evidence of physiological or physical performance differences between consuming a carbohydrate-electrolyte drink and plain water" (p. i). At the time the ACSM position stand was written, few investigators had examined the benefits of carbohydrate ingestion during activities other than prolonged continuous exercise.[42]

A study published by Ball and colleagues in 1995[52] was among the first to provide evidence in favor of ingesting carbohydrate during exercise lasting less than 1 hour. To determine if frequent ingestion of a carbohydrate-electrolyte drink during high intensity cycle ergometer exercise would affect sprint capacity at the end of the exercise session, eight male competitive cyclists completed testing on 3 days. The first day was for assessment of VO_{2max}. The other two test sessions were the counterbalanced 50-minute trials (at 80% VO_{2max}), when subjects ingested 2 ml/kg body weight at 10, 20, 30, and 40 minutes of either a carbohydrate-electrolyte solution or water placebo. Immediately after the 50-minute bout, subjects performed a Wingate anaerobic power test. The tests were performed after a 12-hour fast. Peak power (794 ± 84 vs. 748 ± 97 W), mean power (701 ± 85 vs. 655 ± 74 W), and minimum power (627 ± 101 vs. 585 ± 93 W) during the final sprint were all significantly higher for the carbohydrate-electrolyte solution trials, while the ratings of perceived exertion during the 50-minute bout were lower (5.0 vs 5.6). The authors concluded that cyclists and other athletes may benefit by periodically ingesting a carbohydrate-electrolyte solution during moderate-duration, high intensity competitions after an overnight fast.

Anantaraman et al.[53] studied five moderately trained subjects during a 1-hour high intensity test. Each subject reported to the laboratory in a post-absorptive state, on three different occasions separated by at least 1 week. For each test, they warmed up for 2 minutes and then cycled continuously at an initial intensity of 90% VO_{2max}, trying to maintain power output as close to the initial value as possible for 60 minutes. A glucose-polymer or placebo drink (300 ml) was ingested 2 minutes prior to the start of exercise and at 15, 30, and 45 minutes during the exercise test, in the appropriate combinations to produce a glucose before, placebo during condition (G/P), glucose before, glucose during condition (G/G), or placebo before, placebo during condition (P/P). Both G/P and G/G resulted in a greater total amount of work (619 ± 234 and 599 ± 235 kJ, respectively) compared with P/P (560 ± 198 kJ). The authors stated that no additional benefit of ingesting carbohydrate both prior to and during exercise was obtained compared with carbohydrate ingestion only prior to exercise. They suggested that this might be due to limited gastric emptying during the exercise at such a high intensity. However, their subjects spent much of the 60-minute exercise bout between 70% and 80% VO_{2max}. Gastric emptying should not be substantially impaired at that intensity. Unfortunately, the absence of a placebo/glucose condition in this study precludes any conclusions about the relative contribution of carbohydrate ingestion before vs. during the exercise.

The contribution of carbohydrate ingestion during cycling exercise at 80% VO_{2max} is clear from an elegant study by Below et al.[54] Eight endurance-trained men exercised in a warm environment on a cycle ergometer for 50 minutes at 80% VO_{2max}, followed by a cycling performance test involving the completion of an individually set amount of work in the shortest time possible. This design simulates the actual conditions faced during a 40-km cycling time trial with a finishing sprint. Each subject performed the test under four conditions separated by at least 72 hours:

1. ingestion of fluid plus carbohydrate
2. fluid alone
3. carbohydrate alone
4. placebo

The design allowed for testing the main effects of large vs. small fluid replacement, and carbohydrate (79 ± 4 grams) vs. no carbohydrate, plus the potential interaction between the factors. Subjects performed the final sprint significantly faster with carbohydrate than without (10.23 ± 0.28 vs. 10.92 ± 0.32 minutes). Performance was also significantly faster (10.22 ± 0.27 vs. 10.93 ± 0.32 minutes) with large (79% of fluid loss) than with small (13% of fluid loss) fluid replacement. Furthermore, there was no interaction between the factors, indicating that their effects were independent. Finally, the effects of the factors in this study were additive: performance improvement was twice as large with both carbohydrate and large fluid replacement (time = 9.93 ± 0.28 minutes) than when only one of the factors was present. This is important because, very often, studies will provide carbohydrate in liquid form (i.e., a sports drink), and therefore it could be questioned whether the improvement in performance is due to rehydration rather than carbohydrate ingestion. For example, muscle glycogen use during exercise has been shown to be reduced by ingestion of enough distilled deionized water to prevent a loss of body mass.[55]

Another study looked at a cycling time trial, but focused on performance without any additional measurements in order to reduce the variability of the performance results.[56] Nineteen endurance trained cyclists performed an individually set amount of work as fast as possible on a cycle ergometer. Two tests were performed in random order by each subject, receiving 8 ml/kg body weight as a bolus during the warm-up period, plus 2 ml/kg body weight upon reaching 25%, 50%, and 75% of the prescribed amount of work, of either a 7.6% carbohydrate-electrolyte solution or placebo. Time to complete the set amount of work was significantly lower with carbohydrate ingestion than with placebo (58.74 ± 0.52 vs. 60.15 ± 0.65 minutes, respectively). Because of the nature of this study, the authors were not able to evaluate potential mechanisms for this improvement.

In summary, the few available scientific publications regarding higher intensity, shorter-duration, continuous exercise support the ergogenic effect of carbohydrate feeding, particularly if the exercise test or event involves a final sprint, as is common during time trials and other sports competitions. Provision of fluids is also important in this type of effort, as shown in the study of Below et al.[54]

6.3.4 INTERMITTENT EXERCISE

There has recently been a growing interest in studying the effects of carbohydrate feeding on intermittent exercise of relatively short duration and high intensity. Most team sports are included in this category: soccer, basketball, rugby, American football, volleyball, and hockey all fit this description. Tennis and combat sports are also typically intermittent. Training sessions for swimming, track, cycling, rowing, and general conditioning often include repeated, high intensity efforts alternated with recovery periods. In most cases, high intensity exercise is alternated with short to long periods of rest or reduced intensity exercise.

High intensity exercise (intensity $\geq 90\% VO_{2max}$) without recovery periods results in high concentrations of lactic acid in blood and skeletal muscle, and usually leads to exhaustion rather quickly, regardless of carbohydrate availability.[3] For that reason, whenever possible, athletes will alternate the high intensity efforts with adequate recovery, which enables them to exercise longer and at higher intensities. Typically, exercise duration can vary from 45 minutes to about 2 hours. Under these conditions, energy expenditure is high, and muscle fibers rely heavily on muscle glycogen for ATP production. It is not uncommon to reach very low levels of muscle glycogen at the end of such exercise.[57,58]

Research publications from the past decade show that intermittent high intensity exercise performance is improved by carbohydrate supplementation. Researchers have looked at two separate aspects of carbohydrate supplementation: supplementation of carbohydrates in the regular diet to improve glycogen stores, and ingestion of carbohydrates during exercise. The first application is outside the scope of this chapter; suffice to say that higher dietary carbohydrate intake has been shown to result in higher pre-exercise glycogen stores, which in turn have resulted in improved exercise performance.[18,57,59,60]

The ingestion of carbohydrate during intermittent high intensity exercise deserves specific discussion. A 1984 paper by Hargreaves and colleagues[33] reported an ergogenic effect of carbohydrate feedings during intermittent cycling, but the total duration was 4 hours. Ten male subjects cycled for 20 minutes at 50% VO_{2max}, followed by 10 minutes of intense intermittent cycling (four bouts of 30 seconds of cycling at 100% VO_{2max} followed by 2 minutes of rest). This sequence was repeated each half-hour for 4 hours; the final sprint bout was a timed ride to exhaustion. All subjects performed two trials separated by at least 2 weeks with a crossover design. One trial involved ingesting a solid feeding of 43 grams sucrose, 9 grams fat, and 3 grams protein in 400 ml of water, at 0, 1, 2, and 3 hours of exercise, for a total of 172 grams carbohydrate. The placebo trial used the same pattern, but 400 ml of an artificially sweetened drink was given instead. During the sprint rides to exhaustion, subjects performed 45% longer in the carbohydrate trial (127 ± 25 vs. 87 ± 18 seconds, $p < 0.05$). In addition, blood glucose levels were higher shortly after each carbohydrate feeding, and vastus lateralis glycogen utilization was significantly lower for the carbohydrate than the placebo trials (101 ± 10 vs. 126 ± 6 mmol/kg wet weight). The authors concluded that carbohydrate feeding during prolonged intermittent exercise results in a significant reduction of glycogen utilization and an enhancement of sprint performance at the end of the activity.

In an effort to understand the physiologic and performance responses to intermittent exercise of varied intensity commonly found in some sport training programs, Murray and colleagues[61] studied 13 adult males during cycling exercise in the heat. Subjects performed repeated sub-maximal exercise bouts at 55% to 65% VO_{2max}, alternated with five rest periods of 3 to 15 minutes, plus two brief high intensity performance tests requiring completion of an individually set amount of work as fast as possible. Four different conditions were completed by all subjects in counterbalanced fashion: water placebo (WP), 5% glucose polymer solution (GP), 6% sucrose/glucose solution (SG), or 7% polymer/fructose (PF); 2 ml/kg body weight were ingested during each of the five rest periods. Completion times for the first performance test were not statistically different among conditions. However, the second performance test (at the end of about 2 hours of cycling) showed significantly shorter ($p < 0.001$) times for both the SG and PF treatments (384 ± 39 and 375 ± 30 seconds) when compared with WP (432 ± 43 seconds). Performance time on the GP trial (401 ± 52 seconds) was not significantly different from that on the WP trial. This study involved intermittent exercise, but, throughout the exercise session, used low intensities that would seldom be found in most training sessions or competition in combination with the performance tests used.

Simard et al. (1988) completed a study with seven elite collegiate ice hockey players during an actual hockey game.[62] Each player was studied during two separate matches, one with carbohydrate supplementation and one with placebo, 4.5 hours after a standardized meal. Beverages were consumed before (926 ml of a 10%-glucose or saccharine solution with lemon juice), and during the games (114 ml of the same solutions at 20 and 40 minutes of play). Under the carbohydrate condition, a total of 100 grams of carbohydrate was consumed before and 20 g during the match. Measurements of muscle glycogen before and after the matches were obtained, as well as total time of play, distance skated, and mean speed of each player. The hockey players skated 10.2% more distance, and net glycogen utilization was 10.3% lower, with carbohydrate supplementation. When the glycogen decrease was corrected for distance skated, the net glycogen utilization was significantly lower in the carbohydrate match.

Several interesting field studies on soccer are cited in a review paper by Hawley et al.[63] The combined results illustrate how supplementation with fluids plus carbohydrate during soccer matches has resulted in improved soccer performance, namely greater second-half running distances (greater overall distance but also a higher number of sprints), and a larger number of ball contacts together with a greater involvement in play during the final 30 minutes of the games, compared with matches when only water was consumed. Team performance was also improved, resulting in more goals scored and less conceded with water plus carbohydrate supplementation vs. water alone.

Nicholas and colleagues[51] designed a shuttle running protocol to simulate running during a typical team sport competition such as soccer, rugby, or basketball. They asked nine players to perform two exercise sessions, 7 days apart, each consisting of two parts. First, a 75-minute exercise period of intermittent running in blocks of 15 minutes (sprinting, jogging, and walking) was conducted. This was followed by a period of intermittent running at 55% and 95% VO_{2max} to fatigue. The order of tests was randomized, with the subjects drinking 5 ml/kg body weight before the exercise and 2 ml/kg body weight every 15 minutes thereafter of either a 6.9% carbohydrate-electrolyte solution or a non-carbohydrate placebo. The tests were performed after a 10-hour fast. The carbohydrate electrolyte drink provided an average of 47 grams of carbohydrate/hour, and allowed the subjects to run for 2.2 minutes longer than when drinking a placebo solution (8.9 ± 1.5 vs. 6.7 ± 1.0 minutes). Blood glucose concentrations tended to be higher during the carbohydrate ingestion trial, but the ratings of perceived exertion were not different between trials. The authors concluded that carbohydrate feedings during intermittent exercise improved intermittent running performance and suggested that the 33% increase in endurance capacity obtained might be due to reduced muscle glycogen utilization during the first 75 minutes of exercise in the carbohydrate treatment.

Davis and colleagues[64] also looked at the effects of ingesting carbohydrate drinks on fatigue during intermittent high intensity cycling. Nine men and 7 women, all physically active but untrained, completed three trials with 1 week between exercise sessions. Subjects arrived in the laboratory after a 10-hour fast, having refrained from heavy exercise for 48 hours prior to the experimental trials. The first session was à familiarization trial; in the other two sessions, subjects received 4 ml/kg body weight of either a 6% carbohydrate-electrolyte beverage or an artificially flavored placebo, in counterbalanced fashion, every 20 minutes. They also received either placebo or an 18%-carbohydrate solution before the exercise. The exercise sessions consisted of repeated 1-minute cycling bouts at 120% to 130%VO_{2max} alternated with 3 minutes of rest until fatigue. Total time to fatigue was delayed from a mean of 60 ± 6 minutes with the placebo to 87 ± 13 minutes with the carbohydrate drink. The positive effect of carbohydrate ingestion was the same for the women as for the men. Plasma glucose and insulin concentrations generally increased under both conditions during the intermittent exercise, but the increases were larger for the carbohydrate than for placebo. Plasma glucose was significantly higher at all exercise time points in carbohydrate than placebo. The authors concluded that consumption of carbohydrate drinks at frequent intervals can improve exercise capacity during activities involving repeated intervals of intense exercise and rest that last about 1 hour.

In a study of prolonged intermittent high intensity running, Nassis et al.[65] evaluated the endurance capacity of nine well-trained distance runners who performed the tests on two different occasions, with carbohydrate supplementation or placebo, after an overnight fast. Following a warmup of 5 minutes of continuous running at 60% VO_{2max} plus 5 minutes of intermittent running at 70% and 45% VO_{2max}, subjects rested for 5 minutes of data collection and then started the intermittent running protocol. The subjects repeated 15 second bouts of fast running at 80% (first 60 minutes), 85% (60 to 100 minutes), and 90% VO_{2max} (100 minutes to volitional fatigue), alternated with 10 seconds of running at 45% VO_{2max}, replicating the protocol of Bangsbo et al.[18] Time to fatigue was not different between conditions (placebo = 113 ± 23 minutes; carbohydrate = 110 ± 21 minutes), and blood glucose was similar throughout the tests under both conditions, even though the runners ingested an average of 30 grams carbohydrate/hour throughout the carbohydrate trial. Muscle glycogen was not measured in this study. The authors offer a possible explanation for the lack of an ergogenic effect from the possibility of delayed gastric emptying due to the intensity of the exercise. This is not likely, since the same or higher intensities in other studies did not seem to interfere significantly with gastric emptying and delivery of glucose to the blood (see above). It is possible that 30 grams of carbohydrate per hour is not enough under these circumstances. Another possible explanation is that the recovery periods were too short; other studies have allowed recovery periods that were up to three times as long as the time of intense exercise bouts[64] (see Table 6.1).

An interesting and necessary question relates to the physiologically plausible mechanism for the improvement in performance often noted with the ingestion of carbohydrate during intermittent exercise. As explained above, during prolonged moderate exercise lasting 2 hours or more, regular carbohydrate ingestion helps maintain blood glucose levels later in exercise, enabling a higher power output at that time, or a longer time to fatigue. The proposed mechanism during intermittent exercise involves slower glycogen depletion rates, either because of glycogen sparing, or due to glycogen resynthesis during the recovery periods.

TABLE 6.1
Performance Effects of Carbohydrate Use During Stop and Go Exercise

Ref.	Authors	Exercise	Effort Intensity (% VO_{2max})	Effort Duration	Recovery Intensity (% VO_{2max})	Recovery Duration	Performance Test	Improved Performance?
64	Davis et al., 1997	Cycling	120–130	1 min	Rest	3 min	Time to fatigue	YES
33	Hargreaves et al., 1984	Cycling	100	30 s	Rest[a]	120 s[a]	Time to fatigue	YES
65	Nassis et al., 1998	Running	80, 85, 90	15 s	45	10 s	Time to fatigue	NO
51	Nicholas et al., 1995	Running[b]	95–130	15 s	Walk to jog at 55	45 s	Time to fatigue	YES
			95	20 meters	55	20 meters	Time to fatigue	YES
34	Yaspelkis et al., 1993	Cycling	75	8 min	45	8 min	Time to fatigue at 80% VO_{2max}	YES
			75	3 min	45	3 min		

[a] This sequence was repeated each half hour for 4 hours: 20 minutes at 50% VO_{2max}, 10 minutes of intervals.

[b] The running protocol of Nicholas et al. had two parts, A and B. Part A was performed for 75 minutes; part B, until exhaustion.

According to Shi and Gisolfi,[66] "The positive effect of carbohydrate supplementation during intermittent exercise may be attributed to oxidation of a large percentage of the ingested carbohydrates, thus providing 16 to 20% of the total energy expenditure during exercise" (p. 159). If the energy from oxidation of exogenous carbohydrate exceeds the reduction in energy from oxidation of fats, some of the extra carbohydrate could spare muscle glycogen utilization, delaying fatigue.

In 1993, Tsintzas and colleagues[50] proposed that a 30-km road race performance improvement with ingestion of carbohydrate during exercise was possibly due to sparing of muscle glycogen. To confirm this hypothesis, they performed a study with seven male recreational runners who ran on a treadmill for 60 minutes at 70% VO_{2max} on 2 separate days, drinking either a carbohydrate-electrolyte solution or water.[32] They noted a 28% reduction in total glycogen utilization as a result of carbohydrate ingestion compared with water, but this glycogen sparing occurred only in the slow-twitch, type I fibers. No performance test was included as part of this study.

In a later paper by the same group, on two separate days Tsintzas et al.[24] asked eight subjects to run on a treadmill at 70% VO_{2max} to exhaustion, ingesting either a 5.5% carbohydrate-electrolyte solution or placebo. They reported a 25% reduction in glycogen utilization, again observed only in type I fibers, with carbohydrate supplementation. Carbohydrate ingestion also resulted in a longer ($p < 0.01$) time to exhaustion (132 ± 12 vs. 104 ± 9 minutes). These two studies provide good evidence that carbohydrate ingestion spares muscle glycogen utilization during moderate continuous running. A 1993 paper by Yaspelkis and colleagues[34] suggests that the same thing happens with cycling exercise alternating between low and moderate intensities (45% and 75% VO_{2max}). In this study, muscle glycogen concentration after 190 minutes of exercise was higher when the subjects ingested three feedings of 18 grams of carbohydrate/hour in a 10% carbohydrate liquid supplement than when ingesting an artificially flavored placebo. Performance was significantly improved by carbohydrate supplementation: time to fatigue at 80% VO_{2max} after 200 minutes of low and moderate cycling was longer (33 ± 7 vs. 2 ± 10 minutes). Because they did not find a glycogen concentration difference in the type II muscle fibers toward the end of exercise, the authors discarded the possibility of glycogen resynthesis during the low intensity intervals of exercise. Glycogen sparing in this study is a much more likely mechanism, supported by higher plasma glucose and insulin levels throughout the exercise session with liquid carbohydrate supplementation.

In 1989, Leatt and Jacobs[67] provided evidence for glycogen sparing during a soccer game. Ten young national-level soccer players were assigned to a control (drinking a placebo) or a carbohydrate (7% glucose polymer solution) group. To balance the difference in playing positions, all control (water placebo) players were on one team, and all carbohydrate-treatment players on the other team. A regulation soccer match was played (two 45-minute halves with 10 minutes of rest in between), drinking 500 ml of the assigned solution before the match and 500 ml at half time. Vastus lateralis muscle biopsies were obtained before and after the game. Final muscle glycogen concentrations of the control group were as low as typically found in professional soccer players after a match, and dehydration was 2.8% of body mass, suggesting that the intensity of play was comparable to a professional soccer game. The decrease in glycogen concentration after the match was significant ($p <$

0. 001), but it was greater for the control group than for the carbohydrate group (181 ± 23 vs. 111 ± 24 mmol glucose units/kg dry wt, $P = 0.002$), representing 39% less glycogen utilization in the carbohydrate group. The major shortcoming of this study is that there was no control or even quantification of total amount of work performed or the intensity of exercise. As a result, the possibility that subjects in the control group exercised at a higher average intensity throughout the match, resulting in a larger glycogen utilization, cannot be ruled out.

Therefore, there is evidence of a reduced net utilization of glycogen with carbohydrate ingestion during intermittent, high intensity exercise.[24,32–34,62,67] Coggan and Coyle[2] pointed out that to provide definitive evidence of "glycogen sparing" would require demonstrating that, given the same pre-exercise muscle glycogen concentration and exercise duration, post-exercise glycogen is significantly higher when fed carbohydrate during the exercise. Six of the seven papers published by that time met the first two criteria, but could not meet the last.[2] However, those papers focused on prolonged strenuous exercise; when intermittent high intensity exercise is analyzed, better support is found in favor of "glycogen sparing." Some evidence favors the theory that an important factor for this reduced net utilization of glycogen during intermittent exercise is glycogen resynthesis during periods of rest and low intensity exercise.

A 1987 paper by Kuipers and colleagues[68] shows that glycogen resynthesis can occur during 3 hours of low intensity cycling at 40% of maximal workload, after depletion to an average of 136 ± 66 mmol/kg dry weight, when trained male subjects are supplemented with carbohydrate. This glycogen synthesis was not as high as that obtained at rest, but was still important (average measured net glycogen synthesis rate of 21 mmol/kg dry weight/hour), and occurred mainly in the type II fibers, which were more likely to be inactive during this type of exercise. In a later study, Kuipers et al.[69] showed that this glycogen resynthesis during low intensity exercise did not happen in untrained men. More recently, Price et al.[70] showed that simultaneous glycogen synthesis and degradation were possible in a single exercising muscle of normal, healthy (presumably untrained) subjects, when muscle contractions were performed at 15% of a maximal voluntary contraction. Owing to the incomplete nature of the scientific literature on this topic, the relative importance of muscle glycogen resynthesis during periods of low intensity exercise warrants further evaluation.

An important limitation to the theory that intermittent exercise performance is enhanced by ingestion of carbohydrate during exercise due to a better maintenance of glycogen stores is that glycogen data are reported on mixed muscle; the results of these assays typically indicate that carbohydrate feeding has no glycogen sparing effect. Davis and colleagues[64] have pointed out, however, that the limiting factor for performance in this type of exercise is not mixed muscle glycogen depletion, but glycogen depletion and fatigue in fast-twitch, type II muscle fibers, which may lead to poorer performance. Because glycogen sparing has been documented in type I but not in type II fibers, a more promising underlying mechanism for the ergogenic effect of carbohydrate ingestion during intermittent high intensity exercise is glycogen resynthesis in type II fibers during the low intensity recovery periods. This idea had already been proposed by Davis's group in an earlier abstract publication of the 1997 study.[71]

To summarize, the evidence available to date shows that high intensity intermittent exercise performance is improved by carbohydrate ingestion during the activity, thanks to a reduced net utilization of muscle glycogen. The fact that high-carbohydrate diets, resulting in higher pre-exercise glycogen stores, cause an improved exercise performance during high intensity intermittent running typical of team sports,[18,59,60] or during actual ice hockey games,[57] also supports the importance of maintenance of glycogen stores for this type of exercise performance.

The prevailing scientific consensus is that there is a positive performance response to carbohydrate ingestion during exercise of different types, intensities, and durations. For this ergogenic effect to occur, the exercise must be long enough or intense enough to significantly reduce muscle glycogen stores or challenge plasma glucose concentration. Some subjects have a greater ability to regulate plasma glucose even under adverse conditions, and they may not benefit from carbohydrate ingestion. Untrained individuals may also benefit only marginally from an increased availability of exogenous carbohydrate. However, because there is no clear evidence of a detrimental effect of carbohydrate ingestion during exercise on performance, utilization of properly formulated sports drinks during physical activity should, at worst, be as beneficial as drinking water and, at best, provide enough carbohydrate to produce the type of performance improvements discussed in this section.

6.4 PRACTICAL ISSUES FOR THE USE OF SPORTS DRINKS DURING EXERCISE TO IMPROVE PERFORMANCE

Most of the following recommendations have been obtained from studies on prolonged strenuous exercise. As more studies are published on the other types of exercise discussed in this chapter, more-specific recommendations may be warranted. Meanwhile, large amounts of useful information are available to support these general recommendations.

6.4.1 TYPE OF CARBOHYDRATES

According to the American College of Sports Medicine, "The inclusion of glucose, sucrose, and other complex carbohydrates in fluid replacement solutions have equal effectiveness in increasing exogenous carbohydrate oxidation, delaying fatigue, and improving performance" (p. iv).[42,72] Carbohydrate oxidation is similar when exercising subjects are fed with glucose or glucose polymers (maltodextrins), but fructose results in lower carbohydrate oxidation rates.[25,73,74] Fructose is clearly not as effective in improving performance, and it may even cause gastrointestinal distress leading to impaired performance.[42,43,72] Hawley and colleagues[25] proposed that oxidation rates of ingested maltose, sucrose, and glucose polymer solutions are very similar to those reported for glucose, provided the carbohydrate is ingested in sufficiently large amounts, supposedly to assure enough carbohydrate delivery to the working muscles. As previously mentioned, Adopo et al.[26] have shown that the combination of 50 grams of glucose and 50 grams of fructose enhances exogenous carbohydrate oxidation above that obtained with 100 grams of glucose alone. This supports the formulation found in some sport drinks where several carbohydrate forms are combined. The oxidation rates of different forms of carbohydrate seem to be strongly related to their glycemic index and stimulation of insulin secretion.[2,75]

Liquid and solid forms of carbohydrate seem to be equally effective ways to supply glucose during exercise and improve performance,[34,76-78] but carbohydrate drinks fulfill a double purpose because they replace the loss of fluids from sweat. This is especially important during activities when dehydration may also impair performance. Besides, liquid forms of carbohydrate tend to be easier to ingest. Carbohydrate gels have become recently available; they are very easy to ingest and carry, but supply no fluid. The particular demands of each sport and the environment in which training and competition occur must be considered when choosing a form of carbohydrate supply.

6.4.2 TIMING OF CARBOHYDRATE INGESTION

According to Coyle,[3] the most effective approach is to ingest carbohydrate at regular intervals throughout exercise. Similar results are obtained if sufficient carbohydrate is ingested at least 30 minutes before the point of fatigue,[2] but once fatigue is reached, the only way to restore carbohydrate and continue exercising is by intravenous infusion of glucose.[30] Similarly, if carbohydrate is ingested too late in exercise, performance is not improved regardless of changes in plasma glucose and insulin.[79] Hargreaves notes that athletes cannot predict when they are 30 minutes away from the point of fatigue (or "late in exercise," for that matter), and therefore it is better to begin carbohydrate ingestion early and continue it at regular intervals throughout the exercise.[4] This approach also makes sense from the point of view of fluid ingestion, because adequate hydration occurs when fluid intake begins early during exercise and is repeated at frequent intervals.[42]

6.4.3 AMOUNT OF CARBOHYDRATE INGESTION: UPPER AND LOWER LIMITS

There is not a clear dose–response relationship between the amount of carbohydrate ingestion during exercise and improvements in performance.[4] However, there seems to be an ideal range of carbohydrate supply between about 30 to 60 grams/hour.[2,28,48,80] The upper limit to useful carbohydrate ingestion during exercise is related to both the rate of delivery of glucose from the gastrointestinal tract to exercising skeletal muscles, and the oxidation rate of exogenous glucose by these muscles. Wagenmakers et al.[74] showed that when carbohydrate is ingested at a rate higher than about 60 grams/hour, exogenous glucose oxidation rates do not increase appreciably. In other words, ingested carbohydrate is oxidized at approximately 1 gram/minute during exercise.[81,82]

Intravenous glucose infusion resulting in hyperglycemia is able to increase the oxidation of carbohydrate and disposal of exogenous glucose during prolonged cycling to higher levels than those obtained with carbohydrate feeding.[83,84] These results have been obtained only with well-trained cyclists, but they suggest that the upper limit of exogenous carbohydrate utilization is partly defined by the delivery

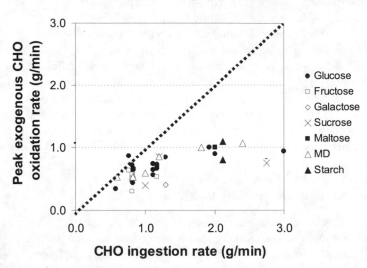

FIGURE 6.4   Peak oxidation rates of ingested carbohydrate. Oxidation rates are depicted against the ingestion rate of different types of carohydrate. Fructose and galactose seem to be oxidized at relatively low rates, whereas glucose, sucrose, maltose, maltodextrins and soluble starch seem to be oxidized at relatively high rates. The horizontal line depicts the absolute maximum for oral carbohydrate oxidation. The dotted line represents the line of identity, where carbohydrate ingestion equals carbohydrate oxidation. (From Jeukendrup and Jentjens, Oxidation of carbohydrate feedings during prolonged exercise: current thoughts, guidelines, and directions for future research. *Sports Med.*, Figure 3, in press. With permission.

of ingested carbohydrate from the gastrointestinal tract to the muscle. In addition, rehydration studies have clearly shown that the rates of gastric emptying and intestinal absorption are impaired by high carbohydrate concentrations (see Chapter 4 for more information on this issue).

The lower limits of carbohydrate ingestion that will improve performance are not as clear. A dose of 13 grams/hour was too low to improve cycling performance at about 67% VO_{2max}[85]. However, a more recent study by Maughan et al.[86] found a significantly improved cycling performance at 70% VO_{2max} with ingestion of only 9.7 grams/hour of carbohydrate in a hypotonic solution (average exercise time to exhaustion = 110 minutes) or 21.6 grams/hour of carbohydrate in an isotonic solution (time = 119 minutes), compared with no fluid (time = 87 minutes). However, ingestion of the same volume of water also resulted in improved performance (time to exhaustion = 101 minutes), and only the isotonic solution with higher carbohydrate content was able to improve performance significantly more than water. The American College of Sports Medicine recommends a minimum of 30 grams of carbohydrate/hour.[42] Hargreaves,[4] however, feels that more research is necessary to better identify the minimum amount of carbohydrate that should be ingested to improve performance. Meanwhile, a reasonable and practical approach is to ingest 30–60 grams of carbohydrate/hour in a properly formulated sports drink, whenever both carbohydrate ingestion and fluid replacement are important.

6.5 SUMMARY

Carbohydrate is an essential fuel for exercise of moderate to high intensity, when ATP must be produced at rates high enough to meet the energy needs of vigorous activity. Carbohydrate intake during exercise has been shown to improve performance during prolonged running and cycling at moderate intensity. Studies from the past 15 years have shown that this performance improvement also occurs during shorter-duration (about 1 hour) exercise of higher intensity (around 80% VO_{2max}), and during intermittent high intensity exercise, both in cycling and running activities. Carbohydrate intake improves performance of prolonged strenuous cycling by contributing to the maintenance of blood glucose levels and carbohydrate oxidation rates late in exercise, when muscle glycogen levels are low. In high intensity intermittent running or cycling, and in prolonged strenuous running, carbohydrate intake supplies large amounts of blood glucose to the muscles, allowing a reduced muscle glycogen utilization or favoring glycogen resynthesis.

Physical activity normally increases sweat output and creates the need for rehydration and replacement of some electrolytes, primarily sodium chloride. Replacing those fluids and electrolytes by ingesting a sports drink at regular intervals, starting early in exercise, is an excellent way to provide carbohydrate to the body, improving the possibility of an enhanced performance.

REFERENCES

1. Lamb, D. R., Basic principles for improving sport performance, *Sports Science Exchange,* 8, 1-6, 1995.
2. Coggan, A. R. and Coyle, E. F., Carbohydrate ingestion during prolonged exercise: effects on metabolism and performance, *Exerc. Sport Sci. Rev.,* 19, 1, 1991.
3. Coyle, E. F., Fuels for sport performance, in *Perspectives in Exercise and Sports Medicine: Optimizing Sport Performance*, Lamb, D. R. and Murray, R., Eds., Cooper Publishing Group, Carmel, IN, 1997.
4. Hargreaves, M., Metabolic responses to carbohydrate ingestion: effects on exercise performance, in *Perspectives in Exercise Science and Sports Medicine: The Metabolic Basis of Performance in Exercise and Sport*, Lamb, D. R. and Murray, R., Eds., Cooper Publishing Group, Carmel, IN, USA, 1999.
5. Maughan, R. J., Carbohydrate-electrolyte solutions during prolonged exercise, in *Perspectives in Exercise Science and Sports Medicine. Ergogenics: Enhancement of Performance in Exercise and Sport* , Lamb, D. R. and Williams, M. H., Eds., Brown and Benchmark, Carmel, IN, 1991.
6. Brooks, G. A., Fahey, T. D., and White T. P., *Exercise Physiology: Human Bioenergetics and Its Applications,* Mayfield Publishing Company, Mountain View, CA, 1996.
7. Lemon, P. W. and Mullin, J. P., Effect of initial muscle glycogen levels on protein catabolism during exercise, *J. Appl. Physiol.,* 48, 624, 1980.

8. Davis, J. M. and Bailey, S. P., Possible mechanisms of central nervous system fatigue during exercise, *Med. Sci. Sports Exerc.,* 29, 45, 1997.

9. Davis, J. M., Carbohydrates, branched-chain amino acids, and endurance: the central fatigue hypothesis, *Int. J. Sport Nutr.,* 5, S29, 1995.

10. Romijn, J. A., Coyle, E. F., Sidossis, L. S., Gastaldelli, A., Horowitz, J. F., Endert, E., and Wolfe, R. R., Regulation of endogenous fat and carbohydrate metabolism in relation to exercise intensity and duration, *Am. J. Physiol.,* 265, E380, 1993.

11. Coyle, E. F., Coggan, A. R., Hemmert, M. K., and Ivy, J. L., Muscle glycogen utilization during prolonged strenuous exercise when fed carbohydrate, *J. Appl. Physiol.,* 61, 165, 1986.

12. Martin, W. H. III, Effects of acute and chronic exercise on fat metabolism, *Exerc. Sport Sci. Rev.,* 24, 203, 1996.

13. Aragón-Vargas, L. F., Effects of fasting on endurance exercise, *Sports Med.,* 16, 255, 1993.

14. Björkman, O. and Eriksson, L. S., Splanchnic glucose metabolism during leg exercise in 60-hour-fasted human subjects, *Am. J. Physiol.,* 245, E443, 1983.

15. Burstein, R., Shpilberg, O., Rubinstein, A., Bashan, N., Falk, B., and Epstein, Y., The effect of prolonged intermittent exercise, combined with food deprivation, on plasma metabolite concentration, *Aviat. Space Environ. Med.,* 62, 555, 1991.

16. Costill, D. L., Coyle E. F., Dalsky, G., Evans, W., Fink, W., and Hoopes, D., Effects of elevated plasma FFA and insulin on muscle glycogen usage during exercise, *J. Appl. Physiol.,* 43, 695, 1977.

17. Montain, S. J., Hopper, M. K., Coggan, A. R., and Coyle, E. F., Exercise metabolism at different time intervals after a meal, *J. Appl. Physiol.,* 70, 882, 1991.

18. Bangsbo, J., Nørregaard, L., and Thorsøe, F., The effect of carbohydrate diet on intermittent exercise performance, *Int. J. Sports Med.,* 13, 152, 1992.

19. Roy, B. D., Tarnopolsky, M. A., MacDougall, J. D., Fowles, J., and Yarasheski, K. E., Effect of glucose supplement timing on protein metabolism after resistance training, *J. Appl. Physiol.,* 82, 1882, 1997.

20. O'Brien, M. J., Viguie, C. A., Mazzeo, R. S., and Brooks, G. A., Carbohydrate dependence during marathon running, *Med. Sci. Sports Exerc.,* 25, 1009, 1993.

21. Bangsbo, J., Madsen, K., Kiens, B., and Richter, E. A., Muscle glycogen synthesis in recovery from intense exercise in humans, *Am. J. Physiol.,* 273, E416, 1997.

22. Bergstrom, J., Hermansen, L., Hultman, E., and Saltin, B., Diet, muscle glycogen and physical performance, *Acta Physiol. Scand.,* 71, 140, 1967.

23. Conlee, R. K., Muscle glycogen and exercise endurance: a twenty-year perspective, *Exerc. Sport Sci. Rev.,* 15, 1, 1987.

24. Tsintzas, O. K., Williams, C., Boobis, L., and Greenhaff, P., Carbohydrate ingestion and single muscle fiber glycogen metabolism during prolonged running in men, *J. Appl. Physiol.,* 81, 801, 1996.

25. Hawley, J. A., Dennis, S. C., and Noakes, T. D., Oxidation of carbohydrate ingested during prolonged endurance exercise, *Sports Med.,* 14, 27, 1992.

26. Adopo, E., Peronnet, F., Massicotte, D., Brisson, G. R., and Hillarie-Marcel, C., Respective oxidation of exogenous glucose and fructose given in the same drink during exercise, *J. Appl. Physiol.,* 76, 1014, 1994.

27. Coyle, E. F., Hagberg, J. M., Hurley, B. F., Martin, W. H., Ehsani, A. A., and Holloszy, J. O., Carbohydrate feeding during prolonged strenuous exercise can delay fatigue, *J. Appl. Physiol.,* 55, 230, 1983.

28. Murray, R., Paul, G. L., Seifert, J. G., and Eddy, D. E., Responses to varying rates of carbohydrate ingestion during exercise, *Med. Sci. Sports Exerc.,* 23, 713, 1991.

29. DeMarco, H. M., Sucher, K. P., Cisar, C. J., and Butterfield, G. E., Pre-exercise carbohydrate meals: application of glycemic index, *Med. Sci. Sports Exerc.*, 31, 164, 1999.

30. Coggan, A. R. and Coyle, E. F., Reversal of fatigue during prolonged exercise by carbohydrate infusion or ingestion, *J. Appl. Physiol.*, 63, 2388, 1987.

31. Hargreaves, M., Interactions between muscle glycogen and blood glucose during exercise, *Exerc. Sport Sci. Rev.*, 25, 21, 1997.

32. Tsintzas, O. K., Williams, C., Boobis, L., and Greenhaff, P., Carbohydrate ingestion and glycogen utilization in different muscle fiber types in man, *J. Physiol.*, 489, 243, 1995.

33. Hargreaves, M., Costill, D. L., Coggan, A., Fink, W. J., and Nishibata, I., Effect of carbohydrate feedings on muscle glycogen utilization and exercise performance, *Med. Sci. Sports Exerc.*, 16, 219, 1984.

34. Yaspelkis, B. B., Patterson, J. G., Anderla, P. A., Ding, Z., and Ivy, J. L., Carbohydrate supplementation spares muscle glycogen during variable intensity exercise, *J. Appl. Physiol.*, 75, 1477, 1993.

35. Tsintzas, O. K. and Williams, C., Human muscle glycogen metabolism during exercise: effect of carbohydrate supplementation, *Sports Med.*, 25, 7, 1998.

36. Dill, D. B., Edwards, H. T., and Talbott, J. H., Studies in muscular activity. vii. Factors limiting the capacity for work, *J. Physiol.*, 77, 49, 1932.

37. Gordon, B., Kohn, L. A., Levine, S. A., Matton, M., Scriver, W. M., and Whiting, W. B., Sugar content of the blood in runners following a marathon race. With special reference to the prevention of hypoglycemia: further observations, *JAMA*, 85, 508, 1925.

38. Levine, S. A., Gordon, B., and Derick, C. L., Some changes in the chemical constituents of the blood following a marathon race. With special reference to the development of hypoglycemia, *JAMA*, 82, 1778, 1924.

39. Neufer, P. D., Costill, D. L., Flynn, M. G., Kirwan, J. P., Mitchell, J. B., and Houmard, J., Improvements in exercise performance: effects of carbohydrate feedings and diet, *J. Appl. Physiol.*, 62, 983, 1987.

40. Coyle, E. F., Jeukendrup, A. E., Wagenmakers, A. J., and Saris, W. H., Fatty acid oxidation is directly regulated by carbohydrate metabolism during exercise, *Am. J. Physiol.*, 273, E268, 1997.

41. Puhl, S. M. and Buskirk, E. R., Nutrient beverages for physical performance, in *Nutrition in Exercise and Sport*, Third Edition, Wolinsky, I., Ed., CRC Press, 1998.

42. American College of Sports Medicine, ACSM position stand on exercise and fluid replacement, *Med. Sci. Sports Exerc.*, 28, i, 1996.

43. Björkman, O., Sahlin, K., Hagenfeldt, L., and Wahren, J., Influence of glucose and fructose ingestion on the capacity for long-term exercise in well-trained men, *Clin. Physiol.*, 4, 483, 1984.

44. Coggan, A. R. and Coyle, E. F., Metabolism and performance following carbohydrate ingestion late in exercise, *Med. Sci. Sports Exerc.*, 21, 59, 1989.

45. Davis, J. M., Bailey, S. P., Woods, J. A., Galiano, F. J., Hamilton, M. T., and Bartoli, W. P., Effects of carbohydrate feedings on plasma free tryptophan and branched-chain amino acids during prolonged cycling, *Eur. J. Appl. Physiol.*, 65, 513, 1992.

46. Sasaki, H., Maeda, J., Usui, S., and Ishiko, T., Effect of sucrose and caffeine ingestion on performance of prolonged strenuous running, *Int. J. Sports Med.*, 8, 261, 1987.

47. Wilber, R. L. and Moffatt, R. J., Influence of carbohydrate ingestion on blood glucose and performance in runners, *Int. J. Sport Nutr.*, 2, 317, 1992.

48. Coggan, A. R. and Coyle, E. F., Effect of carbohydrate feedings during high intensity exercise, *J. Appl. Physiol.,* 65, 1703, 1988.
49. Mitchell, J. B., Costill, D. L., Houmard, J. A., Fink, W. J., Pascoe, D. D., and Pearson, D. R., Influence of carbohydrate dosage on exercise performance and glycogen metabolism, *J. Appl. Physiol.,* 67, 1843, 1989.
50. Tsintzas, O. K., Liu, R., Williams, C., Campbell, I., and Gaitanos, G., The effect of carbohydrate ingestion on performance during a 30-km race, *Int. J. Sport Nutr.,* 3, 127, 1993.
51. Nicholas, C. W., Williams, C., Lakomy, H. K. A., Phillips, G., and Nowitz, A., Influence of ingesting a carbohydrate-electrolyte solution on endurance capacity during intermittent high intensity shuttle running, *J. Sports Sci.,* 13, 283, 1995.
52. Ball, T., Headley, S., Vanderburgh, P., and Smith, J., Periodic carbohydrate replacement during 50 min of high intensity cycling improves subsequent sprint performance, *Int. J. Sport Nutr.,* 5, 151, 1995.
53. Anantaraman, R., Carmines, A. A., Gaesser, G. A., and Weltman, A., Effects of carbohydrate supplementation on performance during 1 h of high intensity exercise, *Int. J. Sport Nutr.,* 16, 461, 1995.
54. Below, P. R., Mora-Rodriguez, R., Gonzalez-Alonso, J., and Coyle, E. F., Fluid and carbohydrate ingestion independently improve performance during 1 h of intense exercise, *Med. Sci. Sports Exerc.,* 27, 200, 1995.
55. Hargreaves, M., Dillo, P., Angus, D., and Febbraio, M. A., Effect of fluid ingestion on muscle metabolism during prolonged exercise, *J. Appl. Physiol.,* 80, 363, 1996.
56. Jeukendrup, A. E., Brouns, F., Wagenmakers, A. J., and Saris, W. H., Carbohydrate-electrolyte feedings improve 1h time trial cycling performance, *J. Sports Med.,* 18, 125, 1997.
57. Akermark, C., Jacobs, I., Rasmusson, M., and Karlsson, J., Diet and muscle glycogen concentration in relation to physical performance in Swedish elite ice hockey players, *Int. J. Sport Nutr.,* 6, 272, 1996.
58. Jacobs, I., Westlin, N., Karlsson, J., Rasmusson, M., and Houghton, B., Muscle glycogen and diet in elite soccer players, *Eur. J. Appl. Physiol.,* 48, 297, 1982.
59. Pizza, F., Flynn, M., Duscha, B., Holden, J., and Kubitz, E., A carbohydrate loading regimen improves high intensity, short duration exercise performance, *Int. J. Sport Nutr.,* 5, 110, 1995.
60. Nicholas, C. W., Green, P. A., Hawkins, R. D., and Williams, C., Carbohydrate intake and recovery of intermittent running capacity, *Int. J. Sport Nutr.,* 7, 251, 1997.
61. Murray, R., Eddy, D. E., Murray T. W., Seifert, J. G., Paul, G. L., and Halaby, G. A., The effects of fluid and carbohydrate feedings during intermittent cycling exercise, *Med. Sci. Sports Exerc.,* 19, 597, 1987.
62. Simard, C., Tremblay, A., and Jobin, M., Effects of carbohydrate intake before and during an ice hockey match on blood and muscle energy substrates, *Res. Q. Exerc. Sport,* 59, 144, 1988.
63. Hawley, J. A., Dennis, S. C., and Noakes, T. D., Carbohydrate, fluid, and electrolyte requirements of the soccer player: a review, *Int. J. Sport Nutr.,* 4, 221, 1994.
64. Davis, J. M., Jackson, D. A., Broadwell, M. S., Queary, J. L., and Lambert, C. L., Carbohydrate drinks delay fatigue during intermittent, high intensity cycling in active men and women, *Int. J. Sport Nutr.,* 7, 261, 1997.
65. Nassis, G. P., Williams, C., and Chisnall, P., Effect of a carbohydrate-electrolyte drink on endurance capacity during prolonged intermittent high intensity running, *Br. J. Sports Med.,* 32, 248, 1998.

66. Shi, X. and Gisolfi, C. V., Fluid and carbohydrate replacement during intermittent exercise, *Sports Med.,* 25, 157, 1998.
67. Leatt, P. B. and Jacobs, I., Effect of glucose polymer ingestion on glycogen depletion during a soccer match, *Can. J. Sports Sci.,* 14, 112, 1989.
68. Kuipers, H., Keizer, H. A., Brouns, F., and Saris, W. H., Carbohydrate feeding and glycogen synthesis during exercise in man, *Pflugers Arch.,* 410, 652, 1987.
69. Kuipers, H., Saris, W. H., Brouns, F., Keizer, H. A., and ten Bosch, C., Glycogen synthesis during exercise and rest with carbohydrate feeding in males and females, *Int. J. Sports Med.,* 10 Suppl 1, S63, 1989.
70. Price, T. B., Taylor, R., Mason, G. F., Rothman, D. L., Shulman, G. I., and Shulman, R. G., Turnover of human muscle glycogen with low intensity exercise, *Med. Sci. Sports Exerc.,* 26, 983, 1994.
71. Jackson, D. A., Davis, J. M., Broadwell, M. S., Query, J. L., and Lambert, C. L., Effects of carbohydrate feeding on fatigue during intermittent high intensity exercise in males and females, *Med. Sci. Sports Exerc.,* 27, S223, 1995.
72. Murray, R., Paul, G. L., Seifert, J. G., Eddy, D. E., and Halaby, G. A., The effects of glucose, fructose, and sucrose ingestion during exercise, *Med. Sci. Sports Exerc.,* 21, 275, 1989.
73. Massicotte, D., Peronnet, F., Brisson, G., Bakkouch, K., and Hillaire-Marcel, C., Oxidation of a glucose polymer during exercise: comparison with glucose and fructose, *J. Appl. Physiol.,* 66, 179, 1989.
74. Wagenmakers, A. J., Brouns, F., Saris, W. H., and Halliday, D., Oxidation rates of orally ingested carbohydrates during prolonged exercise in men, *J. Appl. Physiol.,* 75, 2774, 1993.
75. Saris, W. H., Goodpaster, B. H., Jeukendrup, A. E., Brouns, F., Halliday, D., and Wagenmakers, A. J., Exogenous carbohydrate oxidation from different carbohydrate sources during exercise, *J. Appl. Physiol.,* 75, 2168, 1993.
76. Passias, T. C., Meneilly G. S., and Mekjavic, I. B., Effect of hypoglycemia on thermoregulatory responses, *J. Appl. Physiol.,* 80, 1021, 1996.
77. Lugo, M., Sherman, W. M., Wimer, G. S., and Garleb, K., Metabolic responses when different forms of carbohydrate energy are consumed during cycling, *Int. J. Sport Nutr.,* 3, 398, 1993.
78. Mason, W. L., McConell, G., and Hargreaves, M., Carbohydrate ingestion during exercise: liquid vs. solid feedings, *Med. Sci. Sports Exerc.,* 25, 966, 1993.
79. McConell, G., Kloot, K., and Hargreaves, M., Effect of timing of carbohydrate ingestion on endurance exercise performance, *Med. Sci. Sports Exerc.,* 28, 1300, 1996.
80. Murray, R., Seifert, J. G., Eddy, D. E., Paul, G. L., and Halaby, G., Carbohydrate feeding and exercise: effect of beverage carbohydrate content, *Eur. J. Appl. Physiol.,* 59, 152, 1989.
81. Bosch, A. N., Dennis, S. C., and Noakes, T. D., Influence of carbohydrate ingestion on fuel substrate turnover and oxidation during prolonged exercise, *J. Appl. Physiol.,* 76, 2364, 1994.
82. McConell, G., Fabris, S., Proietto, J., and Hargreaves, M., Effect of carbohydrate ingestion on glucose kinetics during exercise, *J. Appl. Physiol.,* 77, 1537, 1994.
83. Coyle, E. F., Hamilton, M. T., Alonso, J. G., Montain, S. J., and Ivy, J. L., Carbohydrate metabolism during intense exercise when hyperglycemic, *J. Appl. Physiol.,* 70, 834, 1991.
84. Hawley, J. A., Bosch, A. N., Weltan, S. M., Dennis, S. C., and Noakes, T. D., Glucose kinetics during prolonged exercise in euglycaemic and hyperglycaemic subjects, *Pflugers Arch.,* 426, 378, 1994.

85. Burgess, W., Davis, J., Bartoli, W., and Woods, J., Failure of low dose carbohydrate feeding to attenuate glucoregulatory hormone responses and improve endurance performance, *Int. J. Sport Nutr.*, 1, 338, 1991.

86. Maughan, R. J., Bethell, L. R., and Leiper, J. B., Effects of ingested fluids on homeostasis and exercise performance in man, *Exp. Physiol.*, 81, 847, 1996.

7 Post-Exercise Rehydration and Recovery

Susan M. Shirreffs

CONTENTS

0-8493-7008-6/01/$0.00+$.50

7.1 INTRODUCTION

7.1.1 Exercise-Induced Dehydration

For healthy individuals, the stress of physical exercise, especially when undertaken in a hot environment, may pose the greatest challenge to homeostasis that is likely to be encountered. Core temperature must be maintained within the narrow range of around 35° to 40°C, but this is done at the expense of increased body water losses through sweating. If these losses are not corrected or at least minimized, exercise performance will be adversely affected. Potentially more serious, though, is the impact on the body's thermoregulatory effectiveness. Without correction of a body water deficit, sweat production is reduced and core temperature can spiral to dangerously high levels. A rapid and complete rehydration in this situation is therefore of paramount importance.

7.1.1.1 Mechanism of Development

The rise in body temperature that accompanies exercise in the heat can be attenuated by the evaporation of sweat, but large sweat losses result in hypohydration and loss of electrolytes, which may also have serious consequences. In high heat and humidity, working capacity is compromised by the increased heat stress, but the risk to health and well being is a more serious concern. The early onset of fatigue when exercise is undertaken in these conditions is inevitable and may serve to prevent serious health consequences.

7.1.1.2 Effect on Exercise Performance

It is often reported that exercise performance is impaired when an individual is dehydrated by as little as 1–2% of body mass, and that losses in excess of 5% of body mass can decrease the capacity for work by about 30%.[1] Dehydration-induced decrements in performance are common because humans can lose sweat at rapid rates, especially during vigorous exercise in a warm environment. For example, sweat rates of 1 to 2 l/h are common even in mild environmental conditions, with some individuals capable of secreting sweat at rates in excess of 2 to 3 l/h. In a 70-kg (154-lb) person, the loss of just 1.5 l of sweat constitutes a loss of 2.1% of body mass, a level of dehydration that has been shown to compromise physiological function and impair performance. The fact that such losses can occur quickly is clear testament to the need to rapidly replace deficits in body water content.

Undertaking physical activity in a dehydrated state also impairs the capacity to perform high-intensity exercise as well as endurance activities.[2, 3] Nielsen et al.[2] showed that prolonged exercise, which resulted in a loss of fluid corresponding to 2.5% of body mass, resulted in a 45% fall in the capacity to perform high-intensity exercise. A fluid deficit of as little as 1.8% of body mass has been shown to impair exercise tolerance.[4] It may be that even smaller fluid deficits can adversely affect performance in competitive sports where the difference between winning and losing is extraordinarily small, but laboratory methods may not be sufficiently sensitive to detect such small changes in performance.

Fluid losses are distributed in varying proportions among the body fluid compartments: plasma, extracellular water, and intracellular water. The decrease in plasma volume that accompanies dehydration may be of particular importance in influencing an individual's work capacity; blood flow to the muscles must be maintained at a high level to supply oxygen and substrates, but a high blood flow to the skin is also required to convect heat to the body surface where it can be dissipated.[5] When the ambient temperature is high and blood volume has been decreased by sweat loss during prolonged exercise, there may be difficulty in meeting the requirement for a high blood flow to both these tissues. In this situation, skin blood flow is likely to be compromised, allowing central venous pressure and muscle blood flow to be maintained, but reducing heat loss and causing body temperature to rise.[6]

These factors have been investigated by Coyle and his colleagues; their results clearly demonstrate that increases in core temperature and heart rate during prolonged exercise are graded according to the level of hypohydration.[7] They also showed that the ingestion of fluid during exercise increases skin blood flow, and therefore improves thermoregulatory capacity, independent of increases in the circulating blood volume.[8] For example, plasma volume expansion using dextran/saline infusion was less effective in preventing a rise in core temperature than was the ingestion of sufficient volumes of a carbohydrate-electrolyte drink to maintain plasma volume at a similar level.

Because sweat is hypotonic with respect to body fluids, the effect of prolonged sweating is to increase the plasma osmolality, which may have a significant effect on the ability to maintain body temperature. A direct relationship between plasma osmolality and body temperature has been demonstrated during exercise.[9,10] Hyperosmolality of plasma, induced prior to exercise, has been shown to result in a decreased thermoregulatory effector response; the threshold for sweating is elevated and the cutaneous vasodilator response is reduced.[11] In short term (30 min) exercise, however, the cardiovascular and thermoregulatory response appears to be independent of changes in osmolality induced during the exercise period.[12]

7.1.1.3   Role of Post-Exercise Rehydration and Recovery Beverages

Beverages formulated for post-exercise rehydration and recovery generally have two main aims:

1. to replace the water and electrolytes lost in the sweat secreted during exercise
2. to replace the carbohydrate utilized from liver and muscle stores during exercise

The focus of the rest of this chapter is on understanding the physiological mechanisms that underlie the rapid and complete restoration of body water stores and the replenishment of glycogen stores.

7.2 POST-EXERCISE RECOVERY

7.2.1 Fluid Balance Recovery

7.2.1.1 Water Replacement

7.2.1.1.1 Volume required

Obligatory urine losses persist even in the dehydrated state, assuring the elimination of metabolic waste products. It is clear, therefore, that the total fluid intake after exercise-induced or thermal sweating must amount to a volume greater than the volume of sweat that has been lost if effective rehydration is to be achieved. Shirreffs et al.[13] investigated the influence of drink volume on rehydration effectiveness following exercise-induced dehydration equivalent to approximately 2% of body mass. Drink volumes equivalent to 50%, 100%, 150% and 200% of the sweat loss were consumed after exercise. To investigate the possible interaction between beverage volume and its sodium content, a relatively low-sodium drink (23 mmol/l) and a moderately high-sodium drink (61 mmol/l) were compared. By way of comparison, these sodium concentrations are similar to the normal range of sodium concentration in sweat (e.g., 20 to 80 mmol/l).

With the ingestion of both beverages, the urine volume produced was, not surprisingly, related to the beverage volume consumed (Figure 7.1); the smallest urine volumes were produced when 50% of the sweat loss was consumed and the greatest when 200% of the loss was consumed. Subjects did not restore their hydration status when they consumed a volume equivalent to, or only half of, their sweat loss, irrespective of the sodium content of the drink. When a drink volume equal to 150% of the sweat loss was consumed, subjects were slightly hypohydrated 6 h after drinking the test drink with a low sodium concentration, and they were in a similar condition when they drank the same beverage in a volume of twice their sweat loss. With the high-sodium drink, enough fluid was retained to keep the subjects in a state of hyperhydration 6 h after drink ingestion when they consumed either 150% or 200% of their sweat loss. The excess fluid would eventually be lost by urine production or by further sweat loss if the individual resumed exercise or was exposed to a warm environment. Calculated plasma volume changes indicated a decrease of approximately 5.3% with dehydration in all trials. At the end of the study period, the general pattern was for the increases in plasma volume to be a direct function of the volume of fluid consumed. Additionally, the increase in plasma volume tended to be greater after ingestion of the high sodium drink.

7.2.1.2 Electrolyte Replacement

7.2.1.2.1 Sodium

Ingestion of plain water in the post-exercise period results in a rapid fall in the plasma sodium concentration and in plasma osmolality.[14] These changes have the effect of drastically reducing voluntary fluid intake and of stimulating urine output, both of which will delay the rehydration process. In the study of Nose et al.,[14] subjects exercised at low intensity in the heat for 90–110 min, inducing a mean hypohydration of 2.3% of body mass, and then rested for 1 h before beginning to

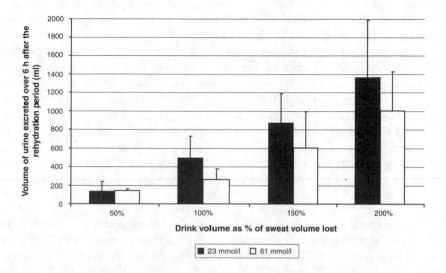

FIGURE 7.1 Total volume of urine excreted over the 6 h after rehydration. The greatest urine volumes were excreted when the largest drink volume was consumed, but smaller urine volumes were excreted after drinking the 61 mmol/l sodium drink in comparison with the 23 mmol/l sodium drink. Values are median and maximum values.

drink. Plasma volume was not restored until after 60 min, when plain water was ingested together with placebo (sucrose) capsules. When sodium chloride capsules were ingested with water to yield a saline solution with an effective concentration of 0.45% (77 mmol/l), plasma volume was restored within 20 min. In the sodium chloride trial, voluntary fluid intake was considerably higher and urine output was less; 71% of the water loss was retained within 3 h, compared with 51% in the plain water trial. The delayed rehydration in the water trial appeared to be a result of a continued net loss of sodium, accompanied by water, in the urine. This was likely caused by reduction in plasma renin activity and aldosterone levels that led to a decrease in water reabsorption.

When a fixed volume of fluid with different sodium concentrations is ingested following exercise-induced hypohydration, the resultant urine output is inversely related to the sodium content of the ingested fluid.[15] In this study, subjects were dehydrated by intermittent exercise in the heat until 2% of body mass was lost. They then consumed a 2050 ml volume of fluid, which was equivalent to 1.5 times their sweat loss. The drinks contained 0, 25, 50 or 100 mmol/l sodium. Over a 5.5-h period after drinking, the smallest urine volume produced was after drinking the 100 mmol/l sodium drink. This amounted to 551ml in comparison with the largest volume of 1316ml, which was produced after drinking the sodium free drink. The volumes produced after the other two drinks were likewise dependent on the quantity of sodium ingested with 958 ml after the 25 mmol/l sodium drink and 627 ml after the 50 mmol/l sodium drink. The significance of these volumes is that while 74% of the 100 mmol/l sodium drink was retained in this period, only 36% of the electrolyte-free drink was retained. The subjects were hypohydrated at this time after drinking the sodium-free and 25 mmol/l sodium drink but were euhydrated after drinking the 50 and 100 mmol/l sodium drink.

Rapid and complete rehydration after exercise can only be achieved if both fluid and electrolyte losses are replaced. Ideally, rehydration drinks should have a sodium concentration similar to that of sweat, but since the sodium content of sweat varies widely among people, no single formulation is possible. The upper end of the normal range for sweat sodium concentration (80 mmol/l), is similar to the sodium concentration of the oral rehydration solution (ORS) recommended by the World Health Organization for rehydration in cases of severe diarrhea (90 mmol/l). By contrast, the sodium concentration of most sports drinks ranges from 10 to 30 mmol/l, and most fruit juices and carbonated soft drinks contain virtually no sodium.

7.2.1.2.2 Potassium

It has been speculated that inclusion of potassium, the major cation in the intracellular space, would enhance the replacement of intracellular water after exercise and thus promote rehydration.[16] Experimental investigation has demonstrated that inclusion of potassium (as 25 mmol/l KCl) may, in some situations, be as effective as sodium (as 60 mmol/l NaCl) in retaining water ingested after exercise-induced hypohydration.[17] In this study, eight male volunteers were dehydrated by 2.1% of body mass by intermittent cycle ergometer exercise in the heat and then ingested either a glucose drink (90 mmol/l), a sodium-containing drink (NaCl 60 mmol/l), a potassium-containing drink (KCl 25 mmol/l) or a drink containing the glucose, sodium, and potassium. The drinks were consumed over a 30-min period beginning 45 min after the end of exercise in a volume equivalent to the volume of sweat lost. This amounted to approximately 1.6 l, and no other food or drink was consumed during the study. All the urine produced and excreted from the end of the rehydration period for the next 6 h was collected. A smaller volume of urine was excreted following rehydration when the electrolyte-containing beverages (248, 303, and 254 ml respectively) were ingested than with the electrolyte-free beverage. Therefore, although different amounts of electrolytes were consumed, there was no difference in the fraction of ingested fluid retained 6 h after finishing drinking the drinks that contained electrolytes. In this situation, therefore, addition of either sodium or potassium has significantly increased the fraction of the ingested fluid that was retained, but there was no additive effect of including both ions, as would be expected if they acted independently on different body fluid compartments. As the beverage volume consumed was equal to the volume of sweat loss, a state of negative fluid balance existed because of the ongoing urine losses, except for a very brief time at the end of the drinking period. Therefore, the volumes of urine excreted were close to basal levels, and further reductions in urine output may not have been possible when both sodium and potassium were ingested together.

With dehydration, water is lost from all the body's fluid compartments. In the study of Maughan et al.,[17] plasma volume was calculated (by the method of Dill and Costill[18]) to have decreased by approximately 4% with dehydration. After drinking, plasma volume increased on all trials to values slightly in excess of baseline, but the rate of recovery was slower when the beverage containing potassium was consumed. After 6 h of rehydration the increase in plasma volume did not differ among trials.

In a rehydration study with rats that were thermally dehydrated by approximately 9% of body mass and then given free access to rehydration solutions consisting of either isotonic NaCl, isotonic KCl, or tap water, Yawata[19] found that the rats drank substantially more NaCl than KCl, but urinated only slightly more after consuming the NaCl. The best rehydration was achieved with the NaCl treatment. In this study, whole-body net fluid balance was influenced by the rat's taste preferences for the beverages, in addition to the drinks' effects on urine production. With the NaCl drink, 178% of the extracellular volume losses were restored but only 50% was restored with the KCl drink. Despite this however, the intracellular fluid restoration was the same with both drinks and was not greater than the control level. The author suggests that, in the extracellular space, restoration sodium concentration is more important than volume restoration but volume restoration has priority in the intracellular fluid.

7.2.1.2.3   Other electrolytes

The importance of the inclusion of magnesium in sports drinks has been the subject of much discussion. Magnesium is lost in sweat and many believe that this causes a reduction in plasma magnesium levels, which are implicated in muscle cramp. Even though there can be a decline in plasma magnesium concentration during exercise, it is most likely due to a redistribution between compartments rather than due to sweat loss. There does not, therefore, seem to be any good reason for including magnesium in post-exercise rehydration and recovery sports drinks.

Sodium, therefore, is the most important electrolyte in terms of recovery after exercise. Without its replacement, water retention is hampered. Potassium is also included in sports drinks in similar concentrations to that which is lost in sweat. Unlike the strong evidence available for the inclusion of sodium, there is not the same for potassium. There is no evidence for the inclusion of any other electrolytes.

7.2.2   SUBSTRATE RECOVERY

7.2.2.1   Carbohydrate

Exercise can lead to a depletion of the body's glycogen stores, particularly those of the liver and the exercising muscle. Glycogen depletion results from the mobilization of glycogen stores to provide energy for muscular contraction, and is a major factor contributing to fatigue. The primary aim of carbohydrate ingestion following exercise is to promote glycogen resynthesis and a rapid restoration of muscle and liver glycogen. This is of particular importance when a further bout of exercise is to be undertaken in the same day and, therefore, is of significance to athletes in training and in competitions where more than one game or round is involved. Several factors influence the rate at which glycogen resynthesis occurs after exercise. The most important factor is undoubtedly the amount of carbohydrate consumed; the type of carbohydrate and the time of ingestion are less important, but do have an effect.

7.2.2.1.1 Type of carbohydrate

Glucose and sucrose ingestion both give rise to similar glycogen synthesis rates when consumed after exercise; these rates typically reach 5–6 mmol $kg^{-1} \cdot h^{-1}$ after the ingestion of 50 grams of glucose or sucrose every 2 h for 6 h after exercise. Fructose alone, however, results in a lower rate of glycogen synthesis, approximately 3 mmol kg/h.[20,21] This lower rate is likely to be due to the relatively slow rate at which the liver converts fructose to glucose. Although the use of fructose as a carbohydrate source is often promoted for athletes, it is poorly absorbed in the small intestine relative to many other sugars, and ingestion of large amounts of fructose is likely to result in diarrhea.[22] There is some evidence that carbohydrates with a high glycemic index — those carbohydrates that result in a large and sustained elevation of the blood glucose concentration after ingestion — are the most effective when rapid glycogen replacement is desired.[23] However, the nature in which carbohydrates with a high- or moderate-glycemic index are consumed after exercise (i.e., as a solid or liquid) appears to have no influence on glycogen synthesis rates.[24,25]

7.2.2.1.2 Quantity of carbohydrate

The rate of glycogen synthesis after exercise reaches a plateau after a certain amount of carbohydrate has been consumed. This has been demonstrated in studies where subjects were fed different amounts of glucose or maltodextrins every 2 h after exercise.[20,26] The results showed that muscle glycogen synthesis occurred at a rate of 2 mmol kg/h when 25 g of carbohydrate was ingested every 2 h, and that the replenishment rate increased to 6 mmol kg/h when 50 g was ingested every 2 h. However, muscle glycogen synthesis did increase to more than about 5 to 6 mmol kg/heven when very large amounts (up to 225 g) of carbohydrate were ingested every 2 h. Further, with intravenous glucose infusion of 100 g every 2 h, muscle glycogen synthesis of about 7 to 8 mmol kg/h has been reported.[25] This rate of glycogen synthesis is not significantly greater than the rates achieved with carbohydrate ingestion, suggesting that glycogen synthesis is not limited by the rate at which substrate is made available by the gastrointestinal tract. Also, increasing the amount of carbohydrate ingested will increase the rate of delivery to the intestine for absorption. Therefore, it seems that the maximum rate of muscle glycogen synthesis after exercise is in the region of 5 to 8 mmol/kg/h, provided that at least 50 g of glucose is ingested every 2 h after exercise.

During the first 2 h after exercise, muscle glycogen resynthesis rates are at their highest, at a rate of around 7 to 8 mmol/kg/h, declining to the more normal value of 5 to 6 mmol/kg/h after this time. One of the benefits of having carbohydrate in sports drinks is that many people find them convenient and appealing at this time when the appetite is blunted.

7.2.2.1.3 Timing of carbohydrate ingestion

The muscle appears to have a particularly high affinity for glucose uptake immediately after exercise, and the greatest rate of muscle glycogen resynthesis occurs over the first 2 h immediately after exercise (i.e., 7 to 8 mmol kg/h vs. the rate after this time of 5 to 6 mmol/kg/h).[27] This increased synthesis rate can only take place if sufficient carbohydrate is ingested. Therefore, to assure maximal glycogen resynthesis rates, carbohydrate should be consumed as soon as possible after exercise. As a practical guide, it is suggested that approximately 0.7 g of glucose per kg of body mass should be consumed every 2 h for the first 4 to 6 h after exercise to maximize the rate of glycogen resynthesis.[20,24] It makes no difference whether this carbohydrate to be consumed is ingested as a few large meals or as many small frequent meals.[28,29]

Liver glycogen restoration occurs less rapidly than muscle glycogen restoration and, indeed, the fast repletion of muscle glycogen stores may be at the expense of liver glycogen levels.[30] However, whereas fructose does not promote as rapid a muscle glycogen restoration as glucose, fructose infusion has been found to give a greater liver glycogen resynthesis than glucose.[31] Some replenishment of the liver glycogen stores occurs by gluconeogenesis of lactate and some amino acids, but this will not provide sufficient substrate to assure complete liver glycogen restoration.

7.2.2.2 Non-Carbohydrate Nutrients

7.2.2.2.1 Protein

Muscle glycogen resynthesis occurs only very slowly when carbohydrate alone is consumed, but there is evidence available to suggest that this rate is enhanced if protein is co-ingested with carbohydrate after exercise. Zawadzki et al.[32] observed a faster rate of muscle glycogen resynthesis after exercise when protein was ingested together with carbohydrate. This effect was deemed to be due to the higher insulin levels produced when the protein was also ingested. Of note, however, is that the glycogen resynthesis rates in this study with the carbohydrate alone were relatively moderate. It leaves open the question as to whether protein ingestion with carbohydrate can elevate muscle glycogen resynthesis rates to values greater than the highest rates of 7–8 mmol kg/h that are generally observed.

7.2.2.2.2 Alcohol and caffeine

Alcohol and caffeine possess well-known diuretic properties and it is usual to advise against the consumption of such drinks when fluid replacement is a priority. However, many people enjoy consuming these beverages, and where large volumes of fluid must be consumed in a relatively short time, a wide choice of drinks will help to stimulate consumption. In many sports, particularly team sports, alcohol intake is a part of the culture of the sport, and athletes are resistant to suggestions that they should abstain completely. However, it is now apparent that the diuretic effect of alcohol, over and above an alcohol-free beverage, is blunted when consumed by individuals who are moderately hypohydrated from exercise in a warm environment.[33] After exercise, subjects consumed a beer shandy (a peculiarly British drink produced by mixing beer with lemonade) containing 0, 1, 2, or 4% alcohol. The volume of urine excreted for the 6 h following drink ingestion was related to the quantity of alcohol consumed, but despite a tendency for the urinary output to increase with increasing alcohol intake, only with the 4% beverage did the increased value approach significance. The calculated decrease in plasma volume with dehydration was approximately 7.6% across all trials. With rehydration, the rate of increase in plasma volume seemed to be related to the quantity of alcohol consumed; 6 h after finishing drinking, the increase in plasma volume relative to the dehydrated

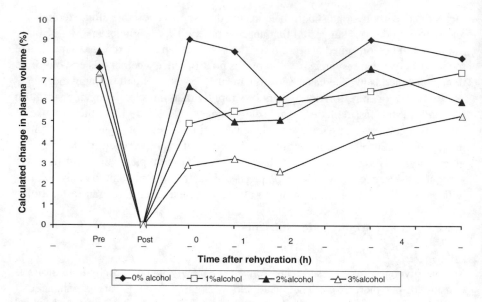

FIGURE 7.2 Calculated change in plasma volume with dehydration equivalent to 2% of body mass and subsequent rehydration with drinks containing 0, 1, 2, and 4% alcohol. The volume of drink consumed was 150% of the sweat loss with dehydration. Values are means.

value was approximately 8% with 0% alcohol, 7% with 1%, 6% with 2%, and 5% with 4% (Figure 7.2). It may be worth noting that the high sugar content of lemonade (10%) means that beer shandy has a carbohydrate content of about 5%, and this carbohydrate may play an important role in the restoration of muscle and liver glycogen stores after exercise. To date, no studies have directly compared the rehydration effectiveness of an alcohol-containing drink with a sports drink consumed after exercise.

González-Alonso et al.[34] in 1992 undertook one of the relatively early studies in the area of post-exercise rehydration and also confirmed that a dilute carbohydrate-electrolyte solution (60 g/l carbohydrate, 20 mmol/l Na^+, 3 mmol/l K^+, 20 mmol/l Cl^-) was more effective in promoting post-exercise rehydration than either plain water or a low electrolyte diet cola: the difference in rehydration effectiveness between the drinks was a result of differences in the volume of urine produced. It is highly likely that the caffeine component of the cola drink had some effect in stimulating the urine formation.

7.2.3 PRIORITIZING POST-EXERCISE RECOVERY

7.2.3.1 Health Considerations

Drinks consumed during or after exercise are generally intended to replace the water and electrolyte losses incurred as a result of sweat secretion, and also to provide carbohydrate to supplement or replenish the glycogen stores in the liver and muscles. The relative importance of providing water or substrate is influenced by many factors.

However, disturbances in body fluid balance and temperature not only can impair exercise performance but also are potentially life threatening. In comparison, the depletion of carbohydrate stores in the liver and working muscles will result in fatigue and a reduction in exercise intensity, but this presents no great risk to health. Therefore, except in situations where depletion of body water has not occurred, the first aim of post-exercise recovery should be to restore any fluid deficit incurred, followed by repletion of liver and muscle glycogen stores.

It must, of course, be recognized that these aims need not be mutually exclusive. Selection of suitable food and drinks should provide both the carbohydrate necessary for optimization of muscle and liver glycogen resynthesis and the water and electrolytes necessary for replacement of sweat losses and restoration of fluid balance.

7.2.3.2 Exercise Performance Considerations

Recently, one study has attempted to distinguish between the effects of carbohydrate provision and the water replacement properties of a drink. Below et al.[35] required eight men to undertake the same cycle ergometer exercise on four separate occasions. After 50 min of exercise at 80% of VO_{2max}, a performance test at a higher exercise intensity (completion of set amount of work as quickly as possible) was completed; this test lasted approximately 10 min. On each of the four trials, a different beverage consumption protocol was followed during the 50-min exercise; nothing was consumed during the performance tests. The beverages were electrolyte containing water in large (1330 ml) and small (200 ml) volumes and carbohydrate electrolyte solutions (79 g) in the same large and small volumes; the electrolyte content of each beverage was the same and amounted to 619 mg (27 mmol) and 141 mg (3.6 mmol) of sodium and potassium, respectively. The results of the study indicated that performance was 6.5% better after consuming the large volume of fluid in comparison with the smaller volume and was 6.3% better after consuming carbohydrate-containing rather than carbohydrate free beverages; the fluid and carbohydrate each independently improved performance and the two improvements were additive. The mechanism for the improvements in performance with the large fluid replacement vs. the small fluid replacement was attributed to a lower heart rate and esophageal temperature when the large volume was consumed. The authors were unable, however, to identify the mechanism by which carbohydrate ingestion improved performance.

7.3 SUMMARY

It is clear that exercise-induced dehydration has a negative impact on exercise performance, and restoration of fluid balance must be achieved after exercise. It is equally well known that muscle glycogen must be restored after exercise if subsequent performance is not to be negatively affected. Sports drinks are formulated to fill both these roles.

Of importance for rehydration purposes is consumption of both an adequate volume (greater than the sweat volume lost) and quantity of sodium. Without both of these, rehydration will be neither rapid nor complete. There is, however, no good evidence for the inclusion of any other electrolytes.

For muscle glycogen resynthesis, carbohydrate consumption in the first 2 h after exercise is of paramount importance to promote a rapid resynthesis. This lends itself well to being achieved through sports drink consumption, as appetite is frequently suppressed immediately after exercise.

REFERENCES

1. Saltin, B., Costill, D. L., Fluid and electrolyte balance during prolonged exercise. In Horton, E. S., Terjung, R. L., (Eds.) *Exercise, Nutrition, and Metabolism*. Macmillan, New York, 150-158, 1988

2. Nielsen, B., Kubica, R., Bonnesen, A., Rasmussen, I. B., Stoklosa, J., Wilk, B., Physical work capacity after dehydration and hyperthermia. *Scand J Sports Sci*, 3, 2-10, 1981

3. Armstrong, L. E., Costill, D. L., Fink, W. J., Influence of diuretic-induced dehydration on competitive running performance. *Med Sci Sports Exerc*, 17, 456-461, 1985

4. Walsh, R. M., Noakes, T. D., Hawley, J. A., Dennis, S. C., Impaired high-intensity cycling performance time at low levels of dehydration. *Int J Sports Med*, 15, 392-398, 1994

5. Nadel, E. R., Circulatory and thermal regulations during exercise. *Fed Proc*, 39, 1491–1497, 1980

6. Rowell, L. B., *Human Circulation*. Oxford University Press, New York, 1986

7. Montain, S. J., Coyle, E. F., Influence of graded dehydration on hyperthermia and cardiovascular drift during exercise. *J Appl Physiol*, 73, 1340-1350, 1992

8. Montain, S. J., Coyle, E. F., Fluid ingestion during exercise increases skin blood flow independent of increases in blood volume. *J Appl Physiol*, 73, 903-910, 1992

9. Greenleaf, J. E., Castle, B. L., Card, D. H., Blood electrolytes and temperature regulation during exercise in man. *Acta Physiologica Polonica*, 25, 397-410, 1974

10. Harrison, M. H., Edwards, R. J., Fennessy, P. A., Intravascular volume and tonicity as factors in the regulation of body temperature. *J Appl Physiol*, 44, 69-75, 1978

11. Fortney, S. M., Wenger, C. B., Bove, J. R., Nadel, E. R., Effect of hyperosmolality on control of blood flow and sweating. *J Appl Physiol*, 57, 1688-1695, 1984

12. Fortney, S. M., Vroman, N. B., Beckett, W. S., Permutt, S., LaFrance, N. D., Effect of exercise hemoconcentration and hyperosmolality on exercise responses. *J Appl Physiol*, 65, 519-524, 1988

13. Shirreffs, S. M., Taylor, A. J., Leiper, J. B., Maughan, R. J., Post-exercise rehydration in man: effects of volume consumed and drink sodium content. *Med Sci Sports Exerc* 28, 1260-1271, 1996

14. Nose, H., Mack, G. W., Shi, X., Nadel, E. R., Involvement of sodium retention hormones during rehydration in humans. *J Appl Physiol*, 65, 332-336, 1988

15. Maughan, R. J., Leiper, J. B., Effects of sodium content of ingested fluids on post-exercise rehydration in man. *Eur J Appl Physiol*, 71, 311-319, 1995

16. Nadel, E. R., Mack, G. W., Nose, H., Influence of fluid replacement beverages on body fluid homeostasis during exercise and recovery. In *Perspectives in Exercise Science and Sports Medicine. Volume 3: Fluid Homeostasis During Exercise* (edited by Gisolfi, C. V. and Lamb, D. B.), pp. 181-205. Benchmark, Carmel, IN, 1990

17. Maughan, R. J., Owen, J. H., Shirreffs, S. M., Leiper, J. B., Post-exercise rehydration in man: effects of electrolyte addition to ingested fluids. *Eur J Appl Physiol*, 69, 209-215, 1994

18. Dill, D. B., Costill, D. L., Calculation of percentage changes in volumes of blood, plasma and red cells in dehydration. *J Appl Physiol*, 37, 247-248, 1974

19. Yawata, T., Effect of potassium solution on rehydration in rats: comparison with sodium solution and water. *Jap J Physiol*, 40, 369-381, 1990

20. Blom, P. C. S., Høstmark, A. T., Vaage, O., Kardel, K. R., Mæhlum, S., Effect of different post-exercise sugar diets on the rate of muscle glycogen synthesis. *Med Sci Sports Exer* 19, 491-496, 1987

21. Jenkins, D. J. A., Wolever, T. M. S., Jenkins, A. L., Josse, R. G., Wong, G. S., The glycemic response to carbohydrate foods. *Lancet* August 18, 388-391, 1984

22. Maughan, R. J., Fenn, C. E., Leiper, J. B., Effects of fluid, electrolyte and substrate ingestion on endurance capacity. *Eur J Appl Physiol* 58, 481-486, 1989

23. Coyle, E. F., Timing and method of increased carbohydrate intake to cope with heavy training, competition and recovery. *J Sports Sci* 9, (Special Issue), 29-52, 1991

24. Keizer, H. A., Kuipers, H., van Kranenburg, G., Geurten, P., Influence of liquid and solid meals on muscle glycogen resynthesis, plasma fuel hormone response, and maximal physical working capacity. *Int J Sports Med*, 8, 99-104, 1986

25. Reed, M. J., Brozinick Jr, J. T., Lee, M. C., Ivy, J. L., Muscle glycogen storage post exercise: Effect on mode of carbohydrate administration. *J Appl Physiol* 66, 720-726, 1989

26. Ivy, J. L., Lee, M. C., Brozinick, J. T., Reed, M. J., Muscle glycogen storage after different amounts of carbohydrate ingestion. *J Appl Physiol* 65, 2018-2023, 1988

27. Ivy, J. L., Katz, A. L., Cutler, C. L., Sherman, W. M., Coyle, E. F., Muscle glycogen synthesis after exercise: effect of time of carbohydrate ingestion. *J Appl Physiol* 64, 1480-1485, 1988

28. Costill, D. L., Sherman, W. M., Fink, W. J., Maresh, C., Witten, M., Miller, J. M., Effects of repeated days of intensified training on muscle glycogen and swimming performance. *Med Sci Sports Exerc* 20, 249-254, 1988

29. Burke, L. M., Collier, G. R., Davis, P. G., Fricker, P. A., Sanigorski, A. J., Hargreaves, M., Muscle glycogen storage after prolonged exercise: effect of the frequency of carbohydrate feedings. *Am J Clin Nutr*, 64, 115-119, 1996

30. Fell, R. D., McLane, J. A., Winder, W. W., Holloszy, J. O., Preferential resynthesis of muscle glycogen in fasting rats after exhaustive exercise. *Am J Physiol* 238, R328-R332, 1980

31. Nilsson, L. H., Hultman, E., Liver and muscle glycogen in man after glucose and fructose infusion. *Scand J Clin Lab Invest*, 33, 5-10, 1974

32. Zawadzki, K. M., Yaspelkis III, B. B., Ivy, J. L., Carbohydrate-protein complex increases the rate of muscle glycogen storage after exercise. *J Appl Physiol*, 72, 1854-1859, 1992

33. Shirreffs, S. M., Maughan, R. J., Restoration of fluid balance after exercise-induced dehydration: effects of alcohol consumption. *J Appl Physiol* 83, 1152-1158, 1997

34. González-Alonso, J., Heaps, C. L., Coyle, E. F., Rehydration after exercise with common beverages and water. *Int J Sports Med* 13, 399-406, 1992

35. Below, R. P., Mora-Rodriguez, R., Gonzalez-Alonso, J., Coyle, E. F., Fluid and carbohydrate ingestion independently improve performance during 1 h of intense exercise. *Med Sci Sports Exerc*, 27: 200-210, 1995

8 Formulating Carbohydrate-Electrolyte Drinks for Optimal Efficacy

Robert Murray and John Stofan

CONTENTS

0-8493-7008-6/01/$0.00+$.50
© 2001 by CRC Press LLC

8.1 INTRODUCTION

8.1.1 The Business of Sports Drinks

As a category of commercial products, sports drinks enjoy considerable public visibility because of their close link with exercise and competitive sports. This is reflected by sports drink sales in the United States, which topped $2.2 billion in 1998, with per capita consumption averaging about eight l.[1] In contrast, the consumption of carbonated soft drinks in the U.S. during 1997 was over 200 l/person, with sales exceeding $14 billion in 1998.[2] Although the sports drink category is dwarfed in comparison with carbonated soft drinks, sports drinks are also a global enterprise and one made all the more interesting because sports drink formulation is rooted in science. Most people are unaware that the basic science underlying the effectiveness of sports drink is an outgrowth of the development of oral rehydration solutions for the treatment of diarrheal disease, a scientific effort that began in earnest in the late 1950s and early 1960s. This chapter summarizes how scientific findings (discussed in detail in the other chapters of this text) provide the basis for the formulation of a physiologically effective sports drink. In many ways, that undertaking pales in comparison with the task of making such a beverage commercially viable. Commercial success requires that a precise balance be struck among product efficacy, product taste, processing limitations, packaging considerations, distribution constraints, and cost containment, not to mention the myriad other requirements to bring a product to market and make it successful. The inherent challenge in such an undertaking is to formulate an efficacious beverage that tastes good during physical activity, is heat tolerant and light stable, can be packaged in recyclable containers appropriate for use during physical activity, and can survive the rigors of a national distribution system.

8.1.2 Sports Drink Composition

Since the mid-1960s, there has been a category of commercial beverages in the U.S. specifically formulated for consumption before, during, and after physical activity. These beverages are often referred to as *sports drinks, carbohydrate-electrolyte beverages*, *electrolyte replacement drinks*, or *isotonic drinks*. Although there is no standard of identity for this category of beverage in the U.S. (other nations have attempted to characterize the formulation specifications for beverages that fall into the *sports drink* category), they are generally composed of varying types of monosaccharides, disaccharides, and sometimes maltodextrins, in concentrations ranging from 6% to 9% weight/volume (by comparison, regular carbonated soft drinks are 10% to 13% carbohydrate wt/vol, and fruit juices range from 11% to 16% carbohydrate wt/vol). Sports drinks typically contain small amounts of minerals (electrolytes) such as sodium, potassium, chloride, and phosphate, and are available in a number of fruit-related flavors. Table 8.1 contains the composition of selected sports drinks and, for comparative purposes, other common beverages.

TABLE 8.1
The Composition of Selected Sports Drinks and Other Beverages

Beverage	Carbohydrate (% wt/vol)	Sodium (mmol/l)	Potassium (mmol/l)	Osmolality (mosm/kg H_2O)
AllSport® (Pepsico)	8 to 9 (varies with flavors)	10	5	516
Cytomax® (Champion Nutrition)	5.5	10	10	208
Gatorade® (The Quaker Oats Co.)	6	20	3	280 (powder) 325–380 (liquid)
Isostar® (Wander)	7.7	30	–	289
MET-Rx ORS® (MET-Rx)	8	23	4	315
Powerade® (Coca-Cola)	8	5	3	381
Perform® (PowerBar)	6.6	20	4	500
Pedialyte® (Ross Labs)	2.5	45	20	250
Rehydralyte® (Ross Labs)	2.5	75	20	325
Coca Cola Classic® (Coca Cola)	11	–	–	700
Orange Juice (Tropicana)	10.8	–	49	663

8.1.3 FORMULATION OBJECTIVES

Ever since work by Adolph and associates[3] in the 1940s, it has become increasingly clear that ingesting fluid during physical activity is *the* central factor in maintaining physiological homeostasis and in sustaining the capacity for sustained physical activity. Recent research by many other investigators[4,5] has strengthened the time-tested conclusions regarding the deleterious influence of dehydration on human function. The bottom line summary is that even a small amount of dehydration (e.g., a 1% loss of body mass) produces negative effects on physiological function and exercise performance. Greater losses of body fluid progressively increase the decrement in function.[6]

In laboratory experiments, it is possible to dictate the composition, timing, and volume of fluid consumption by the subjects and to manipulate their hydration status accordingly. Outside the laboratory, however, there is a wide variety of beverages to choose from, the frequency and volume of fluid ingestion is entirely voluntary, and drinking behavior is influenced by the nature of the physical activity, by social interactions, and by the mere availability of fluid. Regardless of these differences, a sports drink must be formulated to confer meaningful and measurable benefits in a wide variety of circumstances. Depending upon the circumstances of use, a properly formulated sports drink should deliver the following benefits:

- encourage voluntary fluid consumption
- stimulate rapid fluid absorption
- supply carbohydrate for improved performance
- augment physiological response
- speed rehydration

8.1.3.1   Encourage Voluntary Fluid Consumption

It is well known that the taste of a beverage drives voluntary fluid intake, an important factor in the exercise setting. The organoleptic attributes of carbohydrate-electrolyte solutions must take into consideration the changes in sensory responses that accompany physical activity. Perceptions of sweetness, tartness, flavor, mouthfeel, and aftertaste are important sensory parameters that differ between rest and exercise[7] (see Chapter 3 for related information). In addition, the electrolyte composition of the beverage can also affect voluntary fluid intake by influencing the physiological drive for drinking.

Even the production of sports drinks must be compatible with the goal of optimizing product efficacy. For example, pasteurization of carbohydrate-electrolyte solutions is required to avoid the use of chemical preservatives that can impart throat burn and thereby decrease voluntary fluid consumption. This heat processing requires that the product be formulated to withstand exposure to high temperatures (> 170°F, ~80°C) with minimal effect on color and flavor components. This is not an easy undertaking.

The dimensions of the package and the ergonomics of its use are also important considerations, as they influence ease-of-use, voluntary fluid consumption, and consumer acceptance. Consumer demands, the constraints of the distribution system, the limitations of packaging materials and design, and cost factors all interact to influence the type of package required for the product. In most instances, consumers prefer plastic containers and the composition of those containers must meet the limitations imposed by the physical and chemical properties of the product, the rigors of heat processing, and the demands of storage, distribution, consumer use, and recycling.

8.1.3.2   Stimulate Rapid Fluid Absorption

An efficacious sports drink must be formulated to avoid (or to at least drastically minimize) the limitations imposed by gastric emptying and intestinal absorption, while providing fluid, carbohydrate, and electrolytes in amounts and at rates known to induce positive physiological and performance responses. In this regard, the universal standard of comparison is that of the ingestion of water, a solution known to be rapidly absorbed. Small alterations in the carbohydrate concentration of sports drinks can have measurable consequences on gastric emptying and intestinal absorption, as outlined in Chapter 4.

8.1.3.3   Supply Carbohydrate for Improved Performance

Exogenous carbohydrate is available to contracting skeletal muscle and its oxidation is linked to an improved capacity for exercise; Chapter 6 provides a comprehensive review of this research. Sports drink formulation must take into consideration the range of carbohydrate intake and the type of carbohydrates associated with improved performance and balance those requirements with the carbohydrate concentration required for optimal palatability and rapid fluid absorption.

8.1.3.4   Augment Physiological Response

Ingesting ample fluid, carbohydrate, and electrolytes in the form of a sports drink provokes a variety of hormonal responses that influence fluid and electrolyte homeostasis, glucose homeostasis, brain neurotransmitter production, and the function of certain immune cells.[8] The concentration and type of carbohydrate can influence these responses and are, therefore, issues to consider when formulating a sports drink.

8.1.3.5   Speed Rehydration

The types and concentrations of electrolytes in a sports drink play a critical role in determining the rate of rehydration, the completeness of rehydration, and the subsequent distribution of fluid within the body fluid compartments. Although commercial sports drinks commonly contain minerals such as sodium, potassium, and chloride, the concentrations of those electrolytes vary from manufacturer to manufacturer.

Using these five physiological objectives as a framework for discussion, the intent of this chapter is to link current scientific understanding to the formulation requirements of an efficacious sports drink. There is a wealth of science in this area and the interested reader is referred to other chapters in this text and to comprehensive review articles[9,10,11,12,13] for more information.

8.2   ENCOURAGE VOLUNTARY FLUID CONSUMPTION

8.2.1   SCIENTIFIC PRINCIPLES AND PRACTICAL RAMIFICATIONS

Unlike animals such as dogs, donkeys, camels, sheep, and deer, all of which quickly, consistently, and accurately drink to restore fluid deficits,[14] human drinking behavior is often not closely linked to the physiological need for fluid. For example, humans frequently ingest fluid even when there is no physiological need for fluid intake, behavior that is common in social gatherings such as parties and meetings. In contrast, we fail to drink adequately when fluid losses are high, leading to negative fluid balance, as illustrated by the involuntary dehydration that often accompanies physical activity and by the lengthy time normally required to fully rehydrate following exercise.

As detailed in Chapter 3, the onset of thirst is a delayed response; we do not become thirsty until the body is already somewhat fluid deficient, perhaps by as much as 1% to 2% of body mass.[15] To further increase the challenge of remaining euhydrated during physical activity, the nature of the exercise or sporting occasion often results in the ingestion of relatively small volumes of fluid compared with sweat loss, resulting in progressive dehydration.[16,17]

The conscious desire to drink arises from the combined input of osmoreceptors in the hypothalamus that assess the osmolality (primarily the sodium concentration) of the blood, and from baroreceptors in the lungs and major vessels that are sensitive to changes in blood volume and pressure.[18] Dehydration triggers thirst by stimulating both osmoreceptors and baroreceptors in response to the increase in the osmolality of the plasma and the decrease in the circulating blood volume that accompany sweating. An increase in plasma osmolality above the thirst threshold (i.e., > 288 mosm/kg H_2O) results in the release of AVP (arginine vasopressin, also referred to as antidiuretic hormone, ADH) and a concomitant increase in the sensation of thirst.

When fluid is swallowed and enters the bloodstream, plasma osmolality eventually drops below the thirst threshold and blood volume is gradually restored. The restoration of blood volume and osmolality to normal values abolishes the sensation of thirst and voluntary drinking ceases. Interestingly, the simple act of swallowing fluid stimulates an oropharyngeal reflex that also influences thirst and drinking behavior. Figaro and Mack[19] demonstrated the importance of this reflex in a study that used a unique experimental design. On three occasions, subjects dehydrated through exercise and fluid restriction and

1. consumed water *ad libitum* (control)
2. had a similar volume of water infused directly into the stomach (avoiding the oropharyngeal reflex)
3. drank water *ad libitum* but had the water aspirated from the stomach via a nasogastric tube.

When the water was ingested but aspirated from the stomach, inhibition of AVP and thirst occurred within the first 5 minutes of drinking, a response similar to control values. No such changes occurred during the infusion trial in the absence of swallowing, indicating the presence of an oropharyngeal reflex that prompted the release of AVP and stimulated the sensation of thirst. The strength of the oropharyngeal reflex is perhaps best characterized by the aspiration trial in which the subjects voluntarily ingested only 15% more fluid than during the control trial, although none of the fluid reached the bloodstream. These data clearly indicate that the physiological responses to drinking begin when fluid is swallowed and well before any measurable changes in plasma osmolality or plasma volume can occur.

It is not presently known whether the oropharyngeal reflex is sensitive to the composition of the ingested fluid in a way that would influence subsequent drinking behavior, but it is clear that beverage composition has an important effect on drinking behavior. Recent research has also shown that oral administration of a liquid meal and the consequent orosensory mechanisms associated with the liquid meal contribute largely to the suppression of appetite.[20] In the case of thirst, if plasma volume is restored too quickly or if plasma osmolality drops below the thirst threshold prematurely, thirst is ablated and fluid intake is reduced before complete rehydration can occur. This is the scenario that typically occurs when plain water is ingested, and it is for that reason that water is a poor choice when rapid and complete rehydration is the goal.

Not surprisingly, taste and other organoleptic characteristics (e.g., sweetness, mouthfeel, tartness, aftertaste) are important determinants of fluid intake in any setting, but particularly so during exercise. Physical activity alters the hedonic and descriptive characteristics of beverages so that a drink that might be preferred in sedentary circumstances fares poorly in the exercise setting.[21,22] This knowledge is an important consideration whenever fluid intake is of paramount importance, as in military, industrial, or sporting activities, and during leisure-time physical activities in hot and humid weather.[23,24] For these reasons, a properly formulated carbohydrate-electrolyte beverage has organoleptic characteristics that are most highly valued when people are hot, sweaty, and thirsty.[25]

Much remains to be learned about how the organoleptic properties and ingredients of a beverage can be manipulated to maximize voluntary fluid intake. For example, little is known about the mechanisms that underlie the change in taste preference that accompanies exercise, and this effect is difficult to separate because perceptual ratings are often biased by other somatosensory qualities such as beverage, body, and ambient temperatures. Certainly, taste is mediated by other factors such as taste bud density, oral temperature differentials, taste receptors, and solution viscosity, but it is not presently known to what extent these factors interact with exercise.[26,27,28] Also unresolved are the reasons for the change in beverage acceptance that occurs with exercise, although it is clear that this effect is observed among young and old alike. What is well known is that physically active people prefer, and therefore drink more of, beverages that are lightly sweetened, citrus flavored, and moderately tart.[29,30]

Unlike under sedentary circumstances, the presence of carbonation in a beverage consumed during exercise does not stimulate fluid intake, but is instead a significant barrier to voluntary fluid consumption owing to a strong negative impact on acceptability. This effect is primarily due to the sensation of throat burn caused by the presence of high CO_2 volumes in the fluid. Passe et al.[31]examined sensory accept- ability and voluntary fluid intake in 52 adults following 30 minutes of exercise. The presence of sodium benzoate (a preservative) and CO_2 at and above 2.3 volumes (similar to levels in carbonated soft drinks) was associated with reduced fluid intake, stronger perceived throat burn, reduced acceptability and thirst-quenching charac- teristics, and altered perception of sweetness and flavor. All of these factors contrib- uted to the reduction in the desire for that beverage. Also problematic is the fact that the volume of CO_2 in solution decreases as the beverage temperature increases in the stomach; the resulting gas causes bloating, gastric discomfort, and eruction, all of which further reduce voluntary fluid intake. In brief, the presence of carbon- ation is a strong negative organoleptic characteristic in a sports drink.

8.2.2 FORMULATION CONSIDERATIONS

8.2.2.1 Flavors and Colors

Notwithstanding the logistical considerations and physiological constraints that may limit fluid intake during physical activity, a properly formulated sports drink must have the necessary physicochemical characteristics to stimulate and optimize vol- untary drinking. Beverage temperature, color, flavor acceptance, and flavor variety are important factors determining overall acceptability and voluntary consump- tion.[30,31] Olfactory, tactile, and thermal sensitivity also contribute to selection and preferences for particular beverages. Taste, as a perceptual element, is mediated by a number of factors including solution viscosity,[32] oral absorption,[33] temperature,[34] and tastebud density.[26] Thirst, taste, and voluntary fluid intake are influenced by endocrine, neurophysiological, and neuropsychological elements, as discussed in detail in Chapter 3 of this text.

Specific taste preferences and past experiences are also important for the regu- lation of fluid intake. For example, a sports drink made from a homemade recipe is not as acceptable and is not voluntarily consumed in as large a volume as a successful commercial formulation.[35] The lower overall acceptance of a homemade recipe is likely due in part to the subjects' lack of experience with the flavor system and the inherent suboptimal nature of that flavor. Data such as these support the common- sense notion that optimized flavor systems along with the proper balance of ingre- dients encourage voluntary fluid intake. In other words, if a beverage tastes good, people will drink more of it. The interesting twist to this logic is that, as noted in Chapter 3, the drink must be properly formulated for the exercise occasion; that is, the drink must possess the physicochemical characteristics that have great appeal when people are physically active.

8.2.2.2 Carbohydrate Concentration and Type

The types and overall concentration of carbohydrate have an effect on the physio- logical efficacy of a sports drink and on organoleptic characteristics such as flavor balance, sweetness, and palatability. For example, carbohydrate concentration and type influence the rate of water, carbohydrate, and electrolyte absorption, as summarized in Chapter 4 and later in this chapter. Beverages with too much carbohydrate are often perceived as too sweet during exercise, diminishing overall acceptance and negatively affecting voluntary fluid consumption.

Commercially available carbohydrate sources typically include sucrose (from cane or sugar beet), glucose, fructose, corn syrup solids (often referred to as high-fructose corn syrup), maltose, and maltodextrin (frequently, but erroneously referred to as *glucose polymers*). Sports drinks rarely contain complex carbohydrates (e.g., chain lengths > 20 glucose molecules) because of the low sweetness and unacceptably thick mouthfeel characteristics that such carbohydrates impart. Each type of carbohydrate has a different sweetness profile, as characterized by the perceived intensity of the sweetness and by its onset and duration (see Table 8.2). When combinations of carbohydrates are used in a beverage, the resulting sweetness profile is more or less a composite of the constituent carbohydrates at low levels of sweetness, but as sweetness levels increase, the resulting sweetness profile becomes a complex function of the carbohydrate combination.[36]

TABLE 8.2
Relative Sweetness Characteristics of
Various Carbohydrate Types

Carbohydrate	Relative Sweetness*
Fructose, Crystalline	180
High Fructose Corn Syrups	105–130
Sucrose	100
Glucose (2-10% Solution)	50–70
Maltose	50

Note: Sucrose is the standard against which the relative sweetness of other carbohydrates is judged. Adapted from BeMiller, J.N., Sucrose, in *Encyclopedia of Food Science and Technology*: Vol. 4., Hui, Y.H., Ed., John Wiley and Sons, NY, 1992. Reprinted by permission.

It is clear that the proper combination of carbohydrates optimizes sweetness and flavor characteristics, maximizes intestinal water flux, and guarantees adequate energy provision. On the other hand, too much carbohydrate delays both gastric emptying[38] and intestinal fluid absorption,[39,40] increases the risk of gastrointestinal distress,[41,42] and provides no additional benefit to performance.[43] The fructose content of the beverage can be particularly problematic. Drinks containing mostly or solely fructose as a carbohydrate source are contraindicated because the relatively slow, passive transport of fructose in the gut results in slower solute and water absorption,[44] greater decrements in plasma volume,[45] and increased gastrointestinal distress.[45]

8.2.2.3 Sodium Chloride and Other Electrolytes

The presence of sodium chloride affects both the flavor and the functional properties of a sports drink. Typically, a small amount of sodium chloride is added to sports drinks to:

- "round out" flavor profiles
- stimulate fluid consumption by maintaining the osmotic and volume-dependent stimuli for drinking
- ensure ample sodium concentration in the intestinal lumen
- provide an osmotic impetus for the maintenance of extracellular fluid volume
- provoke adequate drinking and rehydration when fluid is consumed following physical activity

Although each possesses different flavor and functional characteristics, sodium chloride, sodium citrate, and sodium acetate are some of the most common forms of sodium used in sports drinks.

As typical sweat sodium concentration ranges from 20 to 80 mmol/l,[46] ingesting sodium helps replace that lost in sweat and stimulates osmotically dependent dipsogenic factors that initiate further drinking. However, too much sodium restores the extracellular fluid space too rapidly, removing the volume-dependent drive to continue drinking. Interestingly, ingesting too much or too little sodium both discourages further drinking and impedes complete rehydration.

Many researchers have systematically evaluated the addition of sodium to sports drinks over the last 15 years. It is now quite clear that some sodium is necessary and sodium-containing fluid provides distinct advantages over plain water and other sodium-free drinks. For example, the addition of a small amount of sodium chloride to a sports drink can markedly influence drinking behavior. Wilk and Bar-Or[47] measured the voluntary fluid intake of pre- and early pubescent boys (ages 9 to 12) during 3 hours of intermittent exercise in a warm environment. Intake of a grape-flavored sports drink was 90% greater than plain water and 45% better than a grape-flavored, artificially sweetened placebo. These results show that the addition of a small amount of sodium chloride ($\sim$ 20 mmol/l) provides a demonstrable impetus for drinking; in fact, the subjects maintained euhydration only on the sports drink trial. The fact that the boys drank 45% more placebo than plain water illustrates the positive impact that flavoring and sweetening have on voluntary fluid intake.

Sodium ingestion during exercise is also critical for the maintenance of plasma sodium levels and in helping to prolong exercise duration, as demonstrated by Vrijens and Rehrer.[48] On two separate occasions, subjects performed cycle ergometer exercise in the heat ($34°C$) for 3 hours while drinking either plain water or a sodium-containing sports drink (18 mmol Na^+/l). Subjects ingested fluid at 15-minute intervals at a rate estimated to be equal to fluid loss. On the water trial, six of the ten subjects were unable to complete three hours of exercise due to volitional exhaustion and one subject developed hyponatremia. With the sports drink, four of ten subjects could not complete 3 hours of exercise. Furthermore, there was a significant negative correlation ($r = -0.674$) for the rate of plasma sodium change and total exercise time. Thus, the maintenance of plasma sodium by ingesting a sports drink at a rate equal to sweat loss helped extend exercise time to exhaustion and prevented hyponatremia.

In addition to stimulating drinking by taking advantage of organoleptic and osmotic factors, a carbohydrate-electrolyte beverage must be formulated to restore plasma volume without promoting a rapid decrease in plasma osmolality and result-ant return to isotonicity. In so doing, more fluid is voluntarily ingested because the osmotic drive to drink is maintained. To accomplish this, the sodium concentration of a sports drink should be at least 20 mmol/l and perhaps as high as 60 mmol/l.[49] However, higher sodium concentrations are not clearly superior in this regard. For example, Greenleaf and colleagues[50] reported that consuming high-sodium beverages (157 mmol/l) prior to exercise had no greater effect in attenuating plasma volume losses during exercise than when low-sodium beverages (20 mmol/l) were consumed prior to exercise. The advantage of both the low- and high-sodium fluids over water, however, was very clear.

The sodium concentration is a critical consideration in sports drink formulation. If the sodium concentration is too high, plasma volume is quickly restored and voluntary drinking is reduced as the osmotic drive to drink is removed. In a study by Wemple et al,[51] following exercise-induced dehydration, consumption of a drink containing 50 mmol/l Na^+ restored plasma volume to control levels within 1 hour compared with slower rates with flavored water and 25 mmol/l Na^+. However, the higher-sodium drink resulted in reduced *ad libitum* fluid intake. The attenuated drinking was likely due to removal of the volume-dependent dipsogenic drive for drinking, but the extent to which the flavor systems and hedonic properties con-tributed to fluid intake remains unclear. It is believed that a lower sodium content (~ 20 to 25 mmol/l) helps restore plasma volume at a slower rate, while maintaining the osmotic drive to drink, resulting in increased fluid consumption.

Although other electrolytes such as potassium and magnesium are sometimes present in sports drinks in small quantities (usually less than 10 mmol/l), they do not appear to play a role in encouraging voluntary consumption or in provoking acute physiological responses, and are added as a means of replacing mineral losses in sweat and urine.[52] Nonetheless, it should be noted that potassium deficiency (hypokalemia) stimulates thirst and might be implicated in the relationship between thirst and fluid intake, although the data in support of this contention are not particularly compelling.[15]

8.2.2.4   Beverage Osmolality

The osmolality of a beverage (i.e., the number of particles in solution) is directly related to the solute composition of the beverage; increasing the amount of carbo-hydrates or electrolytes in a drink (more particles in solution) also increases the osmolality of the drink. Research indicates that sports drinks should be hypotonic or isotonic to ensure rapid gastric emptying[53,54] and intestinal absorption.[55] To date, there is no indication that beverage osmolality, independent of changes in carbohy-drate and electrolyte content, influences voluntary drinking.

8.3   STIMULATE RAPID FLUID ABSORPTION

8.3.1   SCIENTIFIC PRINCIPLES AND PRACTICAL RAMIFICATIONS

As summarized in Chapter 4, the rate of fluid absorption into the bloodstream is determined by the combined rates of gastric emptying and intestinal absorption,[56] responses that are directly influenced by the composition of the ingested beverage. Rapid gastric emptying occurs whenever a large volume of fluid with a low energy density is ingested; for this reason, large volumes of plain water are emptied quite rapidly from the stomach. Solutions containing less than 6% to 7% carbohydrate (e.g., many sports drinks) are also emptied rapidly,[57,58] particularly when compared with soft drinks (10% to 13% carbohydrate wt/vol) and fruit juices (11% to 16% carbohydrate wt/vol). The type of carbohydrates used in the beverage, the beverage osmolality (at least at low levels of carbohydrate), temperature, pH, and mineral content have only minor effects on gastric emptying when compared with the beverage's energy content and the volume ingested. For example, Vist and Maughan[54] demonstrated that beverage osmolality plays a minor role in determining gastric emptying rate compared with the carbohydrate concentration of the beverage, particularly at the lower carbohydrate concentrations of sports drinks.

Of key interest from a formulation standpoint is the knowledge that too much carbohydrate in a beverage will delay gastric emptying. However, gastric emptying characteristics vary widely among individuals (see Chapter 4), as do the responses to different types of carbohydrate. For example, Murray et al.[38] reported that consumption of an 8% carbohydrate beverage (sucrose and maltodextrin) resulted in significantly slower gastric emptying than 4% or 6% carbohydrate solutions (sucrose, glucose, and fructose) during exercise. However, Vist and Maughan[58] showed that a 6% glucose solution emptied slower than water and a 4% glucose solution. These data suggest that there is a breakpoint in carbohydrate concentration above which gastric emptying is significantly slowed and that the breakpoint may be specific to carbohydrate type, with glucose solutions provoking the most powerful inhibitory effect. Additional studies are needed to confirm this finding and to identify the possible physiological consequences of such differences. Nonetheless, these data are instructive in establishing an upper limit for the carbohydrate concentration of a sports drink. However, it should be noted that although the gastric emptying rate of a carbohydrate solution is driven primarily by carbohydrate concentration, the types of carbohydrate, and the osmolality likely interact with carbohydrate concentration to determine gastric emptying rate.

The carbohydrate concentration and the osmolality of the beverage primarily influence the rate at which fluid is absorbed across the intestinal epithelium. Upon passing the pyloric sphincter and entering the duodenum, a drink high in carbohydrate concentration and osmolality and low in sodium chloride (e.g., a carbonated soft drink), is quickly diluted by intestinal secretions that contain sodium and chloride. If this rapid dilution is of great enough magnitude, a transient decrease in plasma volume will occur as fluid temporarily leaves the blood and passes into the intestine.[55]

The presence of carbohydrates (e.g., sucrose and glucose) in the electrolyte replacement beverage stimulate sodium absorption via SGLT-1 membrane transporters in the intestinal epithelium. Water is absorbed through transcellular or paracellular routes to reestablish the osmotic equilibrium that was disrupted by solute absorption. This fundamental knowledge has served as the foundation for the formulation of oral rehydration solutions designed for use in clinical applications (e.g., diarrheal disease) and for beverages formulated for use during physical activity.[56]

8.3.2 FORMULATION CONSIDERATIONS

8.3.2.1 Carbohydrate Concentration and Type

The type of carbohydrate and its concentration are important determinants of fluid absorption. Solutions containing 6% carbohydrate or less are absorbed more rapidly than solutions containing greater amounts of carbohydrate.[59,60] Sucrose, glucose, and maltodextrins share similar rates of absorption.[59] Fructose is absorbed passively and high concentrations of fructose can slow absorption,[44] result in reduced plasma volume,[45] and stimulate gastrointestinal distress.[45] However, fructose ingested in small amounts in combination with sucrose and/or glucose does *not* impede fluid absorption.[55] Providing a blend of carbohydrate types is important to optimize fluid absorption. Shi et al.[55] showed that a solution containing at least two transportable substrates enhances both solute and water flux more than a solution with just one substrate, despite the increased osmolality. Apparently, activation of multiple transport mechanisms plays an important role in optimizing carbohydrate delivery and promoting fluid absorption in the small intestine.

The lature also indicates that the presence of a small amount of fructose in a sports drink may enhance gastric emptying compared with isoenergetic glucose solutions.[61] In addition, fructose confers positive organoleptic properties (as previously mentioned) and may also benefit carbohydrate metabolism, as discussed in the next section of this chapter. For these reasons, properly formulated sports drinks should contain a small amount of fructose (representing less than half of the total carbohydrate content to minimize the risk of gastrointestinal discomfort).

Increasing the carbohydrate concentration of a sports drink beyond 6% to 7% weight/volume has been shown to significantly decrease the rate of fluid absorption, regardless of whether the beverage is infused directly into the small intestine at rest[62] or is consumed by mouth during exercise.[39]

8.3.2.2 Sodium Chloride and Other Electrolytes

Sports drinks usually contain 10 to 30 mmol/l sodium. In contrast, oral rehydration solutions formulated for clinical use typically contain sodium at 45 to 90 mmol/l, with 20 mmol/l potassium. The differences in electrolyte concentration in these two types of beverages appropriately reflect the differences in electrolyte losses in diarrhea and sweat.

The sodium in sports drinks plays a relatively minor role in the absorption process because sodium is quickly added to the intestinal lumen by intestinal secretions, that is, by sodium that passes down the sodium concentration gradient from blood/extracellular fluid into the intestinal lumen.[63] For this reason, sports drinks with higher sodium concentrations require less sodium influx from the blood/extracellular fluid, arguably an advantage when fluid and electrolyte homeostasis is challenged by prolonged exercise in a warm environment.

8.3.2.3   Beverage Osmolality

As noted in Chapter 4, beverage osmolality has only a small influence on gastric emptying, but can have a large influence on fluid absorption in the intestine. Net fluid absorption occurs only when a sufficient osmotic gradient has been established to attract fluid from an area of lower osmolality (the intestinal lumen) to an area of higher osmolality (the intestinal cell and paracellular junctions). Ingesting a drink with high osmolality (e.g., > 400 mosm/kg H_2O) reduces the rate of fluid ingestion simply due to the time required for fluid to be secreted into the intestine to dilute the intestinal contents and create an osmotic gradient that is conducive to fluid absorption. Gisolfi et al.[62] assessed the fluid absorption rates of sucrose, glucose, and maltodextrin solutions of 2%, 4%, 6%, and 8% concentration. Infusion of the 8%-glucose solution (444 mosm/kg H_2O) into the duodeno-jejunum resulted in net fluid secretion; all other solutions prompted net fluid absorption. The only other hypertonic solution tested was a 6% glucose solution (333 mosm/kg H_2O), but it was associated with net fluid absorption rates that were indistinguishable from the other solutions tested. This finding raises the question, "What actually is isotonic in the intestine?" *Isotonic* is most often used to refer to any solution or beverage with an osmolality similar to that of blood, about 280 mosm/kg H_2O. Yet, there is some evidence that the tonicity of the intestinal villi may range between 300 to 700 mosm/kg H_2O.[64] If such an osmotic pressure exists in the proximal small intestine, it could explain why beverages with osmolalities between 300 and 400 mosm/kg H_2O are absorbed at rates indistinguishable from that of water in this portion of the gut.[55,62]

In summary, net absorption of fluid occurs from hypotonic or isotonic solutions; a hypertonic solution is eventually reduced to near isotonicity by intestinal secretions before net fluid absorption can occur. This lowers the absorption rate and increases the risk of gastrointestinal discomfort. The obvious conclusion is that hypertonicity (e.g., > 400 mosm/kg H_2O) is contraindicated for sports drinks.

8.3.2.4   Other Possible Ingredients

There is considerable interest in the identification of different types or combinations of carbohydrate, or ingredients such as amino acids or small peptides that would augment the fluid absorption characteristics of conventional sports drinks and oral rehydration solutions.[65] Rice starch, maltodextrins, glycine, glutamine, and other ingredients have been studied for their ability to induce superior fluid absorption, but so far without compelling success. In brief, the proper balance of carbohydrate content, carbohydrate type, osmolality, and sodium-chloride content can provoke fluid absorption in the proximal small intestine at rates at least as fast as plain water or even more so.

8.4   SUPPLY CARBOHYDRATE FOR IMPROVED PERFORMANCE

8.4.1   SCIENTIFIC PRINCIPLES AND PRACTICAL RAMIFICATIONS

It is now well established that exogenous carbohydrate can be oxidized during exercise at rates approximating 60 to 75 g/hour and that exercise performance is improved as a result,[66] a fact that forms the basis of current practical recommendations for fluid and carbohydrate feeding during physical activity.[25] Carbohydrate intake during exercise raises the blood glucose and insulin concentration, enhances glucose uptake by muscle, maintains carbohydrate oxidation, and possibly benefits central-nervous-system function, all of which promote an improvement in performance.[67]

A current area of interest in many laboratories is the effect of carbohydrate feeding on the type of activity that is common to most typical sporting activities, that is, high-intensity intermittent exercise of relatively short duration. For example, Davis and colleagues[68] have demonstrated that consumption of carbohydrate electrolyte drinks at regular intervals can improve exercise capacity during activities of short-term intense exercise (1-minute bouts of intense cycling separated by 3-minute rest periods, repeated to exhaustion). Many other studies support the beneficial effects of carbohydrate ingestion (particularly in fluid) on high intensity sports activities such as sprinting, shuttle running, basketball, tennis, hockey, and soccer.[69,70,71,72,73,74]

8.4.2   FORMULATION CONSIDERATIONS

8.4.2.1   Carbohydrate Concentration

The carbohydrate concentration of a sports drink must strike a delicate balance among the parameters of sweetness and taste, gastric emptying, intestinal absorption, and fuel supply. Too little carbohydrate will not optimize sweetness and taste characteristics and will not supply enough carbohydrate to improve exercise performance.[75,76] On the other hand, too much carbohydrate disrupts palatability and delays gastric emptying and intestinal absorption.

It is important from a beverage-formulation standpoint to recognize that increasing the concentration of carbohydrate beyond 7% wt/vol provides little additional benefit and does not alter the rate of maximal carbohydrate oxidation.[77] This means that there is potentially greater risk than benefit in increasing carbohydrate content of a sports drink above about 6% to 7% wt/vol. For example, increasing the carbohydrate content of a sports drink risks reducing the gastric emptying and intestinal absorption rates and increasing the risks of gastrointestinal discomfort at no benefit — and perhaps a detriment — to performance.[41,42,78]

8.4.2.2   Carbohydrate Type

Solutions of sucrose, glucose, and maltodextrins ingested during vigorous exercise have been shown to improve the capacity for exercise[66] and, for that reason, are acceptable substrates for inclusion in sports drinks. Solutions containing only fructose, however, do not improve exercise performance,[45,79] ostensibly because fructose cannot be directly oxidized for energy, but must first be converted to glucose in the liver, a relatively slow process that is seemingly unable to adequately supplement the carbohydrate oxidation rate of active skeletal muscle.[67] However, when fructose is ingested with glucose and/or sucrose, the fructose content is not problematic and exercise performance is improved.[80]

8.4.2.3   Amino Acids

There is no compelling evidence that the addition of amino acids to a sports drink confers any benefit to exercise performance. In theory, ingesting branched-chain amino acids (leucine, isoleucine, and valine) will reduce the tryptophan: BCAA ratio in plasma, decrease the uptake of tryptophan by the brain, and thereby improve performance by ensuring that serotonin (the neurotransmitter by-product of tryptophan) production is regulated.[81] Mittleman et al.[82] reported that subjects who ingested a branched-chain amino-acid solution (5.88 grams/l BCAA) were able to cycle significantly longer (153 vs. 137 min) than when they consumed a placebo solution (maltodextrin). The investigators were unable to discern a possible mechanism for this effect and, to date, their findings have not been substantiated by other well-controlled laboratory studies.[74,83,84] Chapter 9 contains more information on this topic.

8.4.2.4   Vitamins

The physiological, metabolic, and performance responses to the ingestion of sports drinks containing vitamins have not been systematically studied, in large part because there is little theoretical indication that such an addition would result in measurable or meaningful benefits. That said, the very fact that this area has not been well studied means that it is impossible to definitively conclude that the addition of a particular vitamin is without benefit. However, the work that has been published is more supportive of the former notion than of the latter; no immediate benefits could be ascribed to including vitamin C,[85] vitamin E and other antioxidants,[86] or nicotinic acid (vitamin B_3)[87] to a sports drink. Perhaps future work will unearth an as yet unexpected benefit for one or more of the vitamins.

8.4.2.5   Other Possible Ingredients

There is a seemingly inexhaustible list of nutrients, some of which are reviewed in detail in Chapter 9, that have been included in sports drinks. This list includes the entire range of vitamins and minerals, metabolic intermediates such as pyruvate, lactate, citrate, and malate, coenzyme Q10, choline, inositol, grape seed extract, glycerol, and many others. Of these dubious candidates for inclusion in a sports drink, glycerol has received perhaps the most attention for its ability to temporarily reduce urine production by transiently increasing the osmolality of body fluids. Ingested in the hours prior to exercise, glycerol intake results in a decrease in urine production and the retention of a variable amount of fluid (e.g., 700 to 1,000 ml).[88]

Theoretically, this *hyperhydration* may have positive effects on cardiovascular and thermoregulatory response, resulting in improved exercise performance. This theory, however, has not been borne out by research; most of the reports indicate no effect of glycerol ingestion prior to exercise.[89] In addition, when glycerol is ingested as part of a sports drink during exercise, there is no physiological or performance advantage.[90]

8.5   AUGMENT PHYSIOLOGICAL RESPONSE

8.5.1   Scientific Principles and Practical Ramifications

Preventing or minimizing dehydration by ingesting adequate volumes of fluid during exercise maintains cardiovascular, thermoregulatory, and performance responses in a dramatic and consistent fashion, as noted in Chapter 5. This protection is similarly conferred by the ingestion of water and properly formulated sports drinks in volumes sufficient to replace most of the sweat loss. In both cases, adequate fluid ingestion results in greater blood volume, greater stroke volume, lower heart rate, greater cardiac output, higher skin blood flow, lower core temperature, lower ratings of perceived exertion, and better performance compared with drinking smaller amounts of fluid.[91] Of course, these positive responses occur only when adequate volumes of fluid are ingested. That is assured in the laboratory setting by dictating the volume and frequency of fluid that subjects must consume. In the field setting, when people are allowed to ingest fluid *ad libitum*, the voluntary consumption of water may be insufficient to keep pace with fluid loss.[18]

Nonetheless, laboratory experiments have illustrated that, in addition to the benefits associated with preventing dehydration, consuming a properly formulated sports drink maintains plasma glucose concentration which, in turn, is associated with blunting of the stress hormone response (adrenocorticotropic hormone, cortisol, epinephrine, growth hormone) seen when only water is ingested.[92] This has important implications for cardiovascular and thermoregulatory control and for the function of various cells of the immune system, the activities of which are influenced by fluctuations in stress hormones.[93] Unfortunately, this work is in its infancy and relatively few studies have been completed, making it difficult to draw conclusions regarding the way in which changes in sports drink formulation may affect these responses.

Nonetheless, the initial results from this work have interesting scientific and practical ramifications. For example, when subjects ingest water during vigorous exercise, plasma epinephrine concentration continues to rise throughout exercise, but this increase is blunted by the ingestion of a sports drink.[94] Attenuating the rise in plasma epinephrine may have beneficial effects on carbohydrate metabolism in liver and muscle by attenuating epinephrine-stimulated glycogenolysis and by reducing the epinephrine-linked impetus for peripheral vasoconstriction. For example, it has been shown that increases in plasma epinephrine, induced by infusing epinephrine into exercising subjects, are associated with significant decreases in skin blood flow and corresponding increases in core temperature.[95] However, it should be noted that plasma epinephrine concentration can be raised to very high levels by epinephrine infusion (over three times greater than may normally occur during exercise while drinking water). More research is required to determine if the magnitude of the blunting of the stress hormone response that occurs with drinking a sports drink results in measurable improvements in cardiovascular and thermoregulatory control.

Carbohydrate ingestion during exercise, by virtue of blunting the stress hormone response, has also been shown to positively affect a number of parameters of immune cell function, including a reduced pro- and anti-inflammatory cytokine response, and lower granulocyte and monocyte phagocytosis and oxidative burst activity.[92,93] However, the practical outcome of these seemingly positive changes awaits determination. For example, how does the timing and dose of carbohydrate affect parameters of immune function? What other nutrients may augment the positive responses? Does ingestion of a sports drink during a marathon run reduce the incidence of upper respiratory tract infection in the days following the event?

8.5.2 FORMULATION CONSIDERATIONS

8.5.2.1 Carbohydrate Concentration and Type

Although there are not enough data to determine how the ingestion of different carbohydrate types affects the cardiovascular, thermoregulatory, and immune responses that are in part mediated by hormonal responses, little is known about the influence of carbohydrate concentration. Burgess et al.[75] demonstrated that a 1.8% carbohydrate beverage failed to blunt the rise in catecholamines, glucagon, ACTH, or cortisol, whereas drinks containing higher carbohydrate concentrations do blunt these responses. All things considered, much remains to be understood about the relationship between carbohydrate intake (e.g., the quantity and frequency of intake, the type of carbohydrate) and cardiovascular, thermoregulatory, and immune responses. In like fashion, there is undoubtedly much more to be learned about the role of carbohydrate intake on neurotransmitter production and function in the brain, responses that could influence both physical and mental performance and mood during vigorous exercise.

8.5.2.2 Sodium Chloride, Other Minerals, and Vitamins

As detailed in this and other chapters, the presence of sodium chloride is a critical element in a sports drink. Sodium plays such an important role in improving beverage taste, stimulating voluntary fluid intake, promoting fluid absorption, maintaining plasma volume, and assuring rapid and complete rehydration, that its presence in a sports drink can rightfully be considered indispensable. Similarly, critical roles have not been identified for other minerals or vitamins. A number of researchers have investigated their potential efficacy, but without compelling results. For example, niacin ingestion was studied to determine if the increase in skin blood flow (the flushing often provoked by niacin ingestion) would improve the thermoregulatory response to heat exposure; it did not.[96] Potassium loss seems to be a common suspect in muscle cramping; witness the numerous times that bananas and orange slices are available after road races and other sporting events. Yet, a relationship between potassium loss and muscle cramping has never been established.[97] Zinc supplementation enjoyed popularity as a nutritional aid to improve immune response, but attempts to substantiate the relationship have been inconclusive.[98]

8.5.2.3 Amino Acids

The theoretical basis for considering the addition of branched-chain amino acids to a sports drink has been discussed above. Even if the science were supportive of a beneficial effect of BCAA ingestion during exercise, a sports drink would not be the ideal means of delivering them. Although small amounts of amino acids can, and have, been added to commercial sports drinks, doing so in anything greater than very small amounts presents nearly insurmountable challenges from a product development standpoint. Amino acids in solution are not shelf-stable for long periods and, even under the best of circumstances, their presence negatively affects palatability and overall beverage acceptance.

Such challenges are particularly true for glutamine, an amino acid that has received considerable recent attention, in part because of its role as a fuel for immune cells such as lymphocytes. Glutamine is notoriously unstable in solution and is quickly degraded, making it an unlikely candidate for inclusion in a sports drink. On the other hand, there is a theoretical rationale for considering its inclusion, in that plasma glutamine levels have been reported to drop during prolonged exercise, which has been implicated in lower lymphocyte proliferation rates.[99] However, research in this area has not demonstrated a beneficial effect of ingesting glutamine on immune function.

8.6 SPEED REHYDRATION

8.6.1 SCIENTIFIC PRINCIPLES AND PRACTICAL RAMIFICATIONS

The rate of rehydration following exercise is of critical importance whenever rapid and complete rehydration is required. That is certainly the case in many sporting, military, industrial, and even routine leisure-time physical activities. A simple example is that of an individual who tends to a garden for a few hours on a hot summer afternoon and finishes the task dehydrated. Normal physical and mental functions are often not regained for hours, until euhydration is restored. A delay in restoring normal hydration could be especially problematic for athletes, soldiers, and workers who must rehydrate rapidly to resume vigorous physical activity.

The addition of caffeine to fluid, as in the case of most diet colas and "herbal energy beverages," limits effective rehydration due to the diuretic effect of caffeine. This effect was demonstrated by Gonzalez-Alonso et al.,[101] who provided dehydrated subjects with a sports drink, water, or diet cola. Following a 2-hour recovery period, the subjects had retained 73% of the sports drink, 65% of water, and only 54% of the diet cola. Due to its diuretic effect, caffeine has also been associated with accelerated mineral loss in urine.[102] Thus, it is counterintuitive to include caffeine in a sports drink.

The sodium concentration of the ingested beverage is a major determinant of the adequacy of rehydration. For most purposes, a sodium concentration between

20 and 50 mmol/l is adequate to aid in restoring plasma volume and fluid balance. Full rehydration cannot occur unless both the sodium and the fluid lost in sweat are replaced.[103] The sodium concentration of an electrolyte-replacement drink should be high enough to maintain voluntary fluid intake and replace the sodium lost in sweat.[103] The primary factor that contributes to the inability to quickly and completely restore body fluids is the excessive loss of plasma volume and sodium that occurs with sweating. Earlier work by Nadel and colleagues[103] indicated that, independent of palatability issues, an effective fluid replacement beverage should contain between 40 and 60 mmol/l of sodium to provide an elevated plasma osmolality, retain the osmotic drive to drink, and replace the sodium lost in sweat, a prerequisite for restoring the extracellular fluid space.[104] More-recent research with similar sodium levels has indicated beneficial effects of relatively high sodium (50 to 60 mmol/l) and large fluid volumes (i.e., at least 125 to 150% of sweat loss) on the maintenance of positive fluid balance and the restoration of hydration for several hours after exercise-induced dehydration.[105,106,107]

From the standpoint of offsetting urinary mineral loss, some investigators have suggested that small amounts of calcium and magnesium might be important additions to a beverage formulated for sports.[52] However, existing data fall short of substantiating the inclusion of electrolytes other than sodium, chloride, and perhaps potassium (the three minerals lost in the greatest quantities in sweat). Verification of the efficacy of including other minerals requires further testing.

8.6.2 FORMULATION CONSIDERATIONS

Striking the optimum balance between sports drink efficacy and palatability is a considerable challenge for sports drink manufacturers. From a food science perspective, sports drinks are relatively simple beverage systems and that fact makes it difficult to manipulate the types and amounts of solutes without having an immediate and noticeable effect on palatability. When palatability is not a major concern, rehydration solutions can be formulated with efficacy foremost in mind. Such is the case with clinical rehydration solutions for which palatability is not a critical consideration. However, the rehydration that is required following physical activity and that required in clinical settings do share some common ground in that rapid fluid replacement is required to restore physiological homeostasis. Clinical dehydration is often complicated by severe metabolic and electrolyte disturbances for which different solution formulations and different modes of administration (oral vs. intravenous) are required. For example, the oral rehydration solutions formulated to treat bouts of childhood diarrhea contain small amounts of carbohydrate (e.g., 2% to 3% wt/vol) and comparatively large amounts of sodium and potassium (e.g., 45 mmol/l and 20 mmol/l, respectively). The oral rehydration solution that is distributed by the World Health Organization to combat severe diarrhea contains 90 mmol/l sodium.[108] The higher electrolyte concentrations and the lower carbohydrate levels of these solutions are consistent with the need to stimulate rapid fluid absorption and to replace the large amounts of electrolytes that can be lost with diarrhea. Due to their low carbohydrate content, high electrolyte content, and poor palatability, such solutions would not be appropriate for the extent of dehydration that is common to physical activity and sport.

8.7 SUMMARY

Sports drinks are among the best-researched food products in the world. There is a wealth of scientific research that can be relied upon to formulate an efficacious beverage that can provide benefits for voluntary fluid intake, rapid fluid absorption, improved performance, and enhanced rehydration. Formulating an efficacious sports drink requires an in-depth knowledge of the physiological and metabolic responses to ingesting fluid, carbohydrates, and electrolytes during exercise, a comprehensive understanding of the interactions between the physicochemical properties of the beverage and the psychosensory responses to exercise and environment, and an ability to apply that knowledge in formulating a beverage that is compatible with the limitations imposed by large scale production, packaging, and product distribution. Relatively small changes in product formulation (e.g., carbohydrate level too high, sodium level too low) and the inclusion of ingredients that are contraindicated (e.g., artificial preservatives) or are of dubious merit (e.g., chromium), can demonstrably alter the physiological and performance responses to ingesting a sports drink during exercise.

REFERENCES

1. *Beverage World Annual Index.* 66-68, May 1999.
2. CSDs, an active market in 1998. *Beverage Industry.* 35-36, March 1999.
3. Adolph EF and associates, Eds. *Physiology of Man in the Desert.* New York, NY: Interscience Publishers, Inc., 1947.
4. Gisolfi CV and Lamb DR, Eds. *Perspectives in Exercise Science and Sports Medicine,* Volume 3: Fluid Homeostasis During Exercise. Carmel, IN: Benchmark Press, 1990.
5. Buskirk ER and Puhl SM, Eds. Body fluid balance. Boca Raton, FL: CRC Press, 1996.
6. Sawka MN and Pandolf KB. Effects of body fluid loss on physiological function and exercise performance. In, Gisolfi CV and Lamb DR, Eds. *Perspectives in Exercise Science and Sports Medicine: Fluid Homeostasis During Exercise.* Indianapolis: Benchmark Press, 1988.
7. Unpublished data, Gatorade Exercise Physiology Laboratory.
8. Nieman DC, Nehlsen-Cannarella SL, Fagoaga, OR, Hensen DA, Davis JM, Williams F, and Butterworth DE. Effects of mode and carbohydrate on the granulocyte and monocyte response to intensive, prolonged exercise. *J. Appl. Physiol.* 84:1252-1259, 1998.
9. Lamb D and Brodowicz GR. Optimal use of fluids of varying formulations to minimize exercise-induced disturbances in homeostasis. *Sports Med.* 3:247-274, 1986.
10. Murray R. The effects of consuming carbohydrate-electrolyte beverages on gastric emptying and fluid absorption during and following exercise. *Sports Med.* 4:322-351, 1987.
11. Maughan RJ and Noakes TD. Fluid replacement and exercise stress. *Sports Med.* 12:16-31, 1991.

12. Maughan RJ, Shirreffs SM, Galloway DR, and Leiper JB. Dehydration and fluid replacement in sport and exercise. *Sports Exercise and Injury.* 1:148-153, 1995.

13. Maughan RJ and Shirreffs SM. Formulating sports drinks. *Chemistry and Industry.* 28-32, January 19, 1998.

14. Grossman, SP. *Thirst and Sodium Appetite.* San Diego: Academic Press, 1990, p. 79.

15. Hubbard RW, Szlyk PC, and Armstrong LE. Influence of thirst and fluid palatability on fluid ingestion during exercise. In *Perspectives in Exercise Science and Sports Medicine: Fluid Homeostasis During Exercise.* C Gisolfi, Lamb D, Eds. Cooper Publishing, Carmel, IN: 1990, 39-95.

16. Noakes, T. D., Fluid replacement during exercise, in *Exercise and Sport Sciences Reviews*, Vol. 21, Holloszy, J. O., Ed. Williams and Wilkins, Baltimore, 1993, 297.

17. Noakes, T.D., Adams, B.A., Myburgh, K.H., Greeff, C., Lotz, T., and Nathan, M. The danger of an inadequate water intake during prolonged exercise, *Eur. J. Appl. Physiol.* 57, 1988, 210.

18. Greenleaf JE. Problem: thirst, drinking behavior, and involuntary dehydration. *Med. Sci. Sports Exerc.* 24:645-656, 1992.

19. Figaro KM and Mack GW. Regulation of fluid intake in dehydrated humans: role of oropharyngeal reflex. *Am. J. Physiol.* (*Regulatory Integrative Comp. Physiol.* 41): R1740-R1746, 1997.

20. Cecil JE, Francis J, and Read NW. Relative contributions of intestinal, gastric, oro-sensory influences and information to changes in appetite induced by the same liquid meal. *Appetite.* 31:377-380, 1998.

21. Greenleaf, JE. Environmental issues that influence intake of replacement beverages. In: *Fluid Replacement and Heat Stress.* Washington, DC: National Academy Press: XV:1-30, 1991.

22. Passe D, Horn M, Murray R. The effects of beverage carbonation on sensory responses and voluntary fluid intake following exercise. *Int. J. Sports Nutr.*7: 286-297, 1997.

23. Sohar E, Kaly J, and Adar R. The prevention of voluntary dehydration. In, *Symposium on Environmental Physiology and Psychology in Arid Conditions.* Paris, France: United Nations Educational, Scientific and Cultural Organization 129-135, 1962.

24. Hubbard RL, Sandick BL, Matthew WT, Francesconi RP, Sampson JB, Durkot MJ, Maller O, and Engell DB. Voluntary dehydration and alliesthesia for water. *J. Appl. Physiol.* 57:868-873, 1984.

25. American College of Sports Medicine. Position stand on exercise and fluid replacement. *Med. Sci. Sports Exerc.* 28:i-vii, 1996.

26. Miller IJ and Reedy FE. Variations in human taste bud density and taste intensity perception. *Physiology and Behavior*, 47(6):1213-1219, 1990.

27. Green B, Frankmann SP. The effect of cooling on the perception of carbohydrate and intensive sweeteners. *Physiology and Behavior*, 43(4):515-519, 1988.

28. Christenson CM. Effects of solution viscosity on perceived saltiness and sweetness. *Perceptual Psychophysics.* 28(4):347-353, 1980

29. Ploutz-Snyder L, Foley J, Ploutz-Snyder R, Kanaley J, Sagendorf K, and Meyer R. Gastric gas and fluid emptying assessed by magnetic resonance imaging. *Eur. J. Appl. Physiol.* 79:212-220, 1999.

30. Engell D, Hirsch E. Environmental and sensory modulation of fluid intake in humans. In Ramsay DJ and Booth DA, Eds. *Thirst: Physiological and Psychological Aspects.* London: Springer-Verlag, 1991, pp. 382-390.

31. Passe D, Horn M, and Murray R. The effect of beverage carbonation on sensory responses and voluntary fluid intake following exercise. *Int. J. Sports Nutr.* 7:286-297, 1997.

33. Calvino AM. Perception of sweetness: the effects of concentration and temperature. *Physiol. Behav.* 36:1021-1028, 1986.
34. Bartoshuk LM, Rennert K, Rodin J, and Stevens JC. Effects of temperature and the perceived sweetness of sucrose. *Physiol. Behav.* 28:905-910, 1982.
35. Passe DP, Horn M, and Murray R. Palatability and voluntary intake of sports beverages, diluted fruit juice, and water during exercise. *Med. Sci. Sports Exerc.* 31:S322, 1999.
36. McBride RL. Sweetness of binary mixtures of sucrose, fructose, and glucose. *J. Exp. Psych.* 12:584-591, 1986.
37. BeMiller JN. Sucrose. In *Encyclopedia of Food Science and Technology: Vol 4*. YH Hui, Ed. John Wiley and Sons, NY: 1992, 2441-2442.
38. Murray R, Bartoli B, Stofan J, Horn M, and Eddy D. A comparison of the gastric emptying characteristics of selected sports drinks. *Int. J. Sports Nutr.*, 9:263-274, 1999.
39. Ryan, AJ, Lambert GP, Shi X, Chang RT, Summers RW, and Gisolfi CV. Effect of hypohydration on gastric emptying and intestinal absorption during exercise. *J. Appl. Physiol.* 84:1581-1588, 1998.
40. Rehrer NJ, Wagenmakers AJM, Beckers EJ, Halliday D, Leiper JB, Brouns F, Maughan RJ, Westerterp K, and Saris WHM. Gastric emptying, absorption, and carbohydrate oxidation during prolonged exercise. *J. Appl. Physiol.* 72:468-475, 1992.
41. Tsintzas OK, Williams C, Singh R, Wilson W, and Burrin J. Influence of carbohydrate-electrolyte drinks on marathon running performance. *Eur. J. Appl. Physiol.* 70:154-160, 1995.
42. Tsintzas OK, Williams C, Wilson W, and Burrin J. Influence of carbohydrate supplementation early in exercise on endurance running capacity. *Med. Sci. Sports Exerc.* 28:1373-1379, 1996.
43. Murray R, Seifert JG, Eddy DE, Paul GL, and Halaby GA. Carbohydrate feeding and exercise: Effect of beverage carbohydrate content. *Eur. J. Appl. Physiol.* 59:152-158, 1989.
44. Shi, X, Schedl HP, Summers RM, Lambert GP, Chang, RT, Xia T, and Gisolfi CV. Fructose transport mechanisms in humans. *Gastroenterology* 113:1171-1179, 1997.
45. Murray R, Paul GL, Seifert JG, Eddy DE, and Halaby GA. The effects of glucose, fructose, and sucrose ingestion during exercise. *Med. Sci. Sports Exerc.* 21(3):275-282, 1989.
46. Maughan RJ. Fluid and electrolyte loss and replacement in exercise. *J. Sports Sci.* 9:117-142, 1991.
47. Wilk B and Bar-Or O. Effect of drink flavor and NaCl on voluntary drinking and hydration in boys exercising in the heat. *J. Appl. Physiol.* 80:1112-1117, 1996.
48. Vrijens DMJ and Rehrer NJ. Sodium-free fluid ingestion decreases plasma sodium during exercise in the heat. *J. Appl. Physiol.* 86:1847-1851, 1999.
49. Nadel ER, Mack GW, and Nose H. Influence of fluid replacement beverages on body fluid homeostasis during exercise and recovery. In *Perspectives in Exercise Science and Sports Medicine: Fluid Homeostasis During Exercise*. Gisolfi C, Lamb D, Eds. Cooper Publishing, Carmel, IN: 1990, 181-198.
50. Greenleaf JE, Jackson CGR, Geelen G, Keil LC, Hinghofer-Szalkay H, and Whittam JH. Plasma volume expansion with oral fluids in hypohydrated men at rest and during exercise. *Aviat. Space Env Med,* 69:837-844, 1998.
51. Wemple RD, Morocco TS, and Mack GW. Influence of sodium replacement on fluid ingestion following exercise-induced dehydration. *Int. J. Sports Nutr.* 7:104-116, 1997.

52. Brouns F, Saris W, and Schneider H. Rationale for upper limits of electrolyte replacement during exercise. *Int. J. Sports Nutr.* 2:229-238, 1992.

53. Maughan RJ and Rehrer NJ. Gastric emptying during exercise. *Sports Sci. Exch.* 6(42):1-5, 1993.

54. Vist GE and Maughan RJ. The effect of osmolality and carbohydrate content on the rate of gastric emptying of liquids in man. *J. Physiol.* 486:523-531, 1995.

55. Shi X., Summers RW, Schedl HP, Flanagan SW, Chang RT, and Gisolfi CV. Effects of carbohydrate type and concentration and solution osmolality on water absorption. *Med. Sci. Sports Exerc.* 27, 1607-1615, 1995.

56. Schedl HP, Maughan RJ, and Gisolfi CV. Intestinal absorption during rest and exercise: implications for formulating an oral rehydration solution (ORS). *Med. Sci. Sports Exerc.* 26(3):267-280, 1994.

57. Murray R, Eddy DE, Bartoli WP, and Paul GL. Gastric emptying of water and isocaloric carbohydrate solutions consumed at rest. *Med. Sci. Sports Exerc.* 26, 725-732, 1994.

58. Vist GE and Maughan RJ. The effect of increasing glucose concentration on the rate of gastric emptying in man. *Med. Sci. Sports Exerc.* 26:1269-1273, 1994.

59. Gisolfi CV, Summers RW, Schedl HP, and Bleiler TL. Intestinal water absorption from select carbohydrate solutions in humans. *J. Appl. Physiol.* 73, 2142-2150, 1992.

60. Davis JM, Burgess WA, Slentz CA, and Bartoli WP. Fluid availability of sports drinks differing in carbohydrate type and concentration. *Amer. J. Clin. Nutr.* 51:1054-7, 1990.

61. Neufer PD, Costill DL, Fink WJ, Kirwan JP, Fielding RA, and Flynn WG. Effects of exercise and carbohydrate composition on gastric emptying. *Med. Sci. Sports Exerc.* 18:658-662, 1986.

62. Gisolfi CV, Summers RW, Schedl HP, Bleiler TL, and Oppliger RA. Human intestinal water absorption: Direct vs. indirect measurements. *Amer. J. Physiol. 258 (Gastrointest. Liver Physiol.)* 21: G216-G222, 1990.

63. Gisolfi CV, Summers RW, Schedl HP, and Bleiler TL. Effect of sodium concentration in a carbohydrate-electrolyte solution on intestinal absorption. *Med. Sci. Sports Exerc.* 27(10):1414-1420, 1995.

64. Dan-Axel Hallack BM, Hulten L, Jodal M, Lindhagen J, and Lundgren O. Evidence for the existence of a countercurrent exchange in the small intestine in man. *Gastroenterology* 74:683:690, 1978.

65. Hirschhorn N and Greenough WB. Progress in oral rehydration therapy. *Sci. American* 264:50-56, 1991.

66. Coggan A and Coyle EF. Carbohydrate ingestion during prolonged exercise: effects on metabolism and performance. In: *Exercise and Sports Science Reviews*, Holloszy, JO, Ed. Baltimore,Williams and Wilkins,1991,19:1-40.

67. Hargreaves M. Metabolic responses to carbohydrate ingestion: Effects on exercise performance. In *Perspectives in Exercise Science and Sports Medicine: The Metabolic Bases of Exercise and Sport Performance*. Carmel, IN: Cooper Publishing, 1999, pp. 93-124.

68. Davis JM, Jackson DA, Broadwell MS, Queary JL, and Lambert CL. Carbohydrate drinks delay fatigue during intermittent high-intensity cycling in active men and women. *Int. J. Sports Nutr.* 7:261-273, 1997.

69. Nicholas CW, Williams C, Lakomy HKA, Phillips G, and Nowitz A. Influence of ingesting a carbohydrate-electrolyte solution on endurance capacity during intermittent high intensity shuttle running. *J. Sports Sci.* 13:283-290, 1995.

70. Hertler-Colbert L, Davis JM, Alderson N, Welsh R, Walters J, and Devolve K. Effects of carbohydrates and chromium ingestion on fatigue during intermittent, high intensity exercise. *Med. Sci. Sports Exer.* 29:S277, 1997.

71. Vergauwen L, Brouns LF, and Hespel P. Carbohydrate supplementation improves stroke performance in tennis. *Med. Sci. Sports Exer.* 30(8): 1289-1295, 1998.

72. Burke ER and Ekblom B. Influence of fluid ingestion and dehydration on precision and endurance performance in tennis. In *Current Topics in Sports Medicine: Proceedings of the World Congress of Sports Medicine.* Bachl N, Prokop L, and Suckert R, Eds. Wien: Urban and Schwarzeberg, 1984, pp379-388.

73. Smith K, Smith N, Wishart C, and Green S. Effect of a carbohydrate-electrolyte beverage on fatigue during a soccer-related running test. *J. Sport Sci.,* 16(5):502-503, 1998.

74. Davis JM, Welsh RS, De Volve, KL, and Alderson NA. Effects of branched-chain amino acids and carbohydrate on fatigue during intermittent, high-intensity running. *Int. J. Sports Med.* 20:309-314, 1999.

75. Burgess WA, Davis JM, Bartoli WP, and Woods JA. Failure of low-dose carbohydrate feeding to attenuate glucoregulatory hormone responses and improve endurance performance. *Int. J. Sports Nutr.* 1:338-352, 1991.

76. Davis JM, Lamb DR, Pate RR, Slentz CA, Burgess WA, and Bartoli WP. Carbohydrate-electrolyte drinks: effects on endurance performance in the heat. *Am. J. Clin. Nutr.* 48:1023-1030, 1988.

77. Wagenmakers AJM, Brouns F, Saris WHM, and Halliday D. Oxidation rates of orally ingested carbohydrates during prolonged exercise in man. *J. Appl. Physiol.,* 75: 2774-2780, 1993.

78. Davis JM, Burgess WA, Slentz CA, Bartoli WP, and Pate RR. Effects of ingesting 6% and 12% glucose/electrolyte beverages during prolonged intermittent cycling in the heat. *Eur. J. Appl. Physiol.* 57:563-569, 1988.

79. Maughan RJ, Fenn CE, and Leiper JB. Effects of fluid, electrolyte and substrate ingestion on endurance capacity. *Eur. J. Appl. Physiol.* 58:481-486, 1989.

80. Murray R, Eddy DE, Murray TW, Seifert JG, Paul GL, and Halaby GA. The effect of fluid and carbohydrate feedings during intermittent cycling exercise. *Med. Sci. Sports Exerc.* 19:597-604, 1987.

81. Blomstrand E, Celsing F, and Newsholme EA. Changes in plasma concentration of aromatic and branched-chain amino acids during sustained exercise in man and their possible role in fatigue. *Acta Physiol. Scand.* 133:115-121, 1988.

82. Mittleman KD, Ricci MR, and Bailey SP. Branched-chain amino acids prolong exercise during heat stress in men and women. *Med. Sci. Sports Exerc.* 30:83-91, 1998.

83. Madsen K, MacLean DA, Kiens B, and Christensen D. Effects of glucose, glucose plus branched-chain amino acids, or placebo on bike performance over 100 km. *J. Appl. Physiol.* 81:2644-2650, 1996.

84. van Hall G, Raaymakers JSH, Saris WHM, and Wagenmakers AJM. Ingestion of branched-chain amino acids and tryptophan during sustained exercise — failure to affect performance. *J. Appl. Physiol.* 486:789-794, 1995.

85. Nieman DC, Henson DA, Butterworth DE, Warren BJ, Davis JM, Fagoaga OR, and Nehlsen-Cannarella SL. Vitamin C supplementation does not alter the immune response to 2.5 hours of running. *Int. J. Sports Nutr.* 7:173-184, 1997.

86. Kanter MM and Williams MH. Antioxidants, carnitine, and choline as putative ergogenic aids. *Int. J. Sports Nutr.* 5:S120-S131, 1995.

87. Murray R, Bartoli WP, Eddy DE, and Horn MK. Physiological and performance responses to nicotinic-acid ingestion during exercise. *Med. Sci. Sports Exerc.* 27:1057-1062, 1995.

88. Lamb DR and Shehata AH. Benefits and limitations to prehydration. *Sports Science Exchange* 73:1-7, 1999.

89. Latzka WA, Sawka MN, Montain SJ, Skrinar GS, Fielding RA, Matott RP, and Pandolf KB. Hyperhydration: tolerance and cardiovascular effects during uncompensable heat stress. *J. Appl. Physiol.* 83:860-866, 1998.

90. Murray R, Eddy DE, Paul GL, Seifert JG, and Halaby GA. Physiological responses to glycerol ingestion during exercise. *J. Appl. Physiol.* 71:144-149, 1991.

91. Coyle EF. Cardiovascular drift during prolonged exercise and the effects of dehydration. *Int. J. Sports Med.* 19:S121-S124, 1998.

92. Nieman DC, Nehlsen-Cannarella SL, Fagoaga OR, Henson DA, Utter A, Davis JM, Williams F, and Butterworth DE. Influence of mode and carbohydrate on the cytokine response to heavy exertion. *Med. Sci. Sports Exerc.* 30:671-678, 1998.

93. Nieman DC. Influence of carbohydrate on the immune response to intensive prolonged exercise. *Exerc. Immun. Rev.* 4:64-76, 1998.

94. Davis JM, Jackson DA, Broadwell MS, Queary JL, and Lambert CL. Carbohydrate drinks delay fatigue during intermittent, high-intensity cycling in active men and women. *Int. J. Sports Nutr.* 7:261-273, 1997.

95. Mora-Rodríguez R, González-Alonso J, Below PR, and Coyle EF. Plasma catecholamines and hyperglycaemia influence thermoregulation in man during prolonged exercise in the heat. *J Physiol.* 491:529-540, 1996.

96. Stephenson LA and Kolka MA. Cardiovascular and thermoregulatory effects of niacin, in *Thermal Physiology.* Mercer JB, Ed. Excerpta Medica, New York, 1989, 279-284.

97. Schwellnus MP, Derman ER, and Noakes TD. Aetiology of skeletal muscle cramps during exercise: a novel hypothesis. *J. Sports Sci.* 15:277-285, 1997.

98. Nieman DC and Pedersen BK. Exercise and immune function: recent developments. *Sports Med.* 27:73-80, 1999.

99. MacKinnon LT and Hooper SL. Plasma glutamine and URTI during intensified training in swimmers. *Med. Sci. Sports Exerc.* 28:285-290, 1996.

100. Rohde T. MacLean DL, and Pedersen BK. Effect of glutamine supplementation on changes in the immune system induced by repeated exercise. *Med. Sci. Sports Exerc.* 30:856-862, 1998.

101. Gonzalez-Alonso J, Heaps CL, and Coyle EF. Rehydration after exercise with common beverages and water. *Int. J. Sports. Med.* 13(5):399-406, 1992.

102. Brouns F, Kovacs EMR, and Senden JMG. The effect of different rehydration drinks on post-exercise electrolyte excretion in trained athletes. *Int. J. Sports Med.* 19:56-60, 1998.

103. Nadel ER, Mack GW, and Takamata A. Thermoregulation, Exercise, and Thirst: Interrelationships in Humans. In *Perspectives in Exercise Science and Sports Medicine: Exercise, Heat, and Thermoregulation.* Gisolfi C, Lamb D, and Nadel ER, Eds. Brown and Benchmark, Dubuque, IA: 1993, 225-249.

104. Maughan RJ, Shirreffs SM, and Leiper JB. Rehydration and recovery after exercise. *Sport Sci. Exch.* 9:1-5, 1996.

105. Maughan RJ and Leiper JB. Sodium intake and post-exercise rehydration in man. *Eur. J. Appl. Physiol* 71:311-319, 1995.

106. Brack AS and Ball D. Dehydration and rapid rehydration: Effects on performance during brief high-intensity exercise. *J. Sport Sciences*, 16:39-40, 1998.
107. Shirreffs S and Maughan RJ. Volume repletion after exercise-induced volume depletion in humans: replacement of water and sodium losses. *Am. J. Physiol.* 274:F868-F875, 1998.
108. Guandalini S. Current controversies in oral rehydration solution formulation. *Clin. Therapeutics* 12:38-50, 1990.

9 Other Ingredients: Role in the Nutrition of Athletes

Craig A. Horswill

CONTENTS

This chapter will briefly review the physiological basis and the performance effects of ingredients that are considered nontraditional in a hydration beverage. The functions of traditional ingredients such as metabolizable carbohydrate, electrolytes such as sodium and potassium, and water are described elsewhere in this text. In describing the nontraditional ingredients, the focus will be on physiology and physical work performance, and on the rationale for their presence in a sports drink. However, it is important to consider that these ingredients may alter the taste, beverage stability, and shelf life, as well as the bioavailability of other (the traditional) ingredients in the beverage. Data on these characteristics are seldom available, thus making it difficult to predict the interactive and comprehensive effects of a novel ingredient on the integrity and efficacy of a sports beverage. Nonetheless, these factors are important and should not be dismissed as insignificant when establishing the effectiveness of a sports drink.

9.1   ENERGY SOURCES

9.1.1   CARBOHYDRATE DERIVATIVES

9.1.1.1   Fiber

Indigestible carbohydrate, or fiber, may play an important role in the health of an individual. A growing body of research shows that soluble fiber may decrease cholesterol levels,[1] reduce the risk of heart disease,[2] and possibly reduce the risk of gastrointestinal cancers,[3] depending on the type of soluble fiber. These benefits are obtained from chronic intake of an adequate amount of fiber.

From a sports performance standpoint, the immediate effect of fiber on glucose absorption and the insulin response has received some attention. In one study,[4] solid foods with soluble fiber and carbohydrate helped increase cycling time to exhaustion by approximately 41 min, or 16%, relative to an isoenergetic feeding trial. Modest changes in plasma insulin concentrations occurred in response to the fiber-containing treatment (rolled oats) vs. the treatments low in fiber (oat flour). In contrast to the hypothesis, no differences existed in the plasma glucose responses. Some have speculated that the insulin response to the ingestion of food with a high glycemic index causes a rebound hypoglycemia that may impair performance,[5] but Kirwan et al. did not detect hypoglycemia after ingestion of either moderate glycemic or high glycemic food.[4]

The few studies specifically on beverages show little evidence of a benefit of adding fiber to a sports drink. MacLaren et al.[6] found no differences in blood glucose responses to solutions containing glucose or maltodextrin when 8% guar gum (a soluble fiber) was added to either beverage. Regardless of the presence of fiber, subjects cycled for longer at 75% VO_{2max} before exhaustion when metabolizable carbohydrate was present in the beverage compared with times for the placebo, which contained no carbohydrate. Purcell and colleagues[7] also failed to find differences in blood glucose and insulin levels 45 min prior to and during 60 min of exercise when subjects drank solutions containing either 75 g of glucose or the same amount of glucose plus 14.5 g of guar gum. The observation that all subjects who suffered gastrointestinal (GI) distress within a group of 55 triathletes consumed a fiber-rich meal before the race raises concerns about adverse effects of adding fiber to a beverage that is consumed during exercise.[8]

Further research may be warranted to clarify the effect of the addition of fiber to sports drinks on the efficacy of such a beverage. Of particular concerns are the possible modifications in blood substrate availability, altered hormonal responses, and the potential for GI distress. The few studies to date have utilized sub-maximal exercise tests in a laboratory environment, and the effects of fiber ingested before and during exercise in competitive conditions need to be addressed.

9.1.1.2 Pyruvate/Dihydroxyacetone

Triose intermediates normally produced during glycolysis have been examined as a possible combined supplement to enhance performance. Two studies from Stanko et al. suggested that pyruvate supplementation at levels of 25 g sodium pyruvate per day, in combination with 75 g dihydroxyacetone, can prolong endurance performance at a constant power output.[9,10] The power output was chosen to elicit an effort of 60% peak oxygen uptake when the upper body was tested[9] and 70% of peak oxygen uptake when the lower body was tested.[10] Initially, the work of Stanko et al. suggested that loading with these intermediates for several days prior to the performance trial may increase muscle glycogen, assuming a standard diet is consumed (55% of energy from carbohydrate, 30% from fat, and 15% from protein).[9] Subsequent research showed that if the diet was high in carbohydrate (70% of total energy), the pyruvate/dihydroxyacetone supplements had no added effect on increasing muscle glycogen levels.[10]

No other laboratory has corroborated the findings of Stanko et al. Stone et al.[11] failed to find an effect of pyruvate/dihydroxyacetone supplementation on performance. Five weeks of pyruvate supplementation (calcium pyruvate at about 19 g/d) showed no differences in strength (one repetition maximum lifts), vertical jump, or body composition compared with the effects of the placebo trial.[11] Enhanced force production is not necessarily expected consequent to using this supplement, but claims have been made that commercially available pyruvate/dihydroxyacetone supplements enhance lipid oxidation and reduce body fatness.[12] Support for this claim was not found within this study.[11]

The limited data on pyruvate/dihydroxyacetone supplementation do not offer a consensus on whether there is an ergogenic effect.[12] The requirement for chronic high dosages and the lack of any data showing an acute benefit from feedings of the triose suggest that the combination is a poor candidate for addition to a sports beverage. In addition, research showing improved performance after high-dose, chronic feedings of pyruvate/dihydroxyacetone also reports that most of the subjects experienced negative gastrointestinal effects.[9,10]

9.1.1.3 Lactate

Lactate has been examined as a supplement that might provide an alternate substrate for oxidative metabolism. Lactate is metabolized during submaximal intensity exercise by skeletal muscle fibers having a high oxidative capacity.[13,14] *In vitro*, lactate may be metabolized at a faster rate than glucose because of enzyme kinetics and the transport of substrate that favor lactate oxidation.[15]

In practice, the addition of lactate to a sports drink has not been demonstrated to enhance performance. Swensen et al.[16] are the only researchers to test for an ergogenic effect. Comparing the performance effects of an isoenergetic beverage of glucose polymers with a beverage containing 6.25% glucose polymer and 0.75% lactate, they reported no difference in cycling time to exhaustion at 70% of VO_{2max}. Previous research indicated that, compared with intake of water alone, a beverage with lactate in the form of Poly L-lactate™ helped maintain blood glucose during 3 h of exercise at 50% VO_{2max}.[17] In contrast, Swensen et al. saw no difference in the blood concentration of carbohydrate substrates, fat substrates, or insulin levels during 3 h of cycling at 70% VO_{2max}.[16] In the latter study, the authors were forced to reduce beverage lactate concentration from 2.5% to minimize the GI, which had been severe in their pilot studies. The dosage required to supply enough lactate to be an alternative source of fuel may produce side effects sufficiently severe to impair performance.

TABLE 9.1
Summary of Carbohydrate Derivatives Added to a Sports Drink

Derivative	Claim	Proposed Mechanism	Substantiation as an Additive
Fiber (guar gum)	Sustained energy	Delayed glucose absorption & blunted insulin response	Two studies to date; effect not detected
Pyruvate/ DHAP	Enhanced endurance	Alternate fuel & enhanced lipid oxidation	Limited supportive data; no studies using sports drinks as delivery vehicle; GI distress likely
Lactate	Enhanced endurance	Alternate fuel for glycogen sparing	No evidence of a performance effect

9.1.2 PROTEINS AND PROTEIN DERIVATIVES

The oxidation of protein provides relatively little energy during exercise.[18,19] Therefore, it is doubtful that the presence of protein in a fluid consumed during exercise offers an ergogenic effect during that activity on the basis of fuel supply alone. A recent study demonstrated that the addition of protein to a carbohydrate beverage consumed during exercise increased the rate of nitrogen excretion but did nothing to alter blood glucose levels or performance of the subjects.[20] Additionally, compared with the carbohydrate-alone trial, the protein treatment did not alter myofibrillar protein breakdown as estimated from 3-methylhistidine excretion.[20] Despite these findings, there are several claims made for the influence of intact proteins, specific amino acids, or protein derivatives in a sports drink. The theory behind the claims and the research findings for these protein compounds are summarized here.

9.1.2.1   Intact Proteins

The benefit of adding protein to a hydration beverage in an attempt to enhance the replenishment of muscle glycogen after exercise has been debated recently. One study suggested that the addition of protein to a carbohydrate meal resulted in greater muscle glycogen stores 4 h after recovery. Although replenishment also occurred during the carbohydrate-only trial, the degree of replenishment appeared to be less than when protein was added.[21] Ingestion of protein alone stimulates insulin secretion and the secretion of gastric inhibitory polypeptide,[22] which can augment insulin action.[23] The rate of glycogen synthesis might therefore be expected to increase if protein were added to a carbohydrate meal. However, the intake of carbohydrate still appears to be the primary factor in glycogen resynthesis. Based on glycogen synthesis rates 1 h after training following isoenergetic feedings[24] and on muscle glycogen levels at the end of 24 h of various dietary recoveries following endurance exercise,[25] an adequate dose of carbohydrate, not the inclusion of protein, dictates recovery. Recent research suggests that, compared with the effects of feedings of protein plus carbohydrate, the rate of resynthesis of muscle glycogen is no different if additional carbohydrate without protein is ingested.[26,27]

9.1.2.2   Branched-Chain Amino Acids (BCAA)

Supplementation of the three BCAA during exercise has been evaluated as a means to counter peripheral fatigue[19] or central fatigue[28] that impairs physical performance. In terms of peripheral fatigue, it has been thought that BCAA may provide a substrate for oxidation during high-intensity exercise, particularly when muscle glycogen levels are low as a result of fasting, insufficient dietary carbohydrate, or during prolonged exercise. Mechanistically, this notion is supported by research[29] showing that the rate of oxidation of BCAA after an overnight fast increases to 4 to 5 times that of the fed state, when muscle glycogen is more abundant. Reduced muscle glycogen content is also a strong stimulus for activation of branched chain α-keto-acid dehydrogenase (BCKADH), the rate-limiting enzyme for BCAA oxidation in muscle during exercise.[30]

At present, though, studies do not demonstrate that BCAA supplementation in a hydration beverage prevents peripheral fatigue during exercise. BCAA oxidation provides, at most, 1% of the total energy used during exercise even with an elevation in the rate of BCAA oxidation.[19] Additionally, the typical practice of athletes is to consume a high-carbohydrate diet and to ingest carbohydrate in fluids during exercise, both of which prevent the activation of BCKADH and thereby limit BCAA oxidation.

BCAA supplementation is theorized to block the uptake into the brain of tryptophan, the precursor of serotonin that is thought to induce central fatigue.[31] During sustained exercise, elevations in free fatty acid levels may displace tryptophan from its binding sites on albumin, the plasma transport protein. Free tryptophan readily crosses the blood–brain barrier and can be converted to serotonin.[32] However, BCAA compete with tryptophan for the same blood–brain barrier transporter [33]; thus, elevation of blood BCAA levels as a result of supplementation might block tryptophan transport and help reduce the onset of central fatigue.

Regardless of the proposed mechanism to counter fatigue, studies on the effects of BCAA ingestion on physical performance show no delay in fatigue during moderate to high-intensity endurance.[34,35,36,37,38] Most recently, this was examined with an exercise protocol that simulated the intermittent high-intensity efforts used in soccer and American football.[37] The researchers found that carbohydrate ingestion in the form of a sports drink increased the duration of an intermittent shuttle-running test performed at the end of the game simulation to nearly 10 min compared with an average of 6.5 min ($p < 0.05$) on the placebo trial. Addition of BCAA to the carbohydrate containing sports drink resulted in a mean time to fatigue of just over 9 min, which was not significantly different from that on the carbohydrate alone trial. Under conditions of heat stress, one study demonstrated that BCAA supplementation increased exercise duration.[39] Subjects cycled at 40% of peak VO_2 for 153 min on average when receiving BCAA in the fluid compared with a time of 137 min on the control beverage ($p = 0.04$). The low intensity used in the exercise protocol renders the findings of questionable relevance to athletes in competition and individuals training at intensities that produce fitness adaptations. Nonetheless, follow-up studies are needed to determine whether athletes obtain similar effects with BCAA ingestion during endurance competition in heat stress.

Ingestion of BCAA during exercise increases ammonia production,[40] but it is unclear whether the increase would reach a level that impacts performance. Under experimental conditions, a feeding induced elevation in plasma ammonia level led to early fatigue during high intensity performance, in part by compromising the buffering capacity.[41,42,43] Also, ammonia accumulation during exercise may advesely affect motor skill function.[44] Based on a consistent lack of evidence of an ergogenic effect during prolonged exercise and intermittent high intensity exercise, it would seem that BCAA supplementation is a metabolically expensive method of providing an alternative substrate to carbohydrate in a hydration solution.

9.1.2.3   Selected Individual Amino Acids

9.1.2.3.1   Glycine

Certain amino acids provide a transportable solute in the gut, so the addition of specific amino acids to a beverage might enhance fluid absorption.[45] As an example, glycine has been examined as a transportable substrate for oral rehydration solutions designed to treat diarrhea-induced dehydration,[46,47,48,49] but only one study to date has examined the potential for glycine in a sports drink.[50] In that study, the addition of glycine (0.4 g/100 ml in a 6% carbohydrate sports drink) produced a mean (±SD) intestinal fluid absorption rate of 511 ± 110 ml/h/40 cm of intestine. This rate was not significantly different from the fluid absorption rate of the same beverage without the addition of glycine (584 ± 184 ml/h/40 cm of intestine).[50]

9.1.2.3.2 Glutamine

Manipulation of glutamine intake has been studied in an attempt to understand and prevent overtraining in athletes. Glutamine is an important fuel for the immune system[51,52,53] and provides the precursor for genetic material in cells, including the white blood cell.[54] It has been speculated that blood glutamine levels decrease with overtraining because of an increased demand for energy through the body when daily energy expenditure is consistently high.[51,55] In theory, addition of glutamine to the diet and, perhaps, in a hydration beverage, might decrease the risk of over-training or impairment to the immune system in the athlete.[56]

Few data exist in support of this theory. One study reported a lower incidence of infections in athletes who consumed a beverage containing glutamine after exercise.[56] However, infection rates were determined from surveys completed by the athletes, and no attempt was made to validate the surveys with clinical assessments. The probability of orally ingested glutamine reaching the plasma and elevating body stores is low for two reasons. Substantial uptake of ingested glutamine occurs at the intestinal cell level because glutamine serves as a fuel for these cells. Additionally, when added to an acidic beverage or when exposed to gastric acids in the stomach, glutamine is rapidly converted to glutamate, which may be poorly tolerated in individuals who experience allergies or chemical sensitivity to monosodium glutamate.[57]

Unrelated to the effects of glutamine supplementation on immune system function is the possibility that glutamine can enhance muscle glycogen recovery after intense exercise. This response has been demonstrated only with intravenous administration of glutamine, which allows the gut to be bypassed.[58] When administered orally, with or without glucose, glutamine does not enhance muscle glycogen recovery moe so than glucose feedings alone,[59] and does not appear to enhance subsequent performance.[60]

9.1.2.3.3 Arginine

The role of arginine as a precursor of nitric oxide, a mediator of vasodilatation, is increasingly receiving research attention, particularly because of the potential impact of nitric oxide on cardiovascular health.[61] At present, two groups have published on the effect of oral arginine supplementation on physical performance or recovery after exercise. Yaspelkis and Ivy failed to find a clear beneficial effect.[62] The authors reported that the addition of arginine to a carbohydrate supplement consumed after exercise did not increase plasma insulin level above that of the carbohydrate-only trial. Consequently, the rate of muscle glycogen synthesis was not different between treatments.[62] In addition to this study, others have reported that arginine supplementation (10 g, three times per day for 14 days preceding a marathon) did not prevent the occurrence of intestinal injury as hypothesized, and instead was associated with impaired performance.[63]

9.1.2.4 Keto-Analogues

Beta-hydroyx-beta-methylbutyrate (HMB) is a recent addition to the list of potential ergogenic aids. This leucine derivative has been proposed to have an anabolic effect that facilitates recovery following intense resistance training. The mechanism by which HMB might work is yet to be determined, but leucine and the keto-analogue of leucine, ketoisocaproic acid, are recognized for their regulatory effects on protein balance during conditions of metabolic stress (burns, surgery, sepsis, and fasting). Additionally, Nissen and Abumrad[64] speculate that cholesterol synthesis is rate limiting during periods of rapid growth (i.e., exercise-induced muscle hypertrophy), and supplementation with HMB might promote production of βhydroxyβmethyl-glutaryl-CoA, which would support cholesterol synthesis.

At present, only two full reports of original research have been published on the effects of HMB as an anabolic agent. Nissen et al.'s lab reported a tendency for a dose-related effect of HMB ingestion on lean body mass accretion during a 7-week period of supplementation and resistance training in untrained individuals.[65] Lean body mass was assessed using the measurement of total body electrical conductivity, which has yet to receive complete validation as a reliable method for determining changes in body composition. Subjects receiving HMB as opposed to placebo had lower plasma concentrations of creatine kinase, a marker of mechanical trauma to skeletal muscle. Kreider et al.[66] failed to find a significant effect of HMB on markers of muscle damage, strength or body composition in resistance-trained athletes under-going a 28-day treatment. Preliminary reports also show mixed results for anabolic and ergogenic effects of HMB. In studies of elderly people, HMB treatments had positive effects of strength gain and increasing fat-free mass.[67,68] In contrast, HMB administration failed to produce effects different from the placebo treatment in intensely training collegiate athletes.[69] If this supplement gains media and marketing exposure, HMB will likely receive a more thorough examination of the accuracy of the claims for promoting muscle growth and recovery after exercise.

9.1.2.5 Creatine

Ingestion of 10 to 25 g of creatine per day for a 5- to 7-day period followed by a maintenance phase of 2 g per day has been investigated for the effects of increasing muscle concentration of creatine and phosphocreatine.[70,71] Elevation of phosphagens could translate into enhanced performance during intense, short-duration physical performance.[71,72] Performance studies suggested that an increase in maximal force generation as indicated by sprint speed, strength as measured by one repetition maximum, or total work or power output during a single exertion is inconsistent and more often not observed.[73,74,75,76,77,78,79,80,81,82,83,84,85] However, other research indicates that the rate of recovery time between repeated sprints or maximal efforts is accel-erated such that fatigue may be reduced in the later (e.g., fourth and fifth) efforts in the series.[84,86,87,88,89,90] This finding has implications for athletes who desire to enhance performance in sports training and competition in which intermittent repeated efforts at very high intensities are critical for success.

Consequent to creatine loading, it has been reported that the body mass may increase by approximately 1–2 kg after the short, 5-day loading phase.[78,86,87,91] Claims have been made that the weight gain is due to an increase in the lean body mass, with the implications that contractile protein mass has increased. However, the rapid gain in weight coupled with a transient reduction in the volume of urine excreted [70] is highly suggestive of water retention, presumably within the muscle cells. Increased body water after creatine loading has been determined using bioelectrical impedance spectroscopy, an imprecise method of estimating body fluid compartments.[92] Future research should possibly incorporate multicomponent methods of assessing body composition to determine whether changes in body composition with creatine supplementation are purely a result of modifications in hydration status or also an increase in contractile proteins. In the event that creatine loading does increase the hydration state, it would be most useful to confirm whether intramuscular fluid volume is increased, and if so, whether an increase above the normal hydration of 73% for the lean body mass[93] has an ergogenic or anabolic effect.

Anecdotal reports from the athletic field raise the question of whether creatine loading increases the risk to muscle of cramping, hamstring pulls, or strains.[94] A recent report indicates that the reduction in plasma volume associated with voluntary dehydration in weight-classification athletes may be magnified if the athletes are loading with creatine.[95] Previously, and unrelated to creatine supplementation, an experimentally induced reduction in plasma volume in athletes was associated with an increased rate of muscle fasciculations that may precede muscle cramps.[96] Clinical trials on the relationship between creatine use and muscle cramping are scarce. A preliminary study involving a small sample size revealed that, during heat stress and exercise-induced dehydration, three of seven athletes receiving creatine but blind to the treatment, experienced muscle cramping. In contrast, one out of nine in the placebo group experienced cramping,[97] Additional double-blind studies with adequate sample sizes are need to clarify whether a cause and effect relationship exists between creatine supplementation and muscle cramps.

There is concern that creatine ingestion could subject the kidney to a taxing nitrogenous load. For example, Vandenberghe et al.[99] reported an increase in urate excretion during the first 3 days of creatine loading in subjects. On a high-protein diet, the production of excess nitrogen induces renal hyperfiltration and hyperfusion, both of which may produce functional and structural degeneration of the nephron.[98] To test whether similar stress is apparent with creatine loading, renal function of five subjects was measured before and after supplementation.[100] The findings indicated that there was not an increase in protein excretion in the urine, nor was renal clearance altered. Although the authors concluded that the creatine loading did not stress the kidneys, it should be noted that the mean urinary excretion rate of total protein after loading was elevated by 50% (60.6 ± 12.3 micrograms/min) compared with 39.4 ± 12.3 micrograms/min for the placebo. The small sample size of five could limit the ability to detect effects of creatine on the kidney, and studies of longer periods of creatine exposure are required before a definitive conclusion can be drawn. The need for further research on adverse effects is urged after two recent case reports of renal dysfunction in otherwise healthy athletes who took loading dosages (about 25 g per day) of creatine for extended periods of time.[101,102] It should be noted that, in recent research, dosages of 10 g per day appeared to be an adequate dose to achieve an increase in the force of maximum voluntary contractions.[73] Lower dosages, if adhered to by the athlete, may reduce the risks of an adverse event.

It has yet to be determined whether the addition of creatine to sports drinks would enhance performance. The acid level of most sports drinks would promote the hydrolysis of creatine and reduce the dosage being delivered. In addition, because all of the research on creatine has allowed at least a 3-day period of loading, it is not clear whether an ergogenic effect of acute feedings would enhance performance that follows immediately (within an hour or two) the administration of creatine in a sports drink.

9.1.2.6 Carnitine

Carnitine is a nitrogenous, vitamin-like compound that is involved in the transport of long-chain fatty acids across the mitochondrial membrane for oxidation. Though some carnitine is obtained from dietary sources, most of the body's carnitine is produced by the liver and released into the bloodstream, where it is actively transported into the muscle.[19,103]

The theory behind carnitine supplementation is that increasing the dietary intake may facilitate fatty acid transport across the inner mitochondrial membrane and enhance the capacity to oxidize fat. To date, research has been unable to demonstrate either effect. Instead, the research shows that additional dietary carnitine does not elevate muscle carnitine concentrations.[104,105,106] Carnitine absorption and transport to the muscle appear to be a barrier, although the exact point of limitation has not been identified.[107,108] Lack of any change in muscle concentrations after loading may explain why exercise performance studies fail to show enhanced fat oxidation, a sparing of muscle glycogen or an ergogenic effect.[106,109,110]

9.1.3 FATS

Fats, primarily endogenous fats, are used as an energy substrate during physical exertion of low to moderately high intensity.[111,112,113] Acute feeding to supply additional lipid is thought to have minimal ergogenic effects on physical performance, and is known to slow gastric emptying due to the high energy density.[114,115] As such, and because of its low solubility in an aqueous solution, fat is generally not considered an appropriate substrate to add to a hydration beverage. Nevertheless, several lipid compounds have been considered as potential additives to sports drinks for reasons reviewed below.

9.1.3.1 Glycerol

As a fuel, glycerol is oxidized slowly. The effect of glycerol as a substrate or ergogen in exercise is minimal compared with the effects of glucose ingestion.[116] However, in an attempt to increase total body water, glycerol loading protocols have been used from 1 to 4 h prior to exercise[117,118] and have even extended over 2 days.[119] Orally ingested glycerol is evenly distributed in the total body water, excluding the central nervous system's fluids. Glycerol increases plasma osmolality and thereby reduces urine output, which causes fluid retention in the body. During exercise that follows glycerol loading, the data are equivocal regarding the effects of glycerol on core temperature, sweat rate, or heart rate.[118,120,121,122] One study suggests that glycerol loading may increase endurance,[118] with loading alone or pre-exercise loading plus the use of fluids with carbohydrate during the cycling. A more recent report, however, indicates that pre-loading with glycerol alone is of no greater benefit than consuming

TABLE 9.2
Summary of Protein Derivatives and Related Compounds Added to a Sports Drink

Derivative	Claim	Proposed Mechanism	Substantiation as an Additive
Intact protein	Enhanced muscle glycogen resynthesis	Protein ingested simultaneously with carbohydrate augments insulin action	One report of support, other studies show carbohydrate dose is critical factor. Effect of protein independent of additional energy needs clarification.
BCAA	Enhanced endurance	Alternate fuel for glycogen sparing	Majority of studies show no effect on endurance.
Glycine	Stimulate fluid absorption	Actively transported solute generates an osmotic pressure that draws fluid across intestinal membrane	Limited data; one study showed no increase in fluid absorption rate of a sports drink.
Glutamine	Boost immune function & accelerate glycogen recovery	Offset glutamine depletion during intense and prolonged training; enhance insulin action glycogen resynthesis	Few studies to date, most show no effect on immune system. Limited data on glycogen resynthesis. No studies on sports drinks.
Arginine	Accelerate recovery after exercise; inhibit protein breakdown during exercise	Precursor of nitric oxide, which regulates vasodilation and local blood flow; also proposed as a conditionally essential amino acid during metabolic stress that accelerates protein turnover	Few studies using arginine in a hydration beverage; data fail to show an effect on performance or recovery.
HMB	Enhance recovery after training	Stimulate rate limiting cholesterol synthesis; provide keto-analogue to spare leucine oxidation	Few studies to date with no clear consensus; no data to clarify mechanism.
Creatine	Enhanced power or sprint capacity	Elevate muscle creatine levels that accelerate recovery of phosphagen concentrations; stimulus for muscle hypertrophy	Loading for several days to elevate muscle level may enhance performance in intermittent anaerobic efforts; not tested for acute effects in a sports drink..
Carnitine	Enhance endurance	Promote intra-mitochondrial lipid transport and oxidation for glycogen sparing effect	Studies fail to show any ergogenic effects.

a carbohydrate-electrolyte beverage during exercise.[122] The lack of an ergogenic effect may be due to the observation that if subjects maintain hydration during exercise, pre-exercise hyperhydration with glycerol offers no added benefit to maintaining cardiovascular function or thermoregulatory responses during exercise.[120]

9.1.3.2   Medium Chain Triglycerides (MCTs)

MCTs have been viewed as a possible ergogen in hydration beverages for several reasons. It has been speculated that MCTs do not slow gastric emptying, that they are absorbed readily, and that they might be oxidized at rates similar to that of carbohydrate. Although the findings in one study suggest that MCTs did not slow gastric emptying,[123] the results should be viewed with caution. The control beverage was a carbohydrate (maltodextrin) solution containing nearly 18 grams per 100 milliliters (18%), which provides two to three times the carbohydrate of the standard sports drink. A high energy density alone could slow gastric emptying and obscure any effect of adding MCT. Maintaining a constant energy density at a lower level (about 240 kcal per liter corresponding to a carbohydrate content of 6 grams per 100 milliliters), we observed in a pilot study on one subject that solutions containing MCTs slowed gastric emptying (data unpublished). One fluid contained 6% carbohydrate, the other 3% carbohydrate and about 1.3% MCT. In the case of the fluid containing MCTs, about 30% of the ingested solution remained in the stomach after 2 h of cycling, whereas less than 8% of the initial volume of fluid remained in the stomach for the fluid containing only carbohydrate. A full-scale study is needed to confirm these results, but it appears that MCTs slow gastric emptying independent of the beverage energy content and more so than would the presence of carbohydrate alone. In agreement, several studies show that the contribution of exogenous MCT to energy metabolism during exercise is relatively small,[111,124,125] even when conditions are manipulated to maximize fat oxidation (i.e., subjects exercise with low muscle glycogen levels).[124] Low intestinal tolerance and rates of absorption are thought to be the limiting factors.[124]

9.1.3.3   Choline

Depletion of choline has been implicated as a cause of fatigue during prolonged physical exertion. Plasma choline levels were reported to decrease significantly between the beginning and end of a marathon in one descriptive study.[126] Subsequently, fluids that provide choline, the precursor of the neurotransmitter acetylcholine, have been examined in clinical trials for an ergogenic effect. The studies report that choline levels can be maintained or elevated by oral administration of choline[127] or lecithin,[128] a precursor of choline, prior to exercise. However, exercise time to fatigue and total work were not increased compared with the control trial.[127]

9.2   SELECTED MICRONUTRIENTS AND ELEMENTS

9.2.1   B Vitamins

Vitamins, particularly the B vitamins, play specific and important roles in the metabolism of carbohydrate, fat, and protein. Vitamins do not provide energy; rather they function as co-factors of enzymes to assist in the release of energy from substrate or in preparing the substrates to deliver energy in a usable form to the muscle. Some of the interest or concern has been driven by the notion that fluid losses during sweating increase the loss of the water-soluble vitamins, ascorbic acid, and the B

TABLE 9.3
Summary of Lipid Derivatives Added to a Sports Drink

Compound	Claim	Proposed Mechanism	Substantiation as an Additive
Glycerol	Elevate total body water to induce hyperhydration for enhanced endurance	Osmotic effect of glycerol decreases renal excretion of fluid for a net increase in total body water; may help maintain thermoregulation during exercise	Several studies demonstrate preloading benefit, but effect is no different than that of matching fluid intake during exercise
MCT	Alternate substrate	MCTs are absorbed and oxidized like a carbohydrate and may spare glycogen	Studies do not show an ergogenic effect; potential for GI distress is great
Choline	Enhance endurance	Precursor of neurotransmitter may become depleted and cause fatigue during prolonged exercise	Studies do not support an ergogenic effect; potential for GI distress exists.

vitamin complex, or that the high metabolic demands of athletes in intense training increase the vitamin requirements. However, available research indicates that sweat is not a significant route of loss of these vitamins,[129] nor can an enhancement in carbohydrate metabolism be demonstrated by supplementing an adequate diet with any of the B vitamins.[130]

Several experimental trials have been conducted to determine whether acute ingestion of water-soluble vitamins enhances performance or affects the metabolic response to exercise. Nicotinic acid, for example, has been tested for potential ergogenic effects. Administered in dosages well above the RDI, nicotinic acid stimulates vasodilatation and increases skin blood flow, which, in theory, might promote thermoregulatory capacity during exercise in the heat,[131] but could simultaneously decrease muscle blood flow. Such an effect could be detrimental to endurance performance. Additionally, dosages of nicotinic acid that inhibit lipid oxidation appeared to accelerate carbohydrate oxidation,[132,133,134] which can accelerate the depletion of muscle glycogen stores.[134] Plasma free fatty acids provide substrate for oxidization during moderately high intensities of exercise and contribute to the sparing of carbohydrate for use late in the performance.[135] The glycogen sparing effect, which may be lost with nicotinic acid loading,[136] is beneficial for sustaining performance.[136,133] Therefore, the potential benefits of enhanced heat dissipation must be weighed against the adverse metabolic effects in deciding whether a B vitamin such as nicotinic acid should be added in large dosages to a sports drink.

9.2.2 ANTIOXIDANT VITAMINS

One of the most intriguing issues for endurance athletes is whether supplementing dietary antioxidants reduces the risk of illness and accelerates the recovery time following intense training. Previously published reviews[137,138,139] provide more details of the antioxidants, but the potential role of vitamin E in the athlete will be briefly summarized here. High rates of energy metabolism or repetitive eccentric contractions that disrupt muscle integrity may increase the rate of formation of oxygen free radicals that promote lipid peroxidation and damage to skeletal muscle.[140,141] Meydani et al.[142] explored the effects of approximately 7 weeks of supplementation of vitamin E (800 IU/day) and found that exercise-induced lipid peroxidation was significantly decreased with the treatment. Supplementation increased muscle levels of the vitamin, but levels were reduced to normal (placebo levels) following stressful exercise. Vitamin E provided an alternative substrate for lipid peroxidation. The muscle loaded with vitamin had less of a decrease of fatty acid concentrations as a result of eccentric exercise (i.e., less lipid peroxidation) and the urinary excretion of thiobarbituric acid adducts (an index of oxidative damage) was reduced compared with the placebo group.

Further research is needed to confirm whether acute vitamin E supplementation is beneficial to the athlete's recovery, particularly if the athlete has adequate vitamin E stores initially. Additional research also needs to demonstrate that a water-soluble beverage such as a sports drink is an effective vehicle for delivering a fat-soluble nutrient in adequate dosages for absorption and elevation of the body's tissue stores.

9.2.3 CHROMIUM AND VANADIUM

Elements such as chromium and vanadium exert insulin-like action under certain conditions. By an as yet unexplained mechanism, these metals may interact with insulin to facilitate the transport of glucose from the blood across cell membranes. Chromium is recognized for its contribution to glucose tolerance and has been assigned an estimated safe and adequate daily dietary intake (ESADDI) of between 50 and 200 micrograms per day for adults.[143] The daily requirement for vanadium as a nutrient is speculative at this point, but the mineral appears to have insulin-like effects when added to the diet of animals with experimentally induced diabetes[144,145] and in clinical trials in patients with non-insulin-dependent diabetes.[146]

Promising effects of chromium supplementation have been reported to occur in populations that are glucose intolerant, in obese, non-insulin-dependent diabetics, and in those who clearly had a chronically inadequate daily intake of chromium.[147,148,149] In these populations, chronic chromium treatments have been observed to increase insulin action and improve glucose tolerance.[150,151,152] Because of the effect of chromium supplementation on insulin action, some have speculated that oral chromium treatments will stimulate lean body mass accretion via the anabolic effects of insulin.[153] Recent well-controlled studies on healthy subjects undergoing physical training have failed to demonstrate this effect.[154,155,156,157]

To date, only one report is available on the acute effect of chromium ingested in conjunction with a hydration beverage on carbohydrate uptake and oxidation and physical performance. Hertler-Colbert et al. employed an exercise protocol of high-intensity intermittent sprint efforts and failed to find a benefit of the addition of chromium to a beverage that provided carbohydrate to the subjects.[158] Ingestion of the sports beverages with carbohydrate enhanced sprinting capacity in the subjects compared with the effects of the placebo (water). Performance was not further enhanced when subjects received a 400-microgram dose of chromium picolinate along with the carbohydrate beverage. Lack of a chromium effect suggests that, in these subjects, the chromium-mediated transport of carbohydrate into the muscle is not a limiting factor in intermittent high-intensity performance.

9.2.4 OXYGENATED FLUIDS

Although published research on the effects of an oxygenated hydration beverage on physical performance is nonexistent, several products described as being super-oxygenated are available on the market. The products claim to help oxygenate the blood by delivering the gas through the intestinal tract. Research suggests that arterial desaturation occurs in some athletes and could contribute to fatigue,[159] but in comparison with the effects of local changes in acid-base status, glycogen availability or dehydration, inadequate oxygen delivery is seldom seen as a major cause of fatigue. Moreover, the effectiveness of intestinal absorption of oxygen to compensate for this potential source of fatigue is questionable. To date, no studies exist to test an effect of ingesting oxygenated fluids on oxygen saturation of the blood.

It is important to note that peroxides are formed when oxygen is dissolved under pressure in an aqueous solution. The level of peroxides is high enough to be detectable to the taste. Peroxides are pro-oxidants, so it is of some concern that individuals would ingest compounds that could potentially have damaging effects on the body's tissues. Vitamins and flavor agents in an oxygenated beverage would also be oxidized, thereby negatively influencing the palatability and nutrient content of a sports drink. In the event that an oxygenated beverage delivers on the claims and produces none of the hypothesized side effects, the actual oxygen content of beverage at the time of consumption is questionable if the beverage is packaged and stored in a gas-permeable container (e.g., plastic).

9.3 NON-NUTRITIVE INGREDIENTS

9.3.1 CAFFEINE

Ingestion of caffeine in dosages from 3 to 9 mg per kg body weight approximately 1 h prior to endurance exercise has been shown to increase the time to exhaustion.[160,161,162] Mechanisms proposed to explain the ergogenic effect include

- a stimulatory effect on the central nervous system (CNS)
- a stimulatory effect on skeletal muscle that results in high cyclic AMP levels or facilitation of regulatory enzymes
- a sparing effect on muscle glycogen via the mobilization of fatty acids from adipose tissue[103]

The majority of data support the glycogen sparing effect, although the findings are not consistent. An ergogenic effect of caffeine ingestion is not seen in studies involving short-duration, high-intensity efforts,[163,164,165] where muscle glycogen is not a limiting factor, but in which direct effects on the CNS or muscle contractility

TABLE 9.4
Summary of Vitamins, Minerals, and Elements Added to a Sports Drink

Compound	Claim	Proposed Mechanism	Substantiation as an Additive
B vitamins	Enhanced substrate oxidation	Mass action: higher intake of vitamins will saturate metabolic pathways involved in carbohydrate and lipid metabolism	Limited data fail to show an ergogenic effect; any effect unlikely due to low probability of developing a dietary deficiency
Antioxidants (AO)	Prevent muscle soreness, speed recovery post-exercise	AO absorb inflammation-promoting free radicals generated during intense exercise or eccentric contractions	Limited biochemical data to support an effect of chronic supplementation of vitamin E on lipid peroxidation; reduction in muscle soreness not observed.
Chromium	Improve carbohydrate metabolism; enhance lipid oxidation; stimulate muscle growth	Enhance anabolic actions of insulin and allow body to reduce insulin secretion	No effect in a sports drink; unlikely to affect carbohydrate metabolism in lean, fit athletes.
Oxygen	Enhance endurance	Elevate oxygen carrying capacity of the blood	No research to date.

could come into play. Although endurance time during prolonged exercise is reported to increase,[160,161,162] research has yet to be conducted to demonstrate a decrease in the time to complete a set distance, i.e., an improvement in race pace.

Addition of caffeine to a sports drink creates the potential for diuresis and a loss of fluids. Research on the recovery from exercise-induced dehydration indicates that nearly 50% of the fluid provided by a caffeinated beverage is lost as urine during a 2-h period following ingestion of 100% of fluid needs.[166] In contrast, approximately 35% of a similar volume of water containing no caffeine was excreted as urine during an identical recovery protocol.[166] In the euhydrated state, the addition of caffeine to a carbohydrate electrolyte beverage stimulated nearly 400 additional milliliters of urine excretion during a 3-h sedentary period than did the same beverage without caffeine.[167] During exercise, it appears that regulatory hormones override the influence of caffeine in an attempt to conserve body fluids.[167] However, if an ergogenic effect were to be attainable, caffeine must be consumed at least 1 h prior to the exercise performance. Hence, the athlete would need to consider the trade-off between the potential metabolic effects on performance and the diuresis and fluid loss before the event begins. In addition, the ingestion of caffeinated beverages during recovery from dehydration promotes the loss of specific minerals, including magnesium and calcium, in the urine and may create a negative balance of some electrolytes after exercise.[168]

Caffeine is cited as an agent that enhances mental focus and possibly cognitive function[169] and is a component in several of the commercially available energy drinks. The beneficial effects of caffeine on cognitive function are controversial and may in fact be due to the chronic, not acute, effects. Recent research suggests acute or habitual caffeine ingestion does not improve mental performance.[169] Possibly the beneficial effect on alertness and mental fatigue observed in some studies may in fact be due to the detrimental effect of caffeine withdrawal during the placebo-control trial rather than a true benefit of the caffeine.[169]

9.3.2 BICARBONATE BUFFERS

The effect of sodium salts of organic acids on anaerobic performance has been investigated in a number of studies. Loading with sodium bicarbonate or sodium citrate has been employed to minimize the decrease in pH that accompanies the accumulation of lactic acid during high-intensity exercise. The most promising findings are typically attained when the exercise protocol comprises a series of sprints with a short rest interval between sprints.[170,171] In theory, the facilitated efflux of hydrogen ions out of the skeletal muscle cells minimizes the proton accumulation that impairs enzyme activity[43,172,173] and cross-bridge formation between contractile proteins.[172,174]

A review of the literature shows that the loading protocols require a 60- to 90-min period between beverage consumption and the exercise for absorption and equilibration of the buffer.[170] Research has not examined the effect of ingesting buffers in a beverage during exercise, in contrast to the protocols of oral loading 60 min before, exercise. Any metabolic benefit would need to be weighed against the negatives of gastrointestinal distress, which has been reported as a side effect of bicarbonate loading.[175,176] Ingesting a dosage of 0.3 g per kg body weight of sodium bicarbonate would deliver almost 6 g of sodium to a 70-kg person. Depending on the volume of fluid that accompanies the sodium load, the sodium concentration entering the intestinal tract could range from 125 to 500 mmol/l, a load that will elevate solution osmolality in the intestinal lumen and could compromise intestinal absorption of fluids[50,177] and promote intestinal distress.

9.3.3 HERBS

The consumer market for dietary supplements used by athlete and fitness enthusiasts has been flooded in recent years with new products, and the industry as a whole has grown dramatically. The driving force for growth is likely to be confusion in the consumer's mind. The perception has been that research and science have recently uncovered herbal compounds and ingredients that provide all the ergogenic and body-building claims made for these products. In fact, little research exists to support most of the claims. Rather, a change in the law that regulates herbals and dietary supplements has unleashed the sales of these products and compounds. Examples of energy drinks and new-age beverages that contain herbs are presented in Table 9.5. The Dietary Supplement and Health Education Act (DSHEA), enacted in 1994 by the U.S. government, deregulated the marketing claims and sales by putting the responsibility on the Food and Drug Administration (FDA) to disprove the claims. Prior to DSHEA, the onus was on the dietary supplement companies to prove their claims by having scientific studies showing evidence of the effect.

TABLE 9.5
Energy Beverages that Contain Herbs

Beverage	Ginseng	Ginko Biloba	Ciwujia	Kava Kava	St. John's Wort	Chamomile
Triumph!	√					
Golf Pro	√	√				
Endurox™			√			
Hansen's	√			√	√	√

9.3.3.1   Ginseng

This herb originates from the dried root of the Araliaceous plant and is purported to enhance endurance capacity and to increase peak oxygen uptake. The mechanism proposed to explain the effect is a stimulatory action of the herb or a metabolite of the herb.

Many anecdotal reports from Asia, where the herb is most popular, provide testimony to an ergogenic effect, but well-designed, well-controlled clinical trials indicate that peak oxygen consumption and endurance at a submaximal workload are not increased.[178,179,180] Because of the risk of side effects such as insomnia, diarrhea, hypertension, agitation, nervousness, and euphoria, and the lack of a clear ergogenic effect in objective studies, addition of ginseng to a hydration beverage is not recommended.

9.3.3.2   Ciwujia

The claims for this herb include enhanced endurance and reduced lactate accumulation because of a decrease in production or an increased metabolism. Limited data from well-controlled clinical trials are available. In two fairly recent reports, ciwujia did not alter metabolism in such a way as to provide a physiological rationale for enhanced performance. The two independent studies[181,182] involved a minimum of 7 days of supplementation with 800 mg of a product (Endurox™) that contained ciwujia. Researchers reported that the metabolic responses at rest and during various intensities of exercise were unchanged, including plasma lactate concentrations, oxygen consumption, and fat and carbohydrate oxidation, as well as heart rate and ventilatory responses. An absence of a change in serum concentrations of glycerol, reported in one study,[182] suggest that ciwujia is ineffective in mobilizing free fatty acids for use as a substrate during submaximal exercise (25% or 65% of peak oxygen uptake).

9.3.3.3   Ginkgo Biloba

Based on positive effects of this herb on cognitive function in patients with early dementia,[183] ginkgo biloba supplements have been marketed to the general population for the same benefits. This may be appealing to the athlete and coach involved in sports where decision making and hand-eye coordination are critical to success. Golf is an example of such a sport, and it is little surprise that a hydration beverage containing ginkgo biloba has been designed for this event (Table 9.5). Studies do not exist to support an enhanced cognitive function as a result of ingesting ginkgo biloba before or during physical efforts of any intensity. Caution is urged for anyone using products with ginkgo because of several case reports of spontaneous bleeding associated with its use in otherwise healthy individuals.[184,185] Ginkgo inhibits the platelet activating factor and increases bleeding time.[186] Such an anticoagulant effect may be magnified with concomitant intake of aspirin, phenolic compounds from red wine, vitamin E, or with routine exercise training, all of which may be a part of the athlete's lifestyle and training program.

9.3.3.4 Hydroxycitric Acid (HCA)

This derivative from the plants *Garcinia cambogia* and *Garcinia indica* may be a competitive inhibitor of the extramitochondrial enzyme ATP-citrate (pro-3S)-lyase. Research using animal models shows that HCA may inhibit the action of the citrate cleavage enzyme, which would uncouple the transfer of energy to ATP.[187] This inhibition might promote a negative energy balance that would contribute to reducing fat mass and assist with body weight control. In animals, HCA may also decrease *de novo* fat synthesis,[188] decrease energy intake,[189] and suppress the rate of weight gain in animals.[190]

Some have speculated that HCA ingestion could enhance endurance and reduce body fat content of athletes.[191] At present, no studies exist to support such effects in healthy fit humans. One clinical trial has examined the effects of HCA supplementation in a group of obese subjects concurrently undergoing a hypoenergetic diet treatment.[192] The researchers found that after 12 weeks of treatment, the patients receiving HCA had no greater reduction in body weight or body fat than did those subjects taking a placebo and maintaining a similar hypoenergetic diet.[192] The study did not include lean athletic subjects nor did it examine the interactive effects of HCA supplementation and exercise. However, obese subjects undergoing energy restriction would presumably be the ideal sample for detecting an effect of HCA, if one existed.

9.4 SUMMARY

A vast array of hydration beverages is available and marketed to the physically active consumer and competitive athlete. Many products have diverged from providing the traditional nutrients of water, carbohydrate, and electrolytes. In general, novel ingredients, or nutraceutical compounds, have been added with little scientific documentation to justify the claims of ergogenicity, enhanced hydration, immune system booster, or anabolism — to list a few. As investigations continue, perhaps some of these unique compounds will be confirmed as efficacious and will gain support of the sport science research community. As discussed elsewhere within this text, the research is fairly clear on what constitutes a sports drink and is required to achieve the primary functions of fluid and energy delivery during exercise. Future studies will help delineate which novel ingredients might be appropriate as functional

TABLE 9.6
Summary of Non-Nutrient Ingredients Added to a Sports Drink

Ingredient	Claim	Proposed Mechanism	Substantiation as an Additive
Caffeine	Enhanced endurance	Mobilizes fatty acids and promotes glycogen sparing; possibly a direct effect on CNS or muscle contractility	Pre-exercise ingestion of caffeine alone may spare glycogen.
Bicarbonate buffers	Enhance sprint capacity	Accelerate the efflux of lactate and H^+ from muscle cell to maintain acid-base balance	Pre-exercise ingestion may enhance sprinting under laboratory conditions; potential for GI distress is significant.
Ginseng	Enhance endurance	Stimulatory effect similar to that of caffeine	No sports drink studies; studies of effect of several days of loading fail to show ergogenicity.
Ciwujia	Speed recovery; enhance lipid oxidation	Not clear, possibly via stimulatory effect similar to caffeine	Two studies to date show no effect.
Ginkgo biloba	Promote cognitive function	Improve blood flow to the brain	No studies on sports drinks or cognitive function during exercise.
Hydroxy-citric acid	Enhance endurance, reduce body fat	Enhance lipid oxidation and elevate resting metabolic rate	No studies using sports drinks or in athletes; limited clinical data suggest no effect.

additives in other beverages including pre-athletic-event beverages, post-training recovery fluids, or as part of the general diet and training table of the athlete.

REFERENCES

1. Dubois, C., Armand, M., Senft, M., Portugal, H., Pauli, A-M, Bernard, P-M, Lafont, H., and Lairon, D., Chronic oat bran intake alters postprandial lipemia and lipoproteins in healthy adults., *Am. J. Clinic. Nutr.,* 61, 325, 1995.
2. Wolk, A., Manson, J. E., Stampfer, M. J., Colditz, G. A., Hu, F. B., Speizer, F. E., Hennekens, C. H., and Willet, W. C., Long-term intake of dietary fiber and decreased risk of coronary heart disease among women., *JAMA,* 281, 1998, 1999.
3. Cummings, J. H., Bingham, S. A., Heaton, K. W., and Eastwood, M. A, Fecal weight, colon cancer risk, and dietary intake of nonstarch polysaccharides., *Gastroenterology,* 103, 1783, 1999.
4. Kirwan, J. P., O'Gorman, D., and Evans, W. J., A moderate glycemic meal before endurance exercise can enhance performance., *J. Appl. Physiol.,* 84, 53, 1998.

5. Thomas, D. E., Brotherhood, J. R., and Brand, J. C., Carbohydrate feeding before exercise: effect of glycemic index., *Int. J. Sports Med.,* 12, 180, 1999.

6. MacLaren, D. P. M., Reilly, T., Campbell, I. T., and Frayn, K. N., Hormonal and metabolite responses to glucose and maltodextrin ingestion with and without the addition of guar gum., *Int. J. Sports Med.,* 15, 466, 1994.

7. Parcell, A. C., Ray, M. L., Moss, K. A., Ruden, T. M., Sharp, R. L., and King, D. S., The effect of encapsulated soluble fiber on carbohydrate metabolism during exercise., *Int. J. Sports Nutr.,* 9, 13, 1999.

8. Rehrer, N. J., van Kemenade, M., Meester, W., Brouns, F., and Saris, W. H. M., Gastrointestinal complaints in relation to dietary intake in triathletes, *Int. J. Sports Nutr.,* 2, 48, 1992.

9. Stanko, R. T., Robertson, R. J., Spina, R. J., Reilly, J. J., Greenawalt, K. D., and Goss, F. L., Enhancement of arm exercise endurance capacity with dihydroxyacetone and pyruvate, *J. Appl. Physiol.,* 68, 119, 1990.

10. Stanko, R. T., Robertson, R. J., Galbreath, R. W., Reilly, J. J., Greenawalt, K. D., and Goss, F. L., Enhanced leg exercise endurance with a high-carbohydrate diet and dihydroxyacetone and pyruvate, *J. Appl. Physiol.,* 69, 1651, 1990.

11. Stone, M. H., Sanborn, K., Smith, L. L., O'Bryant, H. S., Hoke, T., Utter, A. C., Johnson, R. L., Boros, R., Hruby, J., Pierce, K. C., Stone, M. E., and Garner, B., Effects of in-season (5 weeks) creatine and pyruvate supplementation on anaerobic performance and body composition in American football players, *Int. J. Sports Nutr.,* 9, 146, 1999.

12. Sukala, W. R., Pyruvate: beyond the marketing hype, *Int. J. Sports Nutr.,* 8, 241, 1998.

13. Mazzeo, R. S., Brooks, G. A., Schoeller, D. A., and Budinger, T. F., Disposal of blood [1-13C] lactate in humans during rest and exercise, *J. Appl. Physiol.,* 60, 232, 1986.

14. Stanley, W. C., Wisneski, J. A., Gertz, E. W., Neese, R. A., and Brooks, G. A., Glucose and lactate interrelations during moderate intensity exercise in humans, *Metabolism,* 37, 850, 1988.

15. Brooks, G.A. and Donovan, C. M., Effect of endurance training on glucose kinetics during exercise, *Am. J. Physiol.,* 244, E505, 1983.

16. Swensen, T., Crater, G., Bassett, D. R., and Howley, E. T., Adding polylactate to a glucose polymer solution does not improve endurance, *Int. J. Sports Med.,* 15, 430, 1994.

17. Fahey, T. D., Larsen, J. D., Brooks, G A., Henderson, S., and Lary, D., The effects of ingesting polylactate or glucose polymer drinks during prolonged exercise, *Int. J. Sports Nutr.,* 1, 249, 1999.

18. Wilmore, J. H. and Costill, D. L. *Training for Sport and Activity,* Wm C. Brown Publishers, Dubuque, 1988, 1.

19. Wagenmakers, A. J. M., Nutritional supplements: Effects on exercise performance and metabolism, in *Perspectives in Exercise Science and Sports Medicine,* Lamb, D. R. and Murray, R., Eds., Cooper Publishing Group, Carmel, IN 1999, 207.

20. Colombani, P. C., Kovacs, E., Frey-Rindova, P., Frey, W., Langhans, W., Arnold, M., and Wenk, C., Metabolic effects of a protein-supplemented carbohydrate drink in marathon runners, *Int. J. Sports Nutr.,* 9, 181, 1999.

21. Zawadzki, K. M., Yaspelkis, B. B, and Ivy, J. L., Carbohydrate-protein complex increases the rate of muscle glycogen storage after exercise, *J. Appl. Physiol.,* 72, 1854, 1992.

22. Pederson, R. A., Schubert, H. E., and Brown, J. C., Gastric inhibitory polypeptide. Its physiologic release and insulinotropic action in the dog., *Diabetes,* 24, 1050, 1975.

23. Nuttall, F. Q. and Gannon, M. C., Plasma glucose and insulin response to macronutrients in nondiabetic and NIDDM subjects, *Diabetes Care,* 14, 824, 1991.

24. Roy, B. D., Tarnopolsky, M. A., MacDougall, J. D., Fowles, J., and Yarasheski, K. E., Effect of glucose supplement timing on protein metabolism after resistance training, *J. Appl. Physiol.,* 82, 1882, 1997.

25. Burke, L. M., Collier, G. R., Beasely, S. K., Davis, P. G., Fricker, P. A., Heeley, P., Walder, K., and Hargreaves, M., Effect of coingestion of fat and protein with carbohydrate feedings on muscle glycogen storage, *J. Appl. Physiol.,* 78, 2187, 1995.

26. van Loon, L. J. C., Saris, W. H. M., and Kruijshoop, M., Maximizing post exercise glycogen synthesis: carbohydrate supplementation and the application of amino acid or protein hydrolysate mixtures, *Am. J. Clin. Nutr.,* 72, 106, 2000.

27. Carrithers, J.A., Williamson, D.L., Gallagher, P.M., Godard, M.P., Schulze, K.E., and Trappe, S.W., Effects of post exercise carbohydate-protein feedings on muscle glycogen restoration, *J. Appl. Physiol.,* 88, 1976, 2000.

28. Davis, J. M., Carbohydrates, branched chain amino-acids,and endurance: the central fatigue hypothesis, *Int. J. Sports Nutr.,* 5, S29, 1995.

29. Wolfe, R. R., Goodenough, .D., Wolfe, M.H., Royle, G.T. and Nadel, E.R., Isotopic analysis of leucine and urea metabolism in exercising humans., *J. Appl. Physiol.,* 52, 458, 1982.

30. van Hall, G., MacLean, D. A., Saltin, B., and Wagenmakers, A. J. M., Mechanisms of activation of muscle branched-chain alpha-keto acid dehydrogenase during exercise in man., *J. Physiol.,* 494, 899, 1996.

31. Blomstrand, E., Hassmen, P., Ekblom, B., and Newsholme, E. A., Administration of branched-chain amino acids during sustained exercise: effects on performance and on plasma concentrations some amino acids., *Eur. J. Appl. Physiol.,* 63, 83, 1991.

32. Newsholme, E. A., Acworth, I. N., and Blomstrand, B., Amino acids, brain neurotransmitters and a functional link between muscle and brain that is important in sustained exercise., in *Advances in Myochemistry,* Benzi, G., John Libbey Eurotext, London 1987, 127.

33. Hargreaves, K. M. and Pardridge, W. M., Neutral amino acid transport at the human blood-brain barrier, *J. Biol. Chem.,* 263, 440, 1988.

34. Blomstrand, E., Andersson, S., Hassmen, P., Ekblom, B., and Newsholme, E. A., Effect of branched-chain amino acid and carbohydrate supplementation on the exercise-induced change in plasma and muscle concentrations of amino acids in human subjects., *Acta Physiol. Scand.,* 153, 87, 1999.

35. van Hall, G., Raaymakers, J. S. H., Saris, W. H. M., and Wagenmakers, A. J. M., Ingestion of branched-chain amino acids and tryptophan during sustained exercise in man: failure to affect performance., *J. Physiol.,* 486, 789, 1995.

36. Varnier, M., Sarto, P., Martines, D., Lora, L., Carmignoto, F., Leese, G. P., and Naccarato, R., Effect of infusing branched-chain amino acid during incremental exercise with reduced muscle glycogen content., *Eur. J. Appl. Physiol.,* 69, 26, 1994.

37. Davis, J. M., Welsh, R. S., DeVolve, K. L., and Alderson, N. A., Effects of branched-chain amino acids and carbohydrate on fatigue during intermittent, high-intensity running., *Int. J. Sports Med.,* 20, 309, 1999.

38. Madsen, K., MacLean, D. A., Kiens, B., and Christensen, D., Effects of glucose, glucose plus branched-chain amino acids or placebo on bike performance over 100 km., *J. Appl. Physiol.,* 81, 2644, 1996.

39. Mittleman, K. D., Ricci, M. R., and Bailey, S. P., Branched-chain amino acids prolong exercise during heat stress in men and women., *Med. Sci. Sports Exerc.,* 30, 83, 1998.

40. MacLean, D. A. and Graham, T. E., Branched-chain amino acid supplementation augments plasma ammonia responses during exercise in humans, *J. Appl. Physiol.*, 74, 2711, 1999.
41. Jones, N. L., Sutton, J. R., Taylor, R., and Toews, C. J., Effect of the pH on cardio-respiratory and metabolic responses to exercise, *J. Appl. Physiol.*, 43, 959, 1977.
42. Kowalchuk, J. M., Heigenhauser, G. J. F., and Jones, N. L., Effects of pH on metabolic and cardiorespiratory responses during progressive exercise, *J. Appl. Physiol.*, 57, 1558, 1984.
43. Sutton, J. R., Jones, N. C., and Toews, C. J., Effect of pH on muscle glycolysis during exercise, *Clinical Science,* 61, 331, 1981.
44. Bannister, E. W. and Cameron, B. J. C., Exercise-induced hyperammonemia: Peripheral and central effects., *Int. J. Sports Med.,* 11, S129, 1990.
45. Desjeux, J. F., Nath, S. K., and Taminiau, J., Organic substrate and electrolyte solutions for oral rehydration in diarrhea, *Ann. Rev. Nutr.,* 14, 321, 1994.
46. Vesikari, T. and Isolauri, E., Glycine supplemented oral rehydration solutions for diarrhoea, *Arch. Dis. Child.,* 61, 372, 1986.
47. Desjeux, J-F., Tannenbaum, C., Tai, Y-H., and Curran, P. F., Effects of sugars and amino acids on sodium movement across small intestine, *Am. J. Dis. Child.,* 131, 331, 1977.
48. Nalin, D. R., Cash, R. A., Rahman, M., and Yunus, MD., Effect of glycine and glucose on sodium and water absorption in patients with cholera, *Gut,* 11, 768, 1970.
49. Santosham, M., Burns, B. A., Reid, R., Letson, G. W., Duncan, B., Powlesland, J. A., Foster, S., Garrett, S., Croll, L., Wai, N. N., Marshall, W. N., Almeido-Hill, J., and Sack, R. B., Glycine-based oral rehydration solution: reassessment of safety and efficacy, *J. Pediatr.,* 109, 795, 1986.
50. Shi, X., Summers, R. W., Schedl, H. P., Flanagan, S. W., Chang, R., and Gisolfi, C. V., Effects of carbohydration type and concentration and solution osmolality on water absorption, *Med. Sci. Sports Exerc.,* 27, 1607, 1995.
51. Walsh, N. P., Blannin, A. K., Robson, P. J., and Gleeson, M., Glutamine, exercise and immune function: Links and possible mechanisms, *Sports Med.,* 26, 171, 1998.
52. Calder, P. C., Fuel utilization by cells of the immune systems, *Proc. Nutr. Soc.,* 54, 65, 1995.
53. Ardawi, M. S. M. and Newsholme, E. A., Glutamine metabolism in lymphoid tissues, in *Glutamine Metabolism in Mammalian Tissues*, Haussinger, D. and Sies, H., Springer-Verlag, Berlin 1984, 235.
54. Wallace, C. and Keast, D., Glutamine and macrophage function, *Metabolism,* 41, 1016, 1992.
55. Rohde, T., Krzywkowski, K., and Pedersen, B. K., Glutamine, exercise and the immune system — Is there a link?, *Exerc. Immunol. Rev.,* 4, 49, 1998.
56. Castell, L. M., Poortmans, J. R., and Newsholme, E. A., Does glutamine have a role in reducing infections in athletes? *Eur. J. Appl. Physiol.,* 73, 488, 1996.
57. Doble, A., The role of excitotoxicity in neurodegenerative disease: implications for therapy, *Pharmacol. Therap.,* 81, 163, 1999.
58. Varnier, M., Leese, G. P., Thompson, J., and Rennie, M. J., Stimulatory effect of glutamine on glycogen accumulation in human skeletal muscle, *Am. J. Physiol.,* 269, E309, 1995.
59. Bowtell, J. L., Gelly, K., Jackman, M. L., Patel, A., and Rennie, M. J., Oral glutamine stimulates whole body carbohydrate storage during recovery from exhaustive exercise, *FASEB J.* 11, A9, 1997 (Abstract.)

60. Bruce, M., Bowtell, J. L., and Williams, C., Effect of oral glutamine and glucose-polymer supplementation on recovery from exercise, *Eur. Coll. Sports Sci. Abstr.* 4, 48, 1999, (Abstract).

61. Chowienczyk, P. and Ritter, J., Arginine: No more than a simple amino acid? *Lancet,* 350, 901, 1997.

62. Yaspelkis, B. B and Ivy, J. L., The effect of a carbohydrate-arginine supplement on postexercise carbohydrate metabolism, *Int. J. Sports Nutr.,* 9, 241, 1999.

63. Buchman, A. L., O'Brien, W., Ou, C. N., Rognerud, C., Alvarez, M., Dennis, K., and Ahn, C., The effect of arginine or glycine supplementation on gastrointestinal function, muscle injury, serum amino acid concentrations and performance during a marathon run., *Int. J. Sports Nutr.,* 20, 315, 1999.

64. Nissen, S. L. and Abumrad, N. N., Nutritional role of leucine metabolite β-hydroxy β-methylbutyrate (HMB), *J. Nutr. Biochem.,* 8, 300, 1997.

65. Nissen, S., Sharp, R., Ray, M., Rathmacher, J. A., Rice, D., Fuller, J. C., Connelly, A. S., and Abumrad, N., Effect of leucine metabolite β-hydroxy-β-methlbutyrate on muscle metabolism during resistance-exercise training., *J. Appl. Physiol.,* 81, 2095, 1996.

66. Kreider, R. B., Ferreira, M., Wilson, M., and Almada, A. L., Effects of calcium bet-hydroxy-beta-methylbuturate (HMB) supplementation during resistance-training on markers of catabolism, body composition and strength, *Int. J. Sports Med.,* 20, 503, 1999.

67. Nissen, S., Panton, L., Fuller, J., Rice, D., Ray, M., and Sharp, R., Effect of feeding β-hydroxy-β-methylbutyrate (HMB) on body composition and strength changes of women., *FASEB J.* 11, A150, 1997, (Abstract).

68. Vukovich, M. D., Stubbs, N. B., Bohlken, R. M., Desch, M. F., Fuller, J. C., and Rathmacher, J. A., The effect of dietary β-hydroxy-β-methylbutyrate (HMB) on strength gains and body composition changes in older adults, *FASEB J.* 11, A376, 1997, (Abstract.)

69. Kreider, R., Ferreira, M., and Wilson, M., Effects of calcium B-HMB supplementation with and without creatine during training on body composition alterations., *FASEB J.* 11, A374, 1997, (Abstract).

70. Hultman, E., Soderlund, K., Timmons, J. A., Cederblad, G., and Greenhaff, P. L., Muscle creatine loading in men, *J. Appl. Physiol.,* 81, 232, 1996.

71. Harris, R., Soderlund, K., and Hultman, E., Elevation of creatine in resting and exercise muscle of normal subjects by creatine supplementation, *Clinic. Sci.,* 83, 367, 1992.

72. Williams, C., Macronutrients and performance, *J. Sports Sci.,* 13, S1, 1995.

73. Maganaris, C. N. and Maughan, R. J., Creatine supplementation enhances maximum voluntary isometric force and endurance capacity in resistance trained men, *Acta Physiol. Scand.,* 163, 279, 1998.

74. Odland, L. M., MacDougall, J. D., Tarnopolsky, M. A., Elorriaga, A., and Borgmann, A., Effects of oral creatine supplementation on muscle [PCr] and short-term maximum power output., *Med. Sci. Sports Exerc.,* 29, 216, 1997.

75. Burke, L. M., Pyne, D. B., and Telford, R. D., Effect of oral creatine supplementation on single-effort sprint performance in elite swimmers, *Int. J. Sports Nutr.,* 6, 222, 1996.

76. Rossiter, H. B., Cannell, E. R., and Jakeman, P. M., The effect of oral creatine supplementation on the 1000-m performance of competitive rowers, *J. Sports Sci.,* 14, 175, 1996.

77. Redondo, D. R., Dowling, E. A., Graham, B. L., Almada, A. L., and Williams, M. H., The effect of oral creatine monoydrate supplementation on running velocity, *Int. J. Sports Nutr.,* 6, 213, 1999.

78. Mujika, I., Chatard, J. C., Lacoste, L., Barale, F., and Geyssant, A., Creatine supplementation does not improve sprint performance in competitive swimmers, *Med. Sci. Sports Exerc.,* 28, 1435, 1996.

79. Terrillion, K. A., Kolkhorst, F. W., Dolgener, F. A., and Joslyn, S. J., The effect of creatine supplementation on two 700-m maximal running bouts, *Int. J. Sports Nutr.,* 7, 138, 1999.

80. Barnett, C., Hinds, M., and Jenkins, D. G., Effects of oral creatine supplementation on multiple sprint cycle performance, *Austr. J. Sci. and Med. in Sport,* 28, 35, 1996.

81. Cooke, W. H., Grandjean, P. W., and Barnes, W. S., Effect of oral creatine supplementation on power output and fatigue during bicycle ergometry, *J. Appl. Physiol.,* 78, 670, 1995.

82. Cooke, W. H. and Barnes, W. S., The influence of recovery duration on high-intensity exercise performance after oral creatine supplemenation, *Can. J. Appl. Physiol.,* 22, 454, 1997.

83. Snow, R. J., McKenna, M. J., Selig, S. E., Kemp, J., Stathis, C. G., and Zhao, Z., Effect of creatine supplementation on sprint exercise performance and muscle metabolism, *J. Appl. Physiol.,* 84, 1667, 1998.

84. Peyrebrune, M. C., Nevill, M. E., Donaldson, F. J., and Cosford, D. J., The effects of oral creatine supplementation on performance in single and repeated sprint swimming, *J. Sports Sci.,* 16, 271, 1998.

85. Javierre, C., Lizarraga, M. A., Ventura, L. L., Garrido, E., and Segura, R., Creatine supplementation does not improve physical performance in a 150 m race., *J. Physiol. Biochem.,* 53, 343, 1997.

86. Balsom, P. D., Ekblom, B., Soderlund, K., and Hultman, E., Creatine supplementation and dynamic high-intensity intermittent exercise, *Scand. J. Med. and Sci. in Sports,* 3, 143, 1993.

87. Balsom, P. D., Soderlund, K., Sjodin, B., and Ekblom, B., Skeletal muscle metabolism during short-duration high-intensity exercise: influence of creatine supplementation., *Acta Physiol. Scand.,* 154, 303, 1995.

88. Birch, R., Noble, D., and Greenhaff, P. L., The influence of dietary creatine supplemenation on performance during repeated bouts of maxmimal isokinetic cycling in man, *Eur. J. Appl. Physiol.,* 69, 268, 1994.

89. Earnest, C. P., Snell, P. G., Rodriguez, R., Almada, A. L., and Mitchell, T. L., The effect of creatine monohydrate ingestion on anaerobic power indices, muscular strength and body composition, *Acta Physiol. Scand.,* 153, 207, 1995.

90. Greenhaff, P. L., Casey, A., Short, A. H., Harris, R., Soderlund, K., and Hultman, E., Influence of oral creatine supplementation of muscle torque during repeated bouts of maxmimal voluntary exercise in man, *Clinic. Sci.,* 84, 565, 1998.

91. Balsom, P. D., Harridge, S. D. R., Soderlund, K., Sjodin, B., and Ekblom, B., Creatine supplemenation per se does not enhance endurance exercise performance, *Acta Physiol. Scand.,* 149, 521, 1993.

92. Ziegenfuss, T. N., Lemon, P. W. R., Rogers, M. R., Ross, R., and Yarasheski, K. E., Acute creatine ingestion: effects on muscle volume, anaerobic power, fluid volumes, and protein turnover, *Med. Sci. Sports Exerc.* 29, S127, 1997 (Abstract)

93. Moore, F. D. and Boyden, C. M., Body call mass and limits of hydration of the fat-free body: their relation to estimated skeletal weight, *Ann. NY Acad. Sci.,* 110, 62, 1963.

94. Huggins, S. Energy supplement stirs debate, *NCAA News*, 33, 1996.
95. Oopik, V., Paasuke, M., Timpmann, S., Medijainen, L., Ereline, J., and Smirnova, T., Effect of creatine supplementation during rapid body mass reduction on metabolism and isokinetic muscle performance capacity, *Eur. J. Appl. Physiol.*, 78, 83, 1998.
96. Caldwell, J. E., Ahonen, E., and Nousiainen, U., Diuretic therapy, physical performance, and neuromuscular function, *Phys. Sportsmed.*, 12, 73, 1984.
97. Webster, M. J., Vogel, R. A., Erdmann, L. D., and Clark, R. D., Creatine supplementation: effect on exercise performance at two levels of acute dehydration, *Med. Sci. Sports Exerc.*, 31, S265, 1999 (Abstract)
98. Klahr, S., Levey, A., Beck, G., Caggiula, A., Hunsiker, L., Kusek, J., and Striker, G., The effects of dietary protein restriction and blood-pressure control on the progression of chronic renal disease, *New Eng. J. Med.*, 330, 877, 1994.
99. Vandenberghe, K., Goris, M., Van Hecke, P., Van Leemputte, M., Vangerven, L., and Hespel, P., Long-term creatine intake is beneficial to muscle performance during resistance training, *J. Appl. Physiol.*, 83, 2055, 1997.
100. Poortmans, J. R., Auquier, H., Renaut, V., Durussek, A., Saugy, M., and Brisson, G. R., Effect of short-term creatine supplementation on renal responses in men, *Eur. J. Appl. Physiol.*, 76, 566, 1997.
101. Pritchard, N. R. and Kalra, P. A., Renal dysfunction accompanying oral creatine supplements, *Lancet*, 351, 1252, 1998.
102. Koshy, K. M., Griswold, E., and Schneeberger, E. E., Interstitial nephritis in a patient taking creatine, *New Eng. J. Med.*, 340, 814, 1999.
103. Spriet, L. L., Ergogenic aids: recent advances and retreats, in *Perspectives in Exercise Science and Sports Medicine*, Lamb, D. R. and Murray, R., Cooper Publishing Group, Carmel, IN 1997, 185.
104. Lennon, D. F. L., Shrago, E. R., Madden, M., Nagle, F. J., and Hanson, P., Dietary carnitine intake related to skeletal muscle and plasma carnitine concentrations in adult men and women, *Am. J. Clinic. Nutr.*, 43, 234, 1999.
105. Barnett, C., Costill, D. L., Vukovich, M. D., Cole, K. J., Goodpaster, B. H., Trappe, S. W., and Fink, W. J., Effect of L-carnitine supplementation on muscle and blood carnitine content and lactate accumulation during high-intensity sprint cycling, *Int. J. Sports Nutr.*, 4, 280, 1994.
106. Vukovich, M. D., Costill, D. L., and Fink, W. J., Carnitine supplementation: effect on muscle carnitine and glycogen content during exercise, *Med. Sci. Sports Exerc.*, 26, 1122, 1994.
107. Harper, P., Elwin, C. E., and Cederblad, G., Pharmacokinetics of intravenous and oral bolus doses of L-carnitine in healthy subjects, *Eur. J. Clinic. Pharm.*, 35, 555, 1988.
108. Rebouche, C. J., Metabolic fate of dietary carnitine in human adults, *J. Nutr.*, 121, 539, 1991.
109. Oyono-Enguelle, S., Freund, H., Ott, C., Gartner, M., Heitz, A., Marbach, J., Maccari, F., Frey, A., Bigot, H., and Bach, A. C., Prolonged submaximal exercise and L-carnitine in humans, *Eur. J. Appl. Physiol.*, 58, 53, 1988.
110. Colombani, P., Wenk, C., Kunz, I., Krahenbuhl, S., Kuhnt, M., Arnold, M., Frey-Rindova, , P., Frey, W., and Langhans, W., Effects of L-carnitine supplementation on physical performance and energy metabolism of endurance-trained athletes: a double-blind crossover field study, *Eur. J. Appl. Physiol.*, 73, 434, 1996.
111. Decombaz, J., Arnaud, M. J., Milon, H., Moesch, H., Philippossian, G., Thelin, A. L., and Howald, H., Energy metabolism of medium-chain triglycerides vs. carbohydrates during exercise, *Eur. J. Appl. Physiol.*, 52, 9, 1983.

112. Satabin, P., Portero, P., Defer, G., Bricout, J., and Guezennec, C. Y., Metabolic and hormonal responses to lipid and carbohydrate diets during exercise in man, *Med. Sci. Sports Exerc.,* 19, 218, 1987.

113. Peronnet, F., Adopo, E., Massicotte, D., and Hillaire-Marcel, C., Exogenous substrate oxidation during exercise: studies using isotopic labelling, *Int. J. Sports Med.,* 13, S123, 1992.

114. Hunt, J. N. and Knox, M. T., The action of potassium oleate and potassium citrate in slowing gastric emptying, *J. Physiol.,* 171, 247, 1964.

115. Quigley, J. P. and Meschan, I., Inhibition of the pyloric sphincter region by the digestion of products of fat, *Am. J. Physiol.,* 134, 803, 1997.

116. Gleeson, M., Maughan, R. J., and Greenhaff, P. L., Comparison of the effects of pre-exercise feeding of glucose, glycerol and placebo on endurance and fuel homeostasis in man, *Eur. J. Appl. Physiol.,* 55, 645, 1986.

117. Riedesel, M. L., Allen, D. Y., Peake, G. T., and Al-Qattan, K., Hyperhydration with glycerol solutions, *J. Appl. Physiol.,* 63, 2262, 1987.

118. Montner, P., Stark, D. M., Riedesel, M. L., Murata, G., Robergs, R., Timms, M., and Chick, T. L, Pre-exercise glycerol hydration improves cycling endurance time, *Int. J. Sports Med.,* 17, 27, 1996.

119. Koenigsberg, P. S., Martin, K. K., Hlava, H. R., and Riedesel, M. L., Sustained hyperhydration with glycerol ingestion, *Life Sciences,* 57, 645, 1995.

120. Latzka, W. A., Sawka, M. N., Montain, S. J., Skrinar, G. S., Fielding, R. A., Matott, R. P., and Pandolf, K. B., Hyperhydration: thermoregulatory effects during compensable exercise-heat stress, *J. Appl. Physiol.,* 83, 860, 1997.

121. Murray, R., Eddy, D. E., Paul, G. L, Seifert, J. G., and Halaby, G. A., Physiological responses to glycerol ingestion during exercise, *J. Appl. Physiol.,* 71, 144, 1991.

122. Lamb, D. R., Lightfoot, W. S., and Myhal, M., Prehydration with glycerol does not improve cycling performance vs. 6% CHO-electrolyte drink., *Med. Sci. Sports Exerc.,* 29, S249, 1997 (Abstract)

123. Beckers, E. J., Jeukendrup, A. E., Brouns, F., Wagenmakers, A. J. M., and Saris, W. H. M., Gastric emptying of carbohydrate–medium chain triglyceride suspensions at rest., *Int. J. Sports Med.,* 13, 581, 1992.

124. Jeukendrup, A. E., Saris, W. H. M., Van Diesen, R., Brouns, F., and Wagenmakers, A. J. M., Effect of endogenous carbohydrate availability on oral medium-chain triglyceride oxidation during prolonged exercise, *J. Appl. Physiol.,* 80, 949, 1996.

125. Jeukendrup, A. E., Saris, W. H. M., Schrauwen, P., Brouns, F., and Wagenmakers, A. J. M., Metabolic availability of medium-chain triglycerides coingested with carbohydrate during prolonged exercise, *J. Appl. Physiol.,* 79, 756, 1995.

126. Conlay, L. A., Wurtman, R. J., Blusztajn, K., Lopez, G., Coviella, I., Maher, T. J., and Evoniuk, G. E., Decreased plasma choline concentrations in marathon runners, *New Eng. J. Med.,* 315, 892, 1986.

127. Spector, S. A., Jackman, M. R., Sabounjian, L. A., Sakkas, C., Landers, D. M., and Willis, W. T., Effect of choline supplementation on fatigue in trained cyclists, *Med. Sci. Sports Exerc.,* 27, 668, 1995.

128. von Allworden, H. N., Horn, S., Kahl, J., and Feldheim, W., The influence of lecithin on plasma choline concentrations in triathletes and adolescent runners during exercise, *Eur. J. Appl. Physiol.,* 67, 87, 1993.

129. Altman, P. and Dittmer, D. Blood and Other Body Fluids, FASEB, Bethesda, 1961.

130. Fogelholm, M., Ruokonen, I., Laakso, J., Vuorimaa, T., and Himberg, J., Lack of association between indices of vitamin B1, B2 and B6 status and exercise-induced blood lactate in young adults, *Int. J. Sports Nutr.,* 3, 165, 1993.

131. Stephenson, L. and Kolka, M., Cardiovascular and thermoregulatory effects of niacin, in *Thermal Physiology,* Mercer, J., Excerpta, New York, NY 1989, 279.

132. Bergstrom, J., Hultman, E., Jorfeldt, L., Pernow, B., and Wahren, J., Effect of nicotinic acid on physical working capacity and on metabolism of muscle glycogen in man, *J. Appl. Physiol.,* 26, 170, 1969.

133. Pernow, B. and Saltin, B., Availablity of substrates and capacity for prolonged heavy exercise in man, *J. Appl. Physiol.,* 31, 416, 1971.

134. Bergstrom, J., Hultman, E., Jorfeldt, L., Pernow, B., and Wahren, J., Effect of nicotinic acid on physical work capacity and on metabolism in muscle glycogen in man, *J. Appl. Physiol.,* 26, 170, 1969.

135. Romijn, J. A., Coyle, E. F., Sidossis, L. S., Gastaldelli, A., Horowitz, J. F., Endert, E., and Wolfe, R. R., Regulation of endogenous fat and carbohydrate metabolism in relation to exercise intensity and duration, *Am. J. Physiol.,* 265, E380, 1993.

136. Murray, R., Bartoli, W., Eddy, D., and Horn, M., Physiological and performance responses to nicotinic-acid ingestion during exercise, *Med. Sci. Sports Exerc.,* 27, 1057, 1995.

137. Kanter, M., Antioxidants, carnitine,and choline as putative ergogenic aids, *Int. J. Sports Med.,* 5, S120, 1995.

138. Kanter, M., Free radicals, exercise, and antioxidant supplementation, *Int. J. Sports Nutr.,* 4, 205, 1994.

139. Kanter, M. M., Free radicals and exercise: Effect of nutritional antioxidant supplementation, in *Exerc. Sports Sci. Rev.,* <vol> 23, Holloszy, J. O., Williams and Wilkins, Baltimore 1995, 375.

140. Maughan, R., Donnelly, A., Gleeson, M., Whiting, P., Walker, K., and Clough, P., Delayed-onset muscle damage and lipid peroxidation in man after a downhill run, *Muscle Nerve,* 12, 332, 1989.

141. Gee, D. and Tappel, A., The effect of exhaustive exercise on expired pentane as a marker of in vivo lipid peroxidation in the rat, *Life Science,* 28, 2425, 1981.

142. Meydani, M., Evans, W. J., Handelman, G., Biddle, L., Fielding, R. A., Meydani, S. N., Burrill, J., Fiatarone, M. A., Blumberg, J. B., and Cannon, J. G., Protective effect of vitamin E on exercise-induced oxidative damage in young and older adults, *Am. J. Physiol.,* 264, R992, 1993.

143. Committee on Dietary Allowances, Food and Nutrition Board National Research Council. Recommended Daily Allowances, National Academy of Sciences, Washington, D.C., 1989, p 284.

144. Shechter, Y. and Karlish, S. J. D., Insulin-like stimulation of glucose oxidation in rat adipocytes by vanadyl (IV) ions, *Nature,* 284, 556, 1980.

145. Dubyak, G. R. and Kleinzeller, A., The insulin-mimetic effects of vanadate in isloated rat adipocytes, *J. Biol. Chem.,* 255, 5306, 1980.

146. Boden, Guenther, Chen, X., Ruiz, J., van Rossum, G. D. V., and Salvatore, T., Effects of vanadyl sulfate on carbohydrate and lipid metabolism in pateitns with non-insulin-dependent diabetes mellitus, *Metabolism,* 45, 1130, 1996.

147. Offenbacher, E. G. and Pi-Sunyer, F. X., Chromium in human nutrition, *Ann. Rev. Nutr.,* 8, 543, 1988.

148. Anderson, R. A., Chromium, glucose tolerance, and diabetes, *Biol. Trace Elem. Res.,* 32, 19, 1992.

149. Grant, K. E., Chandler, R. M., Castle, A. L., and Ivy, J. L., Chromium and exercise training: effect on obese women., *Med. Sci. Sports Exerc.,* 29, 992, 1997.
150. Anderson, R. A., Polansky, M. M., Bryden, N. A., Roginski, E. E., Mertz, W., and Glinsmann, W. H., Chromium supplementation of human subjects: effects on glucose, insulin and lipid parameters., *Metabolism,* 32, 894, 1983.
151. Anderson, R. A., Bryden, N. A., and Polansky, M. M., Serum chromium of human subjects: effects of chromium supplementation and glucose., *Am. J. Clinic. Nutr.,* 41, 571, 1985.
152. Anderson, R. A., Polansky, M. M., Bryden, N. A., and Canary, J. J., Supplemental-chromium effects on glucose, insulin, glucagon, and urinary chromium losses in subjects consuming controlled low-chromium diets, *Am. J. Clinic. Nutr.,* 54, 909, 1991.
153. Evans, G. W., The effect of chromium picolinate on insulin controlled parameters in humans., *Int. J. Biosocial Med. Res.,* 11, 163, 1989.
154. Lukaski, H. C., Bolonchuk, W. W., Siders, W. A., and Milne, D. B., Chromium supplementation and resistance training: effects on body composition, strength, and trace element status of men., *Am. J. Clinic. Nutr.,* 63, 954, 1996.
155. Hallmark, M., Reynolds, T., DeSouza, C., Dotson, C., Anderson, R., and Rogers, M., Effects of chromium and resistance training on muscle strength and body composition., *Med. Sci. Sports Exerc.,* 28, 139, 1996.
156. Walker, L. S., Bemben, M. G., Bemben, D. A., and Knehans, A. W., Chromium picolinate effect on body composition and muscular performance in wrestlers., *Med. Sci. Sports Exerc.,* 30, 1730, 1998.
157. Campbell, W. W., Beard, J. L., Joseph, L. J., Davey, S. L., and Evans, W. J., Chromium picolinate supplementation and resistive training by older men: effects of iron-status and hematologic indexes., *Am. J. Clinic. Nutr.,* 66, 944, 1997.
158. Hertler-Colbert, L., Davis, J. M., Alderson, N., Welsh, R., Walters, J., and Devolve, K., Effects of carbohydrate and chromium ingestion on fatigue during intermittent, high intensity exercise., *Med. Sci. Sports Exerc.* 29, S277, 1997 (Abstract)
159. Powers, S. K., Martin, D., and Dodd, S., Exercise-induced hypoxemia in elite endurance athletes., *Sports Medicine,* 16, 14, 1993.
160. Graham, T. E. and Spriet, L. L., Performance and metabolic responses to a high caffeine dose during prolonged exercise, *J. Appl. Physiol.,* 71, 2292, 1991.
161. Graham, T. E. and Spriet, L. L., Metabolic, catecholamine and exercise performance responses to varying doses of caffeine., *J. Appl. Physiol.,* 78, 867, 1995.
162. Pasman, W. J., VanBaak, M. A., Jeukendrup, A. E., and DeHaan, A., The effect of different dosages of caffeine on endurance performance time., *Int. J. Sports Med.,* 16, 225, 1995.
163. Collomp, K., Ahmaidi, S., Audran, M., Chanal, J. L., and Prefaut, C., Effects of caffeine ingestion on performance and anaerobic metabolism during the Wingate test., *Int. J. Sports Med.,* 12, 439, 1991.
164. Greer, F., McLean, C., and Graham, T. E., Caffeine, performance, and metabolism during repeated Wingate exercise tests, *J. Appl. Physiol.,* 85, 1502, 1998.
165. Bell, D. G., Jacobs, I., and Zamecnik, J., Effects of caffeine, ephedrine and their combination on time to exhaustion during high-intensity exercise., *Eur. J. Appl. Physiol.,* 77, 427, 1998.
166. Gonzalez-Alonso, J., Heaps, C. L., and Coyle, E. F., Rehydration after exercise with common beverages and water, *Int. J. Sports Med.,* 13, 399, 1992.

167. Wemple, R. D., Lamb, D. R., and McKeever, K. H., Caffeine vs. caffeine-free sports drinks: effects on urine production at rest and during prolonged exercise, *Int. J. Sports Med.*, 18, 40, 1997.

168. Brouns, F., Kovacs, E. M. R., and Senden, J. M. G., The effect of different rehydration drinsk on post-exercise electrolyte excretion in trained athletes, *Int. J. Sports Med.*, 19, 56, 1998.

169. James, J. E., Acute and chronic effects of caffeine on performance, mood, headache, and sleep., *Neuropsychobiology*, 38, 32, 1998.

170. Horswill, C. A., Effects of bicarbonate, citrate, and phosphate loading on performance, *Int. J. Sports Nutr.*, 5, S111, 1995.

171. Matson, L. G. and Tran, Z. V., Effects of sodium bicarbonate ingestion on anaerobic performance: A meta-analytic review, *Int. J. Sports Nutr.*, 3, 2, 1993.

172. Hermansen, L., Effect of metabolic changes on force production in skeletal muscle during maximal exercise, in *Human Muscle Fatigue: Physiological Measurements*, Porter, R. and Whelan, J., Pittman Medical, London 1981, 72.

173. Chasiotis, D., The regulation of glycogen phosphorylase and glycogen breakdown in human skeletal muscle, *Acta Physiologica Scandinavica Supplement*, 518, 1, 1983.

174. Fabiato, A. and Fabiato, F., Effects of pH on the myofilaments and the sarcoplasmic reticulum of skinned cells from cardiac and skeletal muscles, *J. Physiol.*, 276, 233, 1978.

175. Wilkes, D., Gledhill, N., and Smyth, R., Effect of acute induced metabolic alkalosis on 800-m racing time, *Med. Sci. Sports Exerc.*, 15, 277, 1985.

176. Goldfinch, J., McNaughton, L. R., and Davies, P., Bicarbonate ingestion and its effects upon 400-m racing time, *Eur. J. Appl. Physiol.*, 57, 45, 1985.

177. Ryan, A. J., Lambert, G. P., Shi, X., Chang, R. T., Summers, R. W., and Gisolfi, C. V., Effect of hypohydration on gastric emptying and intestinal absorption during exercise, *J. Appl. Physiol.*, 84, 1581, 1998.

178. Allen, J. D., McLung, J., Nelson, A. G., and Welsch, M., Ginseng supplementation does not enhance healthy young adults' peak aerobic exercise performance, *J. Am. Coll. Nutr.*, 17, 462, 1998.

179. Morris, A. C., Jacobs, I., McLellan, T. M., Klugerman, A., Wang, L C H., and Zamecnik, J., No ergogenic effect of ginseng ingestion, *Int. J. Sports Nutr.*, 6, 263, 1996.

180. Bahrke, M. S. and Morgan, W. P., Evaluation of the ergogenic properties of ginseng, *Sports Med.*, 18, 229, 1994.

181. Dustman, K., Plowman, S. A., McCarthy, K., Ehlers, G., Bramer, A., Coreless, C., De Vantier, N., Freimuth, M., and Walicek, H., The effects of Endurox on the physiological responses to stair-stepping exercise, *Med. Sci. Sports Exerc.*, 30, S323, 1998 (Abstract)

182. Cheuvront, S. N., Moffatt, R. J., Biggerstaff, K. D., Bearden, S., and McDonough, P, Effect of EnduroxTM on various metabolic responses to submaximal exercise, *Int. J. Sports Nutr.*, 9, 434, 1999.

183. LeBars, P. L., Katz, M. M., Berman, N., Itil, T. M., Freedman, A. M., and Schatzberg, A. F., A placebo-controlled, double-blind, randomized trial of an extract of gingkgo biloba for dementia., *JAMA*, 278, 1327, 1997.

184. Vale, S., Subarachnoid haemorrhage associated with Gingkgo biloba, *Lancet*, 352, 36, 1998.

185. Rosenblatt, M. and Mindel, J., Spontaneous hyphema associated with ingestion of Gingkgo biloba extract, *New Eng. J. Med.*, 336, 1108, 1997.

186. Chung, K. F., Dent, G., McCusker, M., Guinot, P., Page, C. P., and Barnes, P. J., Effect of ginkgolide mixture (BN 52063) in antagonizing skin and platelet responses to platelet activating factor in man, *Lancet,* 1, 248, 1987.

187. Watson, J. A., Fang, M., and Lowenstein, J. M., Tricarballylate and hydroxycitrate: substrate and inhibitor of ATP: citrate oxaloacetate lyase, *Arch. Biochem. Biophys.,* 35, 209, 1969.

188. Lowenstein, J. M., Effect of (-)-hydroxycitrate on fatty acid synthesis by rat liver *in vivo, J. Biol. Chem.,* 246, 629, 1971.

189. Sullivan, A. C., Riscari, J., Hamilton, J. G., and Neal Miller, O, Effect of (-)-hydroxycitrate upon the accumulation of lipid in the rat appetite, *Lipids,* 9, 129, 1973.

190. Nageswara Rao, R. and Sakeriak, K. K., Lipid-lowering effect and antiobesity effect of (-)-hydroxycitric acid, *Nutr. Res.,* 8, 209, 1999.

191. McCarty, M. F., Inhibition of citrate lyase may aid aerobic endurance, *Medical Hypotheses,* 45, 247, 1995.

192. Heymsfield, S. B., Allison, D. B., Vasselli, J. R., Pietrobelli, A., Greenfield, D., and Nunez, C., Garcinia cambogia (hydroxycitric acid) as a potential antiobesity agent: A randomized controlled trial, *JAMA,* 280, 1596, 1998.

10 Discussion Among Authors

Luis Aragón-Vargas, Craig Horswill,
John Leiper, Ronald Maughan,
Robert Murray, Dennis Passe,
Susan Shirreffs, and John Stofan

When is a sports drink more effective than plain water?

Shirreffs: One of the most noticeable times that a sports drink is more effective than plain water is in the recovery of sweat losses after exercise when no food is consumed before a subsequent exercise bout. The sodium content of the drink provides this benefit. Second, during exercise lasting more than 30 minutes, a sports drink is more effective than plain water because of the carbohydrate substrate it provides.

Leiper: There is no doubt that a well-formulated sports drink is better than water for rehydration following exercise. The sodium content of sports drinks helps to reduce urine formation and stimulate fluid consumption compared with water. Both of these factors assist in the maintenance of hydration status. Plain water is undoubtedly emptied from the stomach faster than many sports drinks; however, overall water absorption is faster from a properly formulated sports drink because of the carbohydrate component. Although many individuals assert that they drink large volumes of plain water daily, studies have shown that the actual volumes consumed are far less than people indicate. This is probably due to the lack of flavoring of plain water and to the thirst-quenching properties of water.

Maughan: Several studies have shown that plain water is effective in improving performance in different types of exercise. Benefits have been reported in prolonged continuous exercise, in varying intensity tests designed to simulate the pattern of activity in team sports, and in both cycling and running time trials. In all of these situations, there is evidence to show that drinking water can improve performance and reduce the disturbances to physiological homeostasis when compared with trials where no drink is consumed. What is most interesting is that in tests where a sports drink has been included in addition to water and a no-drink control, the sports drink almost invariably gives a significantly better performance. In a few studies, there is no statistically significant difference between water and a sports drink. Examination of the data, however, generally shows that, even in these studies, a benefit of the sports drink is apparent. This may not reach the level of statistical significance necessary to be accepted as proof of a benefit, but small numbers of subjects, insensitive tests, and variability in the response of different individuals all combine to make it difficult to achieve this. In some studies, there may be a 10% increase in endurance capacity, with seven out of eight subjects showing improved performance, and yet still no statistically significant benefit. For the athlete, though, a 10% improvement and an almost 90% chance of improvement are well worth having. It is worth remembering, too, that there are no well controlled studies showing that individuals perform better when drinking water than when drinking a well formulated sports drink.

Aragón-V.:   Another thing to keep in mind is that the benefits of a sports drink are proportional to the need for fluid, energy, and electrolytes. When the need is great, as it is during intense exercise in a warm environment, the benefits of a sports drink are significant.

Leiper: That's true. The vast majority of laboratory and field studies have clearly demonstrated that ingestion of properly formulated sports drinks allows exercising individuals to perform better than when they drink plain water. Because intestinal water absorption is faster from dilute carbohydrate solutions than from plain water, hydration status is better maintained, and, therefore, cardiovascular and thermoregulatory responses are less perturbed following the consumption of sports drinks. The carbohydrate content of sport drinks can delay the onset of hypoglycemia during prolonged exercise and thereby improve exercise capacity.

Murray: The simple fact of the matter is that the harder you work, the better a good sports drink will work. And, as Dr. Maughan has said, when it comes to performance, there are many occasions when a sports drink is superior to water but there are no occasions when water is superior to a good sports drink.

What's the most effective way to use sports drinks to improve performance?

Murray: The most effective way of improving performance is to drink a well formulated sports drink during exercise. The preponderance of research shows that performance can be improved if 30 to 60 grams of carbohydrate are ingested during each hour of vigorous exercise. That's the equivalent of about 500 to 1,000 milliliters of sports drink per hour, a very reasonable rate of consumption. As Dr. Maughan will be quick to point out, there are studies that have demonstrated improved performance with a carbohydrate intake of less than 30 grams per hour, evidence that further illustrates the potent effect of carbohydrate consumption on performance. But, when both fluid and carbohydrate intake are important, as is the case in the vast majority of exercise settings, ingesting more fluid, and thereby more carbohydrate, is the best thing to do. Drinking to prevent dehydration should always be the first priority and doing so with a sports drink ensures sufficient carbohydrate intake for improved performance.

Leiper: I would like to add a word of caution regarding drinking during exercise. Recent work in our laboratories and in field studies has identified that intermittent high-intensity exercise can slow gastric emptying. This type of exercise is inherent in most team sports and during many types of competition, increasing the likelihood that athletes will retain more fluid in the stomach than would occur during continuous exercise. The evidence to date suggests that the rate of gastric emptying of most sports drinks is still sufficient, but this finding underscores the need for athletes to practice drinking under game situations.

Can children drink sports drinks?

Maughan: Children should be encouraged to drinks sports drinks whenever they take part in physical activity in a warm environment. Mild levels of dehydration and hyperthermia will reduce exercise capacity, but if a severe fluid deficit is allowed to develop, there is a real risk of heat illness. Because the thirst mechanism is not sufficiently sensitive to ensure that fluid intake will match losses, a conscious effort is necessary if dehydration is to be avoided. Children are particularly likely to forget to drink unless reminded to do so.

Aragón-V.:   There is no clinical or physiological reason to contraindicate drinking a sports drink. The composition of 100 ml of a typical sports drink represents 6 grams of carbohydrate, 46 mg of sodium, and 13 mg of potassium. This is about half the carbohydrate concentration of many soft drinks and fruit juices, and slightly less sodium than in 100 ml of milk.

Horswill: Physically active children should be encouraged to drink a sports drink to stay hydrated. Several studies in the last few years demonstrated that children drank more fluid and stayed better hydrated when consuming a sports drink compared with water. This is an important finding because, in a dehydrated state, a child's core body temperature increases quite rapidly and at a greater rate than that of the adult under similar conditions of exercise and environment. Kids gain heat from the environment more easily than adults due to their larger surface-area to volume ratio, they generate more metabolic heat at the same relative exercise intensity, and they have far less fluid to lose, all of which makes them particularly susceptible to the dangers of dehydration and heat illness.

Why ingest a sports drink during exercise if loss of body mass is the goal?

Maughan: The amount of energy expended in exercise is the key factor in weight loss. The vast majority of the weight lost during an exercise session is from the water that is lost in sweat. Although there may seem to be advantages in increasing the weight loss during each exercise session by restricting fluid intake, this is actually counterproductive. Taking sports drinks during exercise will allow a higher work rate, a greater energy expenditure, and thus more weight loss. In addition, if enough sports drink is consumed, the same amount of work can be performed with less subjective sensation of effort. In other words, the workout feels easier.

Stofan: The bottom line is that, by ingesting a sports drink, you can actually exercise harder and longer, prevent early fatigue, and will likely feel better during and after the exercise. Moreover, the amount of energy ingested is usually negligible in long term energy balance. Weight loss also often requires an understanding that results are not achieved with exercise alone, but that real change in behavior, diet, and physical activity levels are often required. There are no shortcuts.

Horswill: One of the side effects of dieting for body fat reduction is dehydration. Sports drinks are effective in helping individuals, weight-conscious or not, to stay hydrated. Sports drinks provide a small amount of carbohydrate, but the contribution of energy is small compared with the total daily energy intake.

Shirreffs: That's exactly right. People seem to forget that if they don't drink during exercise, the resulting dehydration will force them to work at a lower intensity or for a shorter period of time, both of which will reduce the energy cost of the activity and its potential to help with fat loss. Athletes who want to lose body mass loss to allow them to "make weight" for competition should be counseled to begin their weight reduction as far ahead of time as possible, placing the emphasis on fat loss rather than fluid loss.

Murray: Unless I missed something, the law of conservation of energy hasn't been repealed. Fat loss is a matter of consistently expending more energy than is ingested. It's not a matter of how much energy is lost in a workout or how much energy is ingested in a sports drink during a workout. It's a matter of energy balance at the end of the day. Or, even more relevant, it's a matter of energy balance at the end of the month. But this is a confusing issue for anyone who exercises to lose weight. After all, it seems so counterintuitive to ingest foods or fluids that contain energy when the whole idea is to expend energy through exercise. It's difficult for people to believe that carbohydrates are not converted to fat, that ingesting carbohydrate during exercise can be a real advantage to weight loss for the reasons the rest of you indicated, and that they'll actually feel better, work harder, and recover quicker if they stay hydrated with a sports drink during their workout.

Are there really any meaningful differences among commercial sports drinks?

Murray: Yes, there are meaningful differences among sports drinks, primarily due to difference in carbohydrate concentration. Sports drinks that contain too high a concentration of carbohydrate will result in slower gastric emptying and intestinal fluid absorption. This predisposes to greater gastrointestinal discomfort, as noted by Dr. Clyde Williams' group from the University of Loughborough as an explanation for why ingesting a 6.9% carbohydrate drink did not significantly improve performance compared with water, while a 5.6% carbohydrate drink did result in improved performance. One more factor of note is that the differences among sports drinks will become most evident during intense training and competition when there is a premium placed on rapid fluid and solute absorption. If the carbohydrate concentration is too high, absorption will be slowed and the risk of gastrointestinal discomfort will rise.

Maughan: The athlete has a choice of sports drinks with very different formulations and the carbohydrate content is arguably the most important component to vary. The concentration of carbohydrate has a direct influence on fluid absorption and energy provision. For example, oral rehydration solutions, formulated for correction of the large water and electrolyte losses incurred by children suffering from infectious diarrhea, contain less carbohydrate and higher electrolyte concentrations than sports drinks. In these patients, however, carbohydrate is added only for its effect on stimulating water uptake in the small intestine, not as an energy source. In contrast, the athlete not only wants rapid fluid absorption, but enough carbohydrate to fuel the working muscles. Research clearly shows that very high carbohydrate concentrations, in the range of 10% to 15%, result in dramatic slowing of gastric emptying of ingested fluids. Although these drinks may be more effective in providing carbohydrate, they are likely to compromise fluid replacement when significant sweat losses are incurred.

What are the advantages and disadvantages of intravenous fluid replacement?

Maughan: When sweat losses are very high, some degree of dehydration is almost inevitable, even when there are ample opportunities for fluid ingestion and when a well-formulated and pleasant-tasting drink is available. When opportunities for drinking are limited, dehydration may be severe. Intravenous rehydration has been used for many years to treat collapsed runners suffering from dehydration and hyperthermia after marathon races. In most cases, oral rehydration would have the same effect, but takes much longer. These runners have completed their event, and intravenous rehydration is justified on the grounds of speeding recovery and clearing the aid station faster.

In recent years, intravenous fluid replacement has been used in a variety of different events and has been used in athletes who then return to competition. This is a very different situation and one that raises many questions. It seems likely that benefits can accrue from intravenous administration of fluids at half time in football, field hockey, soccer, or similar team sports. This may be of particular benefit when sweat losses are very high and for individuals prone to gastrointestinal problems when fluid is ingested. There are also some individuals with exceptionally slow rates of gastric emptying, and these individuals may be unable to match sweat losses via the oral route. It takes only a few minutes to replace a liter of fluid, and there are no delays imposed by the gastrointestinal tract. Saline is normally used for this purpose, but glucose may be added for extra benefit.

There are several concerns about the use of intravenous fluids in competitive situations. The risk of infection is small, but is not entirely absent, and is magnified when the procedure is carried out in haste in conditions that are inevitably less than optimal. There must also be a concern that a player returning to the field may have corrected any dehydration incurred but may still be hyperthermic. Restoring the capacity to perform exercise without simultaneously lowering body temperature is not wise.

Murray: I do agree that there are situations when it is impossible to prevent dehydration from occurring. On the other hand, there are all too many situations when the use of intravenous fluid represents nothing more than a failure to follow a sound fluid replacement plan. I've had athletic trainers tell me of athletes who preferred getting IVs before practice because they were too lazy to follow the prehydration guidelines for drinking fluid. As ridiculous as that seems, it's no more disconcerting than triathletes and runners lining up at medical tents after races waiting to get IV fluid, not because there is a medical reason for doing so, but because they think it will help them recover faster. And, I've seen nothing in the scientific literature that shows that intravenous therapy is superior to oral rehydration. In fact, oral rehydration has some advantages over IV fluid use.

Stofan: That's true. One recent study reported a trend for better cardiovascular and thermoregulatory control and for better performance with oral v.s IV fluids. Several other studies have shown that with oral fluid ingestion, subjects felt better during subsequent exercise and had lower RPE values. Let's not forget that the act of drinking stimulates oropharyngeal mechanisms that provoke hormonal responses that help restore normal body fluid balance. That doesn't happen with intravenous therapy. In my mind, the fact that research shows that there are no ergogenic or physiological benefits with intravenous fluids compared with oral fluids is good reason to question the frequency with which intravenous fluids are administered to athletes.

Murray: It's easy to understand the motivation that underlies the use of intravenous fluid administration, but my concern is that it has become too widespread. It's one matter if an athlete can't tolerate oral fluids or is so severely dehydrated that health is potentially jeopardized, but it's quite another matter when intravenous fluid use becomes so commonplace that athletes request it just because they perceive — inaccurately so — that they can recover more quickly than if they drink a similar volume of fluid. Unless fluid is physically forced into a vein, intravenous rehydration is not a rapid process. In fact, I'll wager that most of the perceived benefit comes from lying down.

How much sodium is enough in a sports drink?

Shirreffs: Sodium has a variety of roles in a sports drink and the ideal quantity depends on a number of factors. The inclusion of some sodium in a drink (up to 25 mmol/liter) improves the taste for many people. For drinking before exercise, beverage sodium may help with fluid retention and permit a temporary hyperhydration. During exercise, the inclusion of sodium in a drink may not be necessary except in situations of prolonged exercise if large quantities of a drink are going to be consumed. For post-exercise replacement of sweat losses, the inclusion of sodium in the drink consumed is essential for effective recovery. In addition to helping ensure that sufficient drink volume is consumed, the ideal sodium intake should be moderately high — probably in the order of a concentration of 50 mmol/liter.

Stofan: There is really no consensus regarding the proper level of sodium in a sports drink. While sports drinks typically contain sodium levels between 5 and 25 mmol/liter, differences in sport, environmental conditions, and variability among individuals leads to the conclusion that there is no one level of sodium that is ideal. A sodium level that optimizes flavor characteristics and positively affects fluid balance, yet does not inhibit further fluid intake, is likely to be most nearly ideal.

Murray: I concur with the last comment in that the sodium content of a sports drink has to strike a fine balance between taste and efficacy. Let's not forget that beverage sodium content has a direct effect upon voluntary drinking. Too little sodium in a drink removes the osmotic dependent drive to drink too soon and drinking ceases well before euhydration is reestablished. Too much sodium in a beverage negatively affects taste and removes the volume-dependent drive for thirst, again resulting in the premature cessation of drinking. In practical terms, there is no ideal sodium concentration for a sports drink, but there is an ideal compromise that can be struck between taste and efficacy.

Can physically active people with diabetes use sports drinks?

Aragón-V.: Yes, persons with diabetes can use sports drinks. And there are very good reasons that they should. Maintenance of both blood sugar level and hydration during physical activity can be a challenge for people with diabetes. Ingesting a sports drink can successfully attend to both needs. Those with diabetes should take extra care when exercising in extreme temperatures because of potential problems with thermoregulation related to autonomic neuropathies.

Murray: Physically active people with diabetes should incorporate the use of sports drinks before and during exercise under the guidance of their physicians and in accordance with the carbohydrate exchange plan they normally follow. It is interesting that diabetes normally causes problems due to hyperglycemia, yet it is hypoglycemia that creates problems during and following exercise in people with diabetes. Regular physical activity is a critical element, along with nutrition and insulin therapy or other drugs, in controlling diabetes and lessening the risks of complications. There is no reason that a person with diabetes cannot take part in very vigorous training and competition, provided that adequate planning and care is taken to safeguard against hypoglycemia.

Should physically active people with hypertension drink sports drinks?

Stofan: Anyone who is physically active, and therefore sweating can benefit from a sports drink, even in those cases where the benefit is limited to improved voluntary fluid intake. After all, reducing dehydration is a very real benefit. There is no evidence that sports drink ingestion affects blood pressure. That's because sports drinks contain comparatively little sodium relative to the rest of one's diet. For example, most sports drinks contain no more sodium than an equivalent volume of milk, and I'm not familiar with any restrictions limiting the intake of milk for hypertensive people.

Aragón-V.:   Hypertensive patients using beta-blockers may experience compromised heat dissipation due to reduced skin blood flow, and also an accelerated sweat rate response that could worsen dehydration. Fluid replacement is especially important under these circumstances. Furthermore, diuretic therapy can produce hypokalemia and dehydration, but with adequate fluid intake and potassium supplementation, exercise impairment can be avoided. Hypertensive patients on sodium-restricted diets should have their physicians include the sodium provided by sports drinks into their total intake calculations. The same basic recommendations for average adults apply to physically active hypertensive patients without complications.

Horswill: It's prudent for hypertensive patients to work with their physicians on all aspects of their treatment, including exercise and diet. The specific role of sodium as a cause of hypertension is suspect according to a meta-analysis published in JAMA in 1996. In this examination, only older individuals with hypertension seemed to benefit from controlling dietary sodium. The sodium contribution of a sports drink is deemed small relative to that of the daily intake of food and is typically lower in concentration than that of human sweat.

Why not just make a sports drink at home?

Passe: There are three reasons: flavor, flavor, and flavor. Keep in mind that liking of flavor is a primary driver of voluntary fluid intake during exercise, and suboptimal flavors lead to suboptimal drinking behavior. We've completed a study that contrasted voluntary fluid intake during exercise with four different beverages: water, a commercial sports drink, a homemade sports drink, and orange juice diluted in half with water. All beverages except water were orange flavored. I'll spare you the details of the experimental design, but suffice it to say that the results showed that the commercial sports beverage with its optimized flavor system scored significantly higher than all of the other beverages in overall acceptance and was consumed in significantly greater quantities than all of the other beverages, resulting in significantly lower dehydration.

Maughan: We also found, in a study on rehydration after exercise, that people drank more of the drinks they liked the taste of. This is hardly a surprising finding, but is one that the people who recommend that athletes make up their own drinks seem to forget.

Stofan: As with virtually any commercial beverage, it is nearly impossible to duplicate the flavor systems in your kitchen, not to mention assuring that the remaining ingredients are balanced to provide optimal efficacy. Sports drinks may be relatively simple concoctions in terms of their basic ingredients, but optimizing flavor and other aspects of palatability is far from a simple task.

What can soccer players do to stay hydrated and ingest enough carbohydrate to improve playing performance?

Aragón-V.:   Because the opportunities to drink fluids during games are restricted to the half-time break and occasional stops of the game due to injury, it is important to take advantage of every single one. Players should also begin the game euhydrated. They need to maintain good hydration day after day and ingest around 500 ml of a sports drink about 2 hours before the game to top off the fluid reserves; any excess will be eliminated via urine before the game. Immediately before the game, they should drink 250 ml more of sports drink.

There should be individual sports drink bottles clearly labeled for each player, easily accessible during the break or game stopovers. These bottles are also useful to track the total fluid intake of each player. Each team member should attempt to drink as much fluid as necessary to compensate for sweat loss; this amount should be determined beforehand, weighing each player before and after exercise and estimating average fluid losses for each individual. To improve their tolerance to ingesting large volumes of fluid, it is crucial that players practice drinking frequently during training.

At the end of each game or practice session, every player should ingest an amount of fluid equivalent to 150% of whatever weight deficit exists, to achieve a fast and adequate replenishment of fluid loss. This fluid should have enough sodium to prevent the excess elimination of fluid in the urine.

Leiper: I would like to reemphasize the need for athletes to practice drinking during training sessions and practice matches. This will allow the player to become familiar with the sensation of exercising with fluid in the stomach, help train the stomach to empty faster during exercise, and permit athletes to develop drinking strategies that work best for them.

Why not add creatine or other nutritional supplements to sports drinks?

Murray: First of all, sports drinks are not good vehicles to deliver nutrients because the doses that can be included in a sports drink without adversely affecting the taste and efficacy are quite small. This is particularly true for creatine because it has very poor stability over time in an acid medium.

Horswill: Also, the rationale for using a sports drink is that the ingestion provides acute physiological and performance benefits. The athlete isn't required to consume the beverage for several months or even several days prior to exercise to gain the benefits. For many nutrition supplements, an effect is produced only after consumption of the supplement for a period of time. Acute dosing with creatine has never been shown to be beneficial.

Why not add amino acids to sport drinks?

Horswill: The research on amino-acid ingestion and physical performance fails to show an ergogenic effect. One of the premises in these studies is that a specific group of amino acids, the branched-chain amino acids (BCAA), may provide an alternative source of fuel and help prolong work capacity. In fact, BCAAs are a metabolically expensive alternative to carbohydrate. Why add a fuel that must first be stripped of nitrogen for conversion to a carbon chain (i.e., glucose or a TCA intermediate) instead of ingesting that carbon chain directly? And the nitrogenous waste can add to the drain on the body fluid stores because of the need for increased urine excretion.

Leiper: The most obvious theoretical advantage of including amino acids in sports drinks is that they might potentiate net water absorption in the small intestine. Amino acids that are actively co-transported with sodium by carrier systems other than that of the Na^+-glucose transporter would appear to be ideally suited to promote uptake when glucose transport is at its maximum rate. The majority of intestinal perfusion studies carried out in humans have, however, demonstrated either no improvement or a reduction in the rates of water absorption from carbohydrate drinks containing amino acids. The reason for this finding is not at present known. In addition, because gastric emptying is so tightly controlled, it is unlikely that the Na^+-glucose transporters are normally ever fully saturated in the section of duodeno-jejunum that receives the ingested sports drink from the stomach. The addition of amino acids to a sports drink would also increase the total energy density of the drink, thereby slowing the rate of gastric emptying of the drink and hence reduce the rate of intestinal water absorption.

Murray: There just isn't scientific justification, as yet at least, for including amino acids in a sports drink. Aside from lack of efficacy, the addition of amino acids negatively affects taste and contributes to ammonia production from deamination of the amino acids. There remain some intriguing possibilities regarding the use of amino acids, but none of these possibilities has yet been able to live up to its theoretical potential, as indicated by Drs. Horswill and Leiper. And, the practical fact of the matter is that sports drinks can accommodate only a very small amount of amino acids, perhaps too small to be of any consequence to absorption or metabolism.

Should micronutrients involved in carbohydrate metabolism (for example, B vitamins) be added to sports drinks?

Horswill: The objective of formulating a sports drink is to provide acute effects that support metabolism, physiology, and performance. Certain B vitamins or a mineral such as chromium are involved in the metabolism or transport of glucose, but that doesn't mean that these micronutrients provide more energy and enhance work capacity when ingested with the carbohydrate in a sports drink. In short, the only evidence of improved function and performance from ingesting vitamins and minerals is in individuals who were clearly deficient in those nutrients. In such cases, performance is merely returned to the normal level with supplementation. Although the adequacy of the diet of an athlete may be suspect on any given day, it is nearly impossible to create a frank deficiency in any B vitamin or chromium. Adding micronutrients to a sports drink simply adds micronutrients to the urine.

Murray: Manufacturers who tout the vitamin content of their sports drinks attempt to take advantage of the good-for-you halo that surrounds vitamins in the minds of consumers. This is particularly true of the antioxidant vitamins, even though there is no evidence of an acute benefit from ingesting antioxidants. Perhaps future research will demonstrate a positive effect, but at this time, there is little scientific rationale for including vitamins or minerals other than sodium, chloride, and potassium in a sports drink.

Is it better to mix a sports drink from powder so that it is possible to mix different strengths to suit different activities?

Maughan: In theory, this sounds like a good idea. Athletes could choose different concentrations in hot or cold weather and different individuals could choose a mixture that would best suit their own needs. In practice, however, there are a number of difficulties with this approach. There are difficulties in knowing what the best mix would be, and even if this is known, it is not easy to make this up at home. Although it seems intuitively obvious that a whole spectrum of different formulations could be devised to individualize the sports drink, there is not good evidence that this is the case. And the amount of powder to be mixed would be difficult to measure accurately without access to a very sensitive balance.

Passe: One occasionally hears discussion among athletes about mixing a sports beverage from a dry mix at concentrations higher or lower than the recommended label instructions or changing the concentration of a liquid sports beverage by diluting it. While this may have appeal to some, research suggests that the flavor level identified by the manufacturer is usually optimum and will result in the most acceptable flavor profile. So, from strictly a taste and voluntary intake point of view, it is best not to alter the composition of a properly formulated sports drink. On the other hand, there are likely some sports drinks with flavor profiles that are not optimized. Rather than encouraging athletes to alter the composition of the beverage, the best approach would be to find a sports drink with acceptable hedonic characteristics.

Murray: Athletes should keep in mind that diluting a sports drink to achieve a blunted flavor profile also dilutes its benefits. Diluting the carbohydrate and electrolyte content reduces the end impact that those ingredients are formulated to deliver — not a good idea when improved performance is the goal. Sports drinks come in many different flavors and there are also differences in flavor intensities. Often just switching to a different flavor is enough to solve whatever annoyances have developed with a particular flavor. Finally, there is little evidence that different compositions, such as concentrated formulations for cold-weather activities, are of greater benefit than the standard sports-drink formulation. After all, there is a ceiling on exogenous carbohydrate oxidation of about one gram per minute, so ingesting higher carbohydrate concentrations will not do much more than slow gastric emptying and fluid absorption. And that's not a good thing in any exercise environment.

Does drinking a chilled beverage increase the risk of stomach cramps?

Maughan: It is often recommended that sports drinks should be chilled to improve palatability and to speed the rate of gastric emptying. The former is certainly an advantage, as cool drinks are perceived as being more pleasant to drink and will lead to an increased consumption. There is not good evidence, however, that chilled drinks empty from the stomach at appreciably faster rates than drinks at room temperature. The concern about stomach cramps probably arises from the fact that ingestion of very large volumes of ice-cold fluids can lead to a "dumping syndrome," where the fluids may disturb gastric function. In laboratory studies, however, subjects have been able to ingest rather large volumes of cool fluids without experiencing adverse effects.

Murray: I agree. First of all, our research shows that within 5 minutes after drinking 400 ml of a sports drink, beverage temperature will rise from about 10°C to over 30°C. This is probably why there is little to no effect of beverage temperature on gastric emptying and why there is little likelihood that cramping will occur.

Passe: I should add that, in terms of beverage acceptance, the relationship between drink temperature and overall acceptance approximates an inverted U-shape. That is, at higher beverage temperatures, overall acceptance drops off precipitously. No surprise there; who wants to drink a warm beverage when you are hot, sweaty, and thirsty? At beverage temperatures lower than refrigerator temperature (about 4°C to 7°C), overall acceptance also declines, as physically active people find it difficult to quickly ingest such cold drinks.

What do you predict for the next generation of sports drinks?

Passe: As with so many food and beverage categories, the future of sports drinks is likely to hold significant changes in formulation, flavor development, packaging, and marketing. The trend has been for more choices, higher product quality, and better production efficiency resulting in superior value and availability. For instance, there will be more flavor blends with better "fidelity to standard"; that is, the flavors will be indistinguishable from fresh and natural fruit.

Distribution will be even more efficient than it is today, so that the average age of the product on the shelf will be younger and fresher. It has always been true that one of the best ways to improve a product is to get it to the consumer faster.

The sports drink of the future will likely be formulated for age groups, gender, use occasion, and physical requirement. As research accumulates, a closer correspondence will be achieved between product formulation and consumer needs. Product formulations will be more finely tuned to the unique needs of aging populations, children, gender, weight-management or dietary-management goals, and sport or activity requirement. As justified by empirical research, value-added ingredients will be included to target performance, nutrition, and general health maintenance goals.

Packaging innovation will take advantage of breakthroughs in product development. For instance, individual containers may have multiple flavor options so that, in the same container, a base formulation may have several flavor choices that the consumer activates at the time of use. Container sizes, shapes, and materials will continue to evolve to meet choice, convenience, and cost goals. Much of the packaging innovation will not be visible. Environmentally friendly sourcing of materials, including recycling, will be refined to achieve lower levels of waste.

Aragón-V.:   I agree that different sports drink formulations may evolve to address different needs before, during, and after exercise, or the needs imposed by different environmental conditions. Perhaps I shouldn't lump all of these types of beverages into the "sports-drink" category because they will likely have vastly different compositions. We know, for instance, that a post-exercise drink should have a higher concentration of carbohydrate to promote glycogen resynthesis and sodium to promote fluid conservation in the body. By definition, I suppose that is no longer a sports drink because you wouldn't want to drink it during most types of exercise. Nonetheless, it is an example of how the broad category of products will evolve.

Horswill: At the risk of being somewhat pessimistic, I think one thing we can expect in the future is even more unsubstantiated product claims and confusion among consumers. Because the claims will be wide-ranging and unproven, it will be a challenge to keep consumers educated about the benefits they can truly expect from a well-formulated sports drink. This will be a big challenge because manufacturers will increasingly spike their products with herbs, phytochemicals, and other compounds that have little to do with hydration and performance. Pessimism aside, I do think that whatever advances are made with the formulation of sports drinks, top-notch science will always win out. That was the case 40 years ago when sports drinks were first developed and will remain the case in the future. I guess I'm an optimist, after all.

Stofan: Here's a little speculation: with a great deal of innovation in packaging and fluid delivery systems, the next generation of sports drinks will likely also become more sport- and occasion-specific. As scientists learn more about the specific needs for particular sports and the particular demands that each sport places on the body's physiology, sports drinks will play a more refined role. In the future, I wouldn't be surprised to see the distinction between conventional sports supplements and pharmaceuticals blurred somewhat, as sports drinks incorporate ingredients that are churned out as by-products of pharmaceutical research. These ingredients won't be drugs per se, but natural compounds that provide a nutritional rather than a pharmacological effect. However, I agree with Dr. Horswill's comments that phytochemicals and herbs will also work their way into this category.

We know that the basic components of sports drinks — water, carbohydrates, and electrolytes — are vital to human function during activity in hot environments. It's reasonable to predict that the use of sports drinks will increase in nontraditional areas such as in military situations, among mining, agriculture, and construction workers, and during all types of outdoor recreation.

Maughan: Although I do think that some of this crystal ball thinking is bound to come true, I don't think that the basic formulation of sports drinks is likely to undergo major changes in the foreseeable future. Current formulations are based on sound scientific principles and have been thoroughly researched. A very large number of well-controlled laboratory studies show that the addition of small amounts of carbohydrate and electrolytes confers significant performance advantages over plain water. It is also well established that the sugars used in the current formulations —

glucose, sucrose, and maltodextrin — outperform the other more exotic sugars, such as fructose and galactose, that have been tried. It is equally clear that there is a fairly broad range of concentrations of the main ingredients that are equally effective; too much sugar or salt, however, has negative effects. In addition to the laboratory studies, the benefits of ingesting a dilute carbohydrate-electrolyte drink are well recognized by athletes whose collective experience shows that there are benefits from a well-formulated drink.

It is possible that there will be an attempt to make drinks suited for different situations. A drink with higher sodium levels and a lower carbohydrate content might be appropriate when sweat losses are very high, and a drink with a higher carbohydrate content might be appropriate for recovery after exercise if glycogen resynthesis is a priority. The picture is complicated, however, by the large variability among individuals. A number of different ingredients have been added to sports drinks in an attempt to provide an additional benefit. These ingredients include lactate, branched-chain amino acids, glycerol, and caffeine, as well as an assortment of vitamins and minerals. For the reasons outlined in previous chapters, none of these seems to confer a worthwhile benefit. New flavors and colors will continue to be developed for sports drinks. These provide no direct physiological benefit, but the element of choice and variety is important in encouraging athletes to ingest drinks. It would be nice to think that athletes and coaches will be better informed and will play an active role in the evaluation of existing products and in the development of new products.

Index

C

Caffeine, 17, 31, 191, 239, 270
  abstinence, negative consequences of, 78
  users, mood in, 78
Calcium, 17, 31
Carbohydrate(s), *see* Fluids, carbohydrates, and
      electrolytes, gastric emptying and
      intestinal absorption of
  concentration, 204
  derivatives, 226
  electrolyte beverage, non-carbonated, 71
  as fuel during exercise, 154
  ingestion, timing of, 175, 190
  intake, *see* Exercise, metabolic and
      performance responses to during
  metabolism, 266
  monomers, 108
  normal stores of in typical athletes, 6
  oxidation, 158, 161, 237
  peak oxidation rates of ingested, 176
  requirements, 5, 21
  sources, during exercise, 159
  supplementation, 172
  types, 174, 211
Carbohydrate-electrolyte drinks, formulation of
      for optimal efficacy, 197–223
  business of sports drinks, 198
  carbohydrate for improved performance,
      211–213
    formulation considerations, 211–213
    scientific principles and practical
      ramifications, 211
  formulation objectives, 199–201
    carbohydrate for improved performance,
      201
    physiological response, 201
    rapid fluid absorption, 201
    speed rehydration, 201
    voluntary fluid consumption, 200–201
  physiological response, 213–215
    formulation considerations, 214–215
    scientific principles and practical
      ramifications, 213–214
  rapid fluid absorption, 208–210
    formulation considerations, 209–210
    scientific principles and practical
      ramifications, 208–209
  speed rehydration, 215–217
    formulation considerations, 216–217
    scientific principles and practical
      ramifications, 215–216
  sports drink composition, 198–199
  voluntary fluid consumption, 202–207

formulation considerations, 204–207
scientific principles and practical
      ramifications, 202–204
Carbonation intensity, 70
Cardiac output, 133
Cardiovascular drift, 133
Cardiovascular function, inadequate methodology
      for assessment of, 138
Carnitine, 234, 235
Carrier mediated transporter systems, 113
Catecholamines, 49, 52, 135, 148
Cellular dehydration, 46, 48
Cellular hydration status, minute decreases in, 46
Central fatigue, 155
Chloride, 17, 31
Choline, 212, 236, 237
Chromium, 238, 240
Citrate, 212
Citric acid beverage, 67
Ciwujia, 242, 244
Clinical dehydration, 216
Coca Cola Classic®, 199
Coenzyme Q10, 212
Coffee purchase frequency, 79
Competition
  carbohydrate requirements for, 21
  nutrition for, 12
Corn syrups, high fructose, 205
Cortisol, 213
Creatine, 232, 235, 265
Creatine phosphate, 154
Cycle tour, 4
Cycling to fatigue, 144
Cytomax®, 199

D

Daily water balance, 34, 36
Dehydration, 12, 24, 188, 259
  cellular, 46, 48
  clinical, 216
  drinking to prevent, 258
  exercise-induced, 184, 193
  involuntary, 202
  voluntary, 45, 64
Determination, 2
Diabetes, 263
Diet(s)
  high-carbohydrate, 174
  high-protein, 35
  more-extreme forms of, 20
Dietary recall, 4